Advances in Diagnosis and Management of Pancreatobiliary Disorders

Advances in Diagnosis and Management of Pancreatobiliary Disorders

Guest Editor

Francesca Lodato

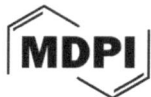

Basel • Beijing • Wuhan • Barcelona • Belgrade • Novi Sad • Cluj • Manchester

Guest Editor
Francesca Lodato
Department of
Gastroenterology and
Interventional Endoscopy
Maggiore Hospital Bologna
Bologna
Italy

Editorial Office
MDPI AG
Grosspeteranlage 5
4052 Basel, Switzerland

This is a reprint of the Special Issue, published open access by the journal *Journal of Clinical Medicine* (ISSN 2077-0383), freely accessible at: https://www.mdpi.com/journal/jcm/special_issues/8H3J192QOL.

For citation purposes, cite each article independently as indicated on the article page online and as indicated below:

Lastname, A.A.; Lastname, B.B. Article Title. *Journal Name* **Year**, *Volume Number*, Page Range.

ISBN 978-3-7258-3409-9 (Hbk)
ISBN 978-3-7258-3410-5 (PDF)
https://doi.org/10.3390/books978-3-7258-3410-5

© 2025 by the authors. Articles in this book are Open Access and distributed under the Creative Commons Attribution (CC BY) license. The book as a whole is distributed by MDPI under the terms and conditions of the Creative Commons Attribution-NonCommercial-NoDerivs (CC BY-NC-ND) license (https://creativecommons.org/licenses/by-nc-nd/4.0/).

Contents

Min Je Sung, Sung Yong Han, Jong Hyun Lee, Tae In Kim, Dong Uk Kim, Chang-Il Kwon, et al.
Combinatorial Effects of Terpene, Chenodeoxycholic Acid, and Ursodeoxycholic Acid on Common Bile Duct Stone Recurrence and Gallbladder Stone Dissolution
Reprinted from: J. Clin. Med. 2024, 13, 7414, https://doi.org/10.3390/jcm13237414 1

Tamara F. Kahan, Matthew Antony Manoj, Ankit Chhoda, Anabel Liyen Cartelle, Kelsey Anderson, Shaharyar A. Zuberi, et al.
Impact of Interhospital Transfer on Outcomes in Acute Pancreatitis: Implications for Healthcare Quality
Reprinted from: J. Clin. Med. 2024, 13, 6817, https://doi.org/10.3390/jcm13226817 15

Suh-Won Lee, Cheng-Han Tsai, Hui-An Lin, Yu Chen, Sen-Kuang Hou and Sheng-Feng Lin
Pericholecystic Fat Stranding as a Predictive Factor of Length of Stays of Patients with Acute Cholecystitis: A Novel Scoring Model
Reprinted from: J. Clin. Med. 2024, 13, 5734, https://doi.org/10.3390/jcm13195734 24

Ali Atay and Ilhami Yuksel
The Experience of a Tertiary Referral Center with Endoscopic Management and Combining Percutaneous Intervention for the Treatment of Walled-Off Necrosis: A Stepwise Approach
Reprinted from: J. Clin. Med. 2024, 13, 4916, https://doi.org/10.3390/jcm13164916 34

Martina Di Franco, Emilia Fortunati, Lucia Zanoni, Norma Bonazzi, Cristina Mosconi, Claudio Malizia, et al.
β1600 Q.Clear Digital Reconstruction of [^{68}Ga]Ga-DOTANOC PET/CT Improves Image Quality in NET Patients
Reprinted from: J. Clin. Med. 2024, 13, 3841, https://doi.org/10.3390/jcm13133841 45

Ching-Tang Tseng, Yi-Jun Liao, Cheng-Li Lin and Yen-Chun Peng
Implications of Serum IgG4 Levels for Pancreatobiliary Disorders and Cancer
Reprinted from: J. Clin. Med. 2024, 13, 3651, https://doi.org/10.3390/jcm13133651 55

Francesco Panzuto, Elisa Andrini, Giuseppe Lamberti, Sara Pusceddu, Maria Rinzivillo, Fabio Gelsomino, et al.
Sequencing Treatments in Patients with Advanced Well-Differentiated Pancreatic Neuroendocrine Tumor (pNET): Results from a Large Multicenter Italian Cohort
Reprinted from: J. Clin. Med. 2024, 13, 2074, https://doi.org/10.3390/jcm13072074 68

Francesca Lodato, Stefano Landi, Marco Bassi, Stefania Ghersi and Vincenzo Cennamo
Urgent Endoscopic Biliary Procedures: "Run Like the Wind"?
Reprinted from: J. Clin. Med. 2025, 14, 1017, https://doi.org/10.3390/jcm14031017 82

Chiara Coluccio, Stefania Cappetta, Giovanna Romagnoli, Valentina Di Giorgio, Paolo Giuffrida, Stefano Fabbri, et al.
Endoscopic-Ultrasound-Guided Radiofrequency Ablation for Pancreatic Tumors
Reprinted from: J. Clin. Med. 2025, 14, 495, https://doi.org/10.3390/jcm14020495 96

Amar Vedamurthy, Rajesh Krishnamoorthi, Shayan Irani and Richard Kozarek
Endoscopic Management of Benign Pancreaticobiliary Disorders
Reprinted from: J. Clin. Med. 2025, 14, 494, https://doi.org/10.3390/jcm14020494 120

Carmen Blanco Abad, Paula Gomila Pons, Sara Campos Ramírez, María Álvarez Alejandro, María Irene Torres Ramón, María Dolores Miramar Gallart, et al.
Hereditary Pancreatic Cancer: Advances in Genetic Testing, Early Detection Strategies, and Personalized Management
Reprinted from: *J. Clin. Med.* **2025**, *14*, 367, https://doi.org/10.3390/jcm14020367 . . . . **141**

Giovanna Impellizzeri, Maria Vittoria Grassini, Giulio Donato, Claudio Giovanni De Angelis and Nico Pagano
An Approach to and Treatment of Indeterminate Biliary Strictures: A Comprehensive Review of the Literature
Reprinted from: *J. Clin. Med.* **2025**, *14*, 29, https://doi.org/10.3390/jcm14010029 . . . . **160**

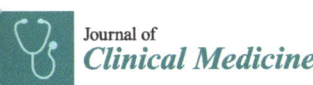

Article

Combinatorial Effects of Terpene, Chenodeoxycholic Acid, and Ursodeoxycholic Acid on Common Bile Duct Stone Recurrence and Gallbladder Stone Dissolution

Min Je Sung [1,†], Sung Yong Han [2,†], Jong Hyun Lee [2], Tae In Kim [2], Dong Uk Kim [2], Chang-Il Kwon [1], Jae Hee Cho [3], Jung Wan Choe [4], Jong Jin Hyun [4], Jae Kook Yang [5], Tae Hoon Lee [5], Jungnam Lee [6], Sung Ill Jang [3,*,‡] and Seok Jeong [6,*,‡]

1. Digestive Disease Center, CHA Bundang Medical Center, CHA University School of Medicine, Seongnam 13496, Republic of Korea; mj1744@cha.ac.kr (M.J.S.); endoscopy@cha.ac.kr (C.-I.K.)
2. Department of Internal Medicine, Pusan National University School of Medicine, Biomedical Research Institute, Pusan National University Hospital, Busan 49241, Republic of Korea; mirsaint@hanmail.net (S.Y.H.); keiasikr@nate.com (J.H.L.); zeitgeister88@daum.net (T.I.K.); amlm3@hanmail.net (D.U.K.)
3. Department of Internal Medicine, Gangnam Severance Hospital, Yonsei University College of Medicine, Seoul 06273, Republic of Korea; jhcho9328@yuhs.ac
4. Department of Internal Medicine, Korea University Ansan Hospital, Ansan 15355, Republic of Korea; jwchoe@korea.ac.kr (J.W.C.); sean4h@korea.ac.kr (J.J.H.)
5. Department of Internal Medicine, Soonchunhyang University Hospital Cheonan, Cheonan 31151, Republic of Korea; c96396@schmc.ac.kr (J.K.Y.); taewoolee9@gmail.com (T.H.L.)
6. Department of Internal Medicine, Inha University Hospital, Inha University College of Medicine, Incheon 22332, Republic of Korea; jungnamlee@inha.ac.kr
* Correspondence: aerojsi@yuhs.ac (S.I.J.); inos@inha.ac.kr (S.J.); Tel.: 82-2-2019-3310 (S.I.J.); 82-32-890-2548 (S.J.)
† These authors contributed equally to this work.
‡ These authors contributed equally to this work.

Abstract: Background: Ursodeoxycholic acid (UDCA), chenodeoxycholic acid (CDCA) plus UDCA (C&U), and terpene are widely administered to prevent common bile duct (CBD) stone recurrence and dissolve gallbladder (GB) stones. We evaluated and compared the combined effects of these agents on CBD stone recurrence and GB stone resolution. **Methods:** This study included patients who underwent endoscopic retrograde cholangiopancreatography (ERCP) at six referral centers, retrospectively. A total of 940 patients who underwent cholecystectomy before or after CBD stone removal by ERCP were evaluated to assess CBD stone recurrence (the CBD recurrence cohort), and 98 patients with GB stones were assessed by abdominal or endoscopic ultrasonography before and 6 months after ERCP to evaluate GB stone resolution (GB cohort). Patients were divided into no-medication, single-agent treatment (UDCA, C&U, or terpene), or dual-agent treatment (terpene plus UDCA or C&U) groups for the analysis. **Results:** In the CBD recurrence cohort, baseline characteristics were similar in the three groups. CBD stone recurrence rates were 41.5%, 12.7%, and 9.8% in the no-medication, single-agent, and dual-agent groups, respectively ($p < 0.001$), and the recurrence rate was significantly lower for those administered C&U plus terpene (5.2% vs. 13.2%, $p = 0.002$). In the GB cohort, baseline characteristics were also similar in the groups. GB stone resolution rates of >30% were observed in 5.3%, 14.3%, and 34.8% of patients in the no-medication, single-agent, and dual-agent groups, respectively ($p = 0.028$). **Conclusions:** C&U plus terpene was significantly more effective for preventing CBD stone recurrence and achieving GB stone resolution than no medication or single agents.

Keywords: choledocholithiasis; recurrence; cholelithiasis

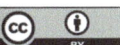

1. Introduction

The migration of gallbladder (GB) stones from the GB to the biliary tree is the main etiology of common bile duct (CBD) stones [1,2], and symptomatic GB stones are accompanied by coexisting CBD stones in 3–16% of patients [3,4]. CBD stones are usually managed with endoscopic procedures, including endoscopic sphincterotomy (EST) [5], endoscopic papillary balloon dilation (EPBD) [6], and stone extraction. After the endoscopic removal of CBD stones, prophylactic cholecystectomy is routinely offered [7], but stones recur in up to 24% of patients [8–10].

The preventative role of oral dissolution therapy based on ursodeoxycholic acid (UDCA) or other choleretic agents in recurrent CBD stones after endoscopic removal has not been established. One randomized control trial (RCT) reported that UDCA is marginally effective at preventing CBD stone recurrence [11], and Somerville et al. concluded that terpene plus UDCA and chenodeoxycholic acid (CDCA) are effective dissolution therapies for CBD stones [12]. Although the combination of UDCA, terpene, and endoscopic biliary stenting was found to be an effective treatment for CBD stones [13], two RCTs showed that adding UDCA to endoprosthetic treatment did not reduce CBD stone size [14,15]. Furthermore, two other studies demonstrated that UDCA and/or terpene did not prevent CBD stone recurrence [16,17].

Nonsurgical management, such as dissolution therapy, is an option for patients with symptomatic GB stones who are either unable or unwilling to undergo cholecystectomy, but dissolution therapy is associated with an overall low curative success rate and a high probability of stone recurrence [18–20]. Although the effectiveness of dissolution therapy was not significant, one study found that UDCA had a small (<20 mm) gallstone dissolution efficacy of 30–50% [21]. In addition, a meta-analysis of 23 RCTs reported GB stone dissolution rates of 37% for ursodiol and 62.8% for CDCA plus UDCA (C&U) combination therapy [18]. Other studies have confirmed higher GB stone dissolution rates for combination therapy than monotherapy. In one study, C&U and UDCA achieved complete small stone dissolution rates of 52% and 24%, respectively [22], and another study reported complete stone dissolution rates for UDCA alone and UDCA plus menthol of 38% and 53%, respectively [23].

It is important to determine which drugs are more effective at reducing CBD stone recurrence and dissolving GB stones. Therefore, we evaluated the effects of UDCA, C&U, and terpene (alone and in combination) on CBD stone recurrence and GB stone dissolution.

2. Materials and Methods

2.1. Patients

The patient flow chart is provided in Figure 1. The records of 21,012 patients who underwent endoscopic retrograde cholangiopancreatography (ERCP) at six referral hospitals during 2011–2015 were screened, retrospectively. Inclusion criteria were ERCP for CBD stone removal and cholecystectomy before or after CBD stone removal by ERCP (the CBD recurrence cohort) or no cholecystectomy and GB stones identified by abdominal ultrasonography or endoscopic ultrasonography (EUS) before and 6 months post-ERCP (the GB cohort). Exclusion criteria were ERCP for malignant obstruction, another bile duct pathology (e.g., benign biliary stricture or intrahepatic duct stone), or a pancreatic duct procedure; EST performed because of previous ERCP; surgically altered anatomy; failure to attend an outpatient follow-up appointment or lost to follow-up within 3 months post-ERCP; or CBD stone recurrence within 3 months post-ERCP.

This study was conducted in accordance with the guidelines of the Declaration of Helsinki (revised in 2013), and the study protocol was approved beforehand by our Institutional Review Board (Approval No. 2021-11-011).

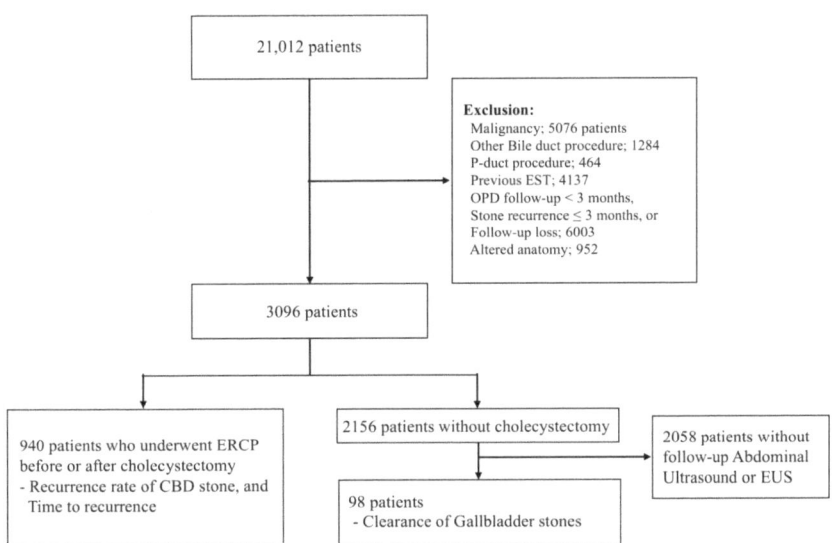

Figure 1. Study flow chart.

2.2. Patient Cohorts

The CBD recurrence cohort included 940 patients who underwent cholecystectomy before or after ERCP. ERCP-related CBD stone recurrence factors, viz. periampullary diverticulum, bile duct stenosis, bile duct diameter, bile duct angle (as defined by Keizman et al. [24,25]), procedure type (EST, EPBD, and mechanical lithotripsy), type of CBD stone removed, and patient data (sex, age, body mass index, and co-morbidities), were evaluated. Recurrent CBD was defined as confirmation by computed tomography, magnetic resonance cholangiopancreatography, or ERCP.

The GB cohort was composed of 98 patients who did not undergo cholecystectomy but underwent ultrasonography before and 6 months after ERCP. The same ultrasound modality (transabdominal or endoscopic) was used pre- and post-ERCP. We assumed that CBD stones and the remaining GB stones were of the same type. Patient data were recorded, and ultrasound images were used to calculate changes in GB stone sizes post-ERCP.

2.3. Medication Groups

Recorded patient usages of UDCA (Ursa®, Daewoong Pharm. Co., Ltd., Seoul, Republic of Korea), C&U (CnU®, Myungmoon Pharm. Co., Ltd., Seoul, Republic of Korea, composed of CDCA 114 mg and UDCA 114 mg), and terpene (Rowahcol®, Pharmbio Korea Co., Ltd., Seoul, Republic of Korea) were as follows: UDCA 600 mg/day (200 mg three times daily after meals), C&U 750 mg/day (250 mg three times daily after meals), and terpene 3 capsules daily (1 capsule three times daily before meals). Medication use was defined as being prescribed medication for ≥3 months during follow-up. Patients whose medication regimen changed during follow-up were classified according to the medication received for the longest time. Patients were divided into three groups: no medication, single agents (UDCA, C&U, or terpene), or dual agents (UDCA or C&U plus terpene).

2.4. GB Stone Resolution Rate

GB stone resolution was defined based on the percentage change in GB stone size from baseline to 6 months post-ERCP, as determined by ultrasonography. When distinct GB stones were present, stone sizes were measured using the ultrasound length measurement tool, and gallstone size was recorded as the maximum diameter of the largest stone. When only gallbladder sludge was present, sludge volume was calculated using $4/3\pi \times r^3$ (r = radius).

2.5. Statistical Analysis

The analysis was performed using IBM SPSS Statistics (version 21.0, IBM Corp. Armonk, NY, USA). Categorical data were expressed as frequencies and percentages and the significances of intergroup differences were determined using the chi-square test. Continuous data were expressed as means ± standard deviations, and the significances of intergroup differences were determined using the independent Student t-test. Statistical significance was accepted for p values < 0.05. Univariate and multivariate analyses were conducted to identify factors associated with CBD stone recurrence. Variables with p values of <0.100 via univariate analysis were included in the multivariate analysis. Kaplan–Meier plots were used to determine cumulative recurrence rates, and recurrence rates were compared using the log-rank test.

3. Results

3.1. Baseline Characteristics

Table 1 summarizes the baseline characteristics of the 940 patients between the no medication group and the medication group in the CBD recurrence cohort. Baseline characteristics were similar between two groups, except for hypertension rates (no medication vs. medication: 49.5% vs. 40.9%, $p = 0.032$), diabetes (27.1% vs. 20.2%, $p = 0.039$) dyslipidemia (14.6% vs. 8.0%, $p = 0.006$), bile duct angle (137.5° ± 18.1° vs. 141.9° ± 19.5° $p = 0.005$), and mechanical lithotripsy (19.2% vs. 27.3%, $p = 0.021$).

Table 1. Baseline characteristics by medication type.

Baseline Characteristics	No Medication $n = 193$	Medication $n = 747$	p Value
Sex, male	106 (55.2)	364 (49.0)	0.125
Age (years)	65.4 ± 14.5	64.2 ± 14.9	0.325
BMI (kg/m^2)	24.1 ± 3.9	24.0 ± 3.6	0.762
Hypertension	95 (49.5)	305 (40.9)	0.032
Diabetes	52 (27.1)	151 (20.2)	0.039
Dyslipidemia	28 (14.6)	60 (8.0)	0.006
Periampullary diverticulum	73 (37.8)	247 (33.2)	0.232
Bile duct diameter (mm)	12.5 ± 4.9	13.1 ± 6.0	0.117
Bile duct angle (°)	137.5 ± 18.1	141.9 ± 19.5	0.005
Procedure			
EST	188 (97.4)	710 (95.0)	0.157
EST + EPBD	81 (42.0)	303 (40.6)	0.723
EST + EPLBD	30 (15.5)	124 (16.6)	0.724
Mechanical lithotripsy	37 (19.2)	203 (27.3)	0.021
Type of removed CBD stone			
Brown	106 (55.2)	446 (60.4)	0.229
Black	56 (29.2)	172 (23.3)	0.083
Cholesterol	30 (15.6)	121 (16.4)	0.825
Duration of medication use (months)	–	9.5 ± 14.0	-

Data are mean ± standard deviation, number, or number (percentage). BMI, body mass index; CBD, common bile duct; EPBD, endoscopic papillary balloon dilation; EPLBD, endoscopic papillary balloon dilation (≥12 mm). EST, endoscopic sphincterotomy.

Table 2 summarizes the baseline characteristics of the 747 patients between the single-agent group and the dual-agent group in the CBD recurrence cohort. Baseline characteristics were similar between the two groups, except for EST + EPBD rates (single agent vs. dual agent: 55.6% vs. 30.2%, $p < 0.001$), mechanical lithotripsy (37.2% vs. 20.5%, $p < 0.001$), brown pigment stone (56.2% vs. 63.2%, $p = 0.026$), and cholesterol stone (21.4% vs. 13.0%, $p = 0.004$).

Table 2. Baseline characteristics by medication type.

Baseline Characteristics	Single Agent n = 306	Dual Agent [#] n = 441	p Value
Sex, male	147 (48.0)	217 (49.7)	0.664
Age (years)	64.8 ± 15.2	63.8 ± 14.6	0.359
BMI (kg/m^2)	24.0 ± 3.4	24.1 ± 3.7	0.835
Hypertension	136 (44.6)	169 (38.3)	0.087
Diabetes	71 (23.2)	80 (18.1)	0.090
Dyslipidemia	18 (5.9)	42 (9.5)	0.074
Periampullary diverticulum	99 (32.6)	148 (33.7)	0.744
Bile duct diameter (mm)	13.2 ± 5.3	13.1 ± 6.4	0.686
Bile duct angle (°)	143.2 ± 17.3	141.0 ± 20.9	0.114
Procedure			
EST	292 (95.4)	418 (94.8)	0.692
EST + EPBD	170 (55.6)	133 (30.2)	<0.001
EST + EPLBD	45 (14.7)	79 (17.9)	0.247
Mechanical lithotripsy	113 (37.2)	90 (20.5)	<0.001
Type of removed CBD stone			
Brown	168 (56.2)	278 (63.2)	0.026
Black	67 (22.4)	105 (23.9)	0.541
Cholesterol	64 (21.4)	57 (13.0)	0.004
Duration of medication use (months)	10.6 ± 16.6	8.7 ± 11.9	0.086

Data are mean ± standard deviation, number, or number (percentage). [#] Dual agent = terpene plus UDCA (ursodeoxycholic acid) or terpene plus C&U (chenodeoxycholic acid [CDCA]). BMI, body mass index; CBD, common bile duct; EPBD, endoscopic papillary balloon dilation; EPLBD, endoscopic papillary balloon dilation (≥12 mm); EST, endoscopic sphincterotomy.

3.2. CBD Stone Recurrence

CBD stone recurrence rates differed significantly between the no-medication group and the medication group (no medication vs. medication: 41.5% vs. 11.0%, $p < 0.001$) and within a year (12.4% vs. 5.2%, $p < 0.001$) (Table 3). Time to recurrence was similar in the groups (24.0 ± 18.6 vs. 23.3 ± 22.3 months, $p = 0.842$). Follow-up duration was significantly longer in the no-medication group (37.7 ± 33.7 vs. 26.0 ± 30.7 months, $p < 0.001$).

Table 3. Common bile duct stone recurrence results by medication type.

Recurrence Results	No Medication n = 193	Medication n = 747	p Value
Recurrence	80 (41.5)	82 (11.0)	<0.001
Recurrence within 1 year	24 (12.4)	39 (5.2)	<0.001
Recurrence frequency 1/2/3+	51/21/8	50/22/10	0.891
Time to recurrence (months)	24.0 ± 18.6	23.3 ± 22.3	0.842
Duration of follow-up (months)	37.7 ± 33.7	26.0 ± 30.7	<0.001

Data are mean ± standard deviation, number, or number (percentage).

Recurrence rates were significantly lower in the medication group than in the no-medication group from 12 months (14.5% vs. 5.0%, $p < 0.001$) to 60 months (39.9% vs. 10.3%, $p = 0.002$) (Figure 2).

However, CBD stone recurrence rates did not differ significantly between the single-agent group and the dual-agent group (single agent vs. dual agent: 12.7% vs. 9.8%, $p = 0.198$) and within a year (4.6% vs. 5.7%, $p = 0.509$) (Supplementary Table S1). This analysis was performed in response to the diverse range of drugs and their combinations. Time to recurrence was similar in the groups (22.4 ± 17.2 vs. 24.2 ± 26.2 months, $p = 0.708$). Also, follow-up duration was similar in the groups (25.5 ± 29.2 vs. 26.3 ± 31.8 months, $p = 0.724$).

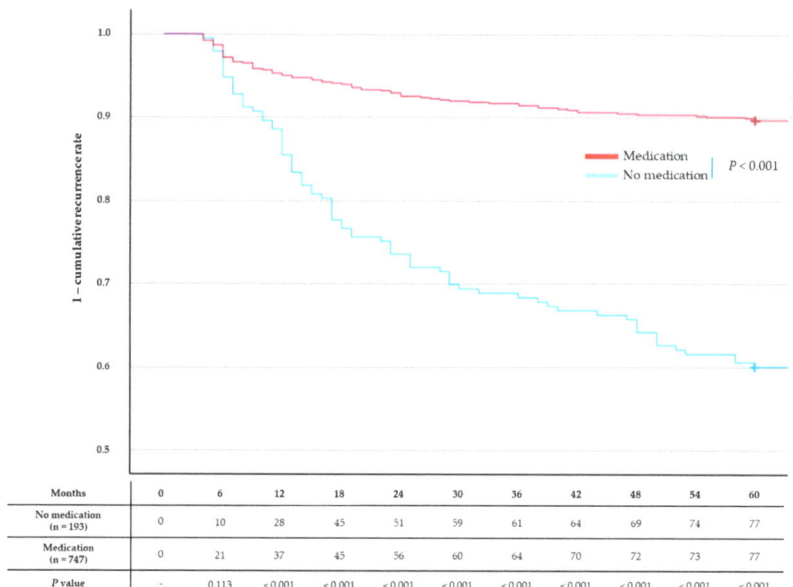

Figure 2. Factors associated with common bile duct stone recurrence. The no-medication group had a significantly higher cumulative recurrence rate than the single-agent or dual-agent groups ($p < 0.001$) However, no significant difference was observed between the two groups at 6 months.

Recurrence rates did not differ significantly between the single-agent group and the dual-agent group (12.7% vs. 9.8%, $p = 0.085$) (Figure 3).

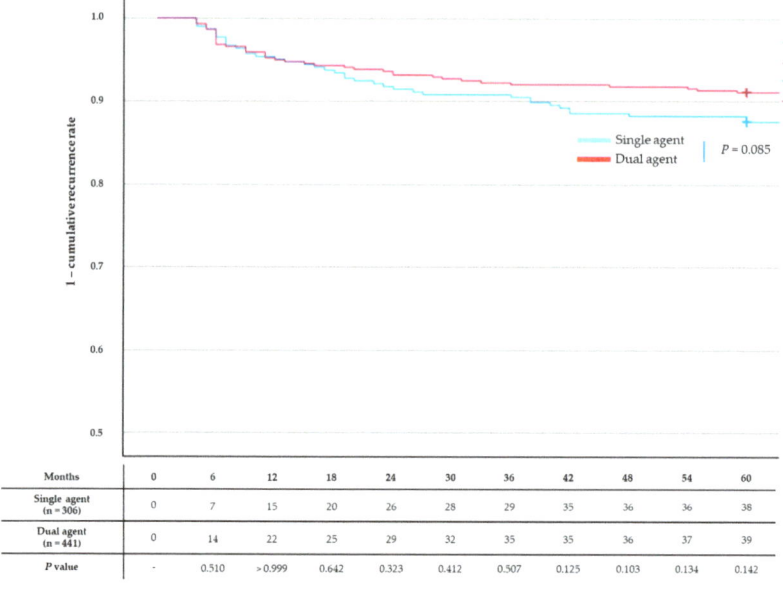

Figure 3. Kaplan–Meier curves for common bile duct stone recurrence. Recurrence rates did not differ significantly between the single-agent group and the dual-agent group ($p = 0.085$).

Subgroup analysis revealed that CBD stone recurrence rates for the medication regimens differed (UDCA vs. C&U vs. terpene vs. UDCA + terpene vs. C&U + terpene: 11.5% vs. 13.3% vs. 19.4% vs. 14.0% vs. 5.2%, $p = 0.016$) (Table 4). A comparative analysis of CBD stone recurrence across various medication subgroups was conducted. In this analysis, the combination of C&U and terpene demonstrated a statistically significant difference compared to other treatments (Supplementary Figure S1). The mean duration of follow-up was similar between the medication regimens ($p = 0.655$). Time to recurrence was significantly different in the medication subgroups (21.2 ± 18.9 vs. 31.8 ± 12.9 vs. 11.2 ± 6.8 vs. 29.2 ± 28.6 vs. 9.6 ± 6.8 months, $p = 0.011$). In the comparative analysis of time to recurrence across various medication subgroups, C&U, as well as the combination of C&U and terpene, demonstrated a statistically significant difference compared to other treatments (Supplementary Figure S2). Also, the duration of medication use was significantly different in the groups (11.1 ± 17.7 vs. 11.7 ± 16.2 vs. 5.1 ± 6.4 vs. 8.5 ± 12.8 vs. 9.0 ± 10.9 months, $p < 0.001$). In the comparison of the duration of medication use across medication subgroups, terpene and UDCA showed a statistically significant difference when compared to other treatments (Supplementary Figure S3).

Table 4. CBD stone recurrence results of the medication subgroups.

	UDCA $n = 200$	C&U $n = 75$	Terpene $n = 31$	UDCA + Terpene $n = 228$	C&U + Terpene $n = 213$	p Value
Recurrence	23 (11.5)	10 (13.3)	6 (19.4)	32 (14.0)	11 (5.2)	0.016
Duration of follow-up	28.7 ± 32.5	20.3 ± 21.5	17.8 ± 17.9	29.2 ± 33.6	23.3 ± 29.5	0.655
Time to recurrence	21.2 ± 18.9	31.8 ± 12.9	11.2 ± 6.8	29.2 ± 28.6	9.6 ± 6.8	0.011
Duration of medication use	11.1 ± 17.7	11.7 ± 16.2	5.1 ± 6.4	8.5 ± 12.8	9.0 ± 10.9	<0.001

Data are means ± standard deviations or numbers (percentages). UDCA, ursodeoxycholic acid; C&U, chenodeoxycholic acid plus ursodeoxycholic acid.

Recurrence rates were significantly lower in the C&U plus terpene group than in the other medication groups ($p = 0.034$) (Figure 4).

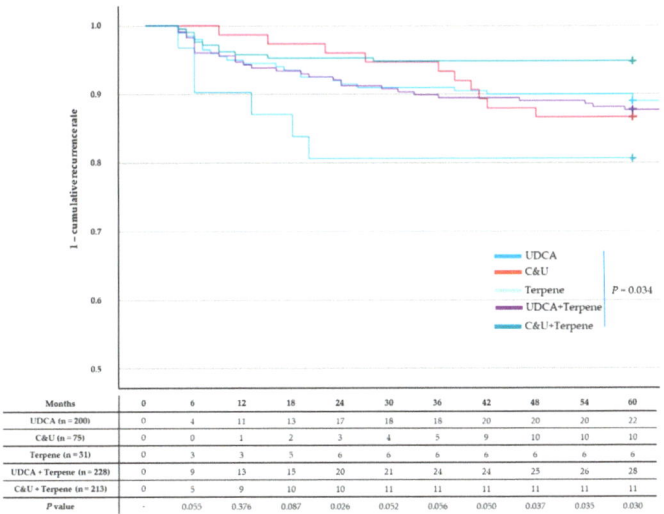

Figure 4. Kaplan–Meier curves for common bile duct stone recurrence. Compared to the other medication groups, the chenodeoxycholic acid and ursodeoxycholic acid (C&U) plus terpene group had significantly lower cumulative recurrence rates ($p = 0.034$).

Age, rates of hypertension, periampullary diverticulum, bile duct diameter, bile duct angle, EST, EST + EPBD, EST + EPLBD, mechanical lithotripsy, brown pigment stones, medication, and medication duration in the recurrence and no-recurrence groups were significantly different (Supplementary Table S2). Significant risk factors for recurrence as determined by multivariate regression analysis were age > 70 years (hazard ratio [HR] 2.041; 95% confidence interval [CI], 1.313–3.172; p = 0.002), bile duct diameter > 13 mm (HR, 1.802; 95% CI, 1.177–2.759; p = 0.007), EST (HR, 0.445; 95% CI, 0.199–0.995; p = 0.049) EST + EPBD (HR, 2.061; 95% CI, 1.267–3.352; p = 0.004), single agents (HR, 0.122; 95% CI 0.069–0.215; p < 0.001), and dual agents (HR, 0.109; 95% CI, 0.064–0.188; p < 0.001) (Table 5).

Table 5. Factors associated with common bile duct stone recurrence.

Factors	HR (95% CI)	p Value for Univariate Analysis	HR (95% CI)	p Value for Multivariate Analysis
Sex, male	1.064 (0.758–1.495)	0.720		
Age > 70 years	2.457 (1.733–3.484)	<0.001 *	2.041 (1.313–3.172)	0.002 *
BMI ≥ 25 kg/m²	0.740 (0.512–1.069)	0.108		
Hypertension	1.498 (1.066–2.106)	0.020 *	0.926 (0.607–1.413)	0.721
Diabetes	1.054 (0.700–1.585)	0.802		
Dyslipidemia	0.991 (0.553–1.776)	0.975		
Periampullary diverticulum	1.452 (1.027–2.055)	0.035 *	1.135 (0.741–1.739)	0.559
Type I	reference	reference		
Type II	0.433 (0.196–0.953)	0.038 *		
Type III	0.585 (0.256–1.338)	0.204		
Type II + III				
Bile duct diameter > 13 mm	1.940 (1.378–2.732)	<0.001 *	1.802 (1.177–2.759)	0.007 *
Bile duct angle < 145°	0.743 (0.529–1.045)	0.088	0.676 (0.447–1.021)	0.063
Procedure				
EST only	0.395 (0.203–0.768)	0.006 *	0.445 (0.199–0.995)	0.049 *
EST + EPBD	3.743 (2.594–5.402)	<0.001 *	2.061 (1.267–3.352)	0.004 *
EST + EPLBD	1.850 (1.238–2.765)	0.003 *		
Mechanical lithotripsy	2.008 (1.402–2.875)	<0.001 *	1.528 (0.923–2.527)	0.099
Type of removed CBD stone				
Brown	reference	reference		
Black	0.704 (0.460–1.077)	0.105		
Cholesterol	0.709 (0.431–1.168)	0.177		
Black + Cholesterol	0.687 (0.482–0.979)	0.038 *	0.871 (0.562–1.352)	0.538
Medication group				
No medication	reference	reference	reference	reference
Single agent	0.206 (0.133–0.321)	<0.001 *	0.122 (0.069–0.215)	<0.001 *
Dual agent	0.153 (0.100–0.234)	<0.001 *	0.109 (0.064–0.188)	<0.001 *
Medication > 7 months	0.555 (0.364–0.847)	0.006 *	1.079 (0.662–1.757)	0.760

Data are means ± standard deviations, numbers, or numbers (percentages). * Statistically significant. Bl, black pigment stone; BMI, body mass index; CBD, common bile duct; CI, confidence interval; EPBD, endoscopic papillary balloon dilation; EPLBD, endoscopic papillary balloon dilation (≥12 mm); EST, endoscopic sphincterotomy; HR, hazard ratio.

3.3. GB Stone Resolution

Baseline characteristics and GB stone resolution results were not significantly different between medication groups in the GB cohort (Table 6). The resolution rate was highest for brown pigment stones, followed by black pigment stones. Mean medication durations were similar for the single-agent and dual-agent groups (12.0 ± 20.8 vs. 11.1 ± 15.3 months, p = 0.870). However, the proportions of patients with a stone resolution rate of >30% were significantly different in the medication groups (no medication vs. single agent vs. dual agent: 5.3% vs. 14.3% vs. 34.8%, p = 0.028). Complete resolution was achieved in 12.5% of patients (7/56) in the single-agent group and 21.7% of patients (5/23) in the dual-agent group (Figure 5).

Table 6. Baseline characteristics and gallbladder stone resolution results by medication group.

	No Medication $n = 19$	Single Agent $n = 56$	Dual Agent $n = 23$	p Value
Baseline characteristics				
Sex, male	8 (42.1)	28 (50.0)	12 (52.2)	0.788
Age (years)	66.3 ± 16.5	70.1 ± 14.2	64.8 ± 14.4	0.297
BMI (kg/m^2)	23.2 ± 6.3	22.9 ± 3.9	24.4 ± 3.3	0.396
Hypertension	9 (47.4)	29 (51.8)	10 (43.5)	0.789
Diabetes	4 (21.1)	13 (23.2)	2 (8.7)	0.326
Dyslipidemia	2 (10.5)	6 (10.7)	1 (4.3)	0.656
Type of removed CBD stone				
Brown/black/cholesterol	11/6/1	37/13/6	11/11/1	0.275
Duration of medication use (months)	-	12.0 ± 20.8	11.1 ± 15.3	0.870
Results				
Stone size change				
Decrease/no change/increase	6/5/8	16/12/28	8/8/7	0.592
Stone size pre-ERCP (cm)	0.95 ± 0.38	1.10 ± 0.74	1.10 ± 0.77	0.702
Stone size post-ERCP (cm)	1.01 ± 0.50	1.18 ± 0.89	0.85 ± 0.71	0.250
Change in stone size (%)	7.69 ± 27.7	24.1 ± 107.1	−1.3 ± 83.9	0.426
>30% stone resolution	1 (5.3)	8 (14.3)	8 (34.8)	0.028 *†

Data are means ± standard deviations, numbers, or numbers (percentages). * Statistically significant. † $p = 0.043$ for the single-agent vs. dual-agent comparison. BMI, body mass index; CBD, common bile duct.

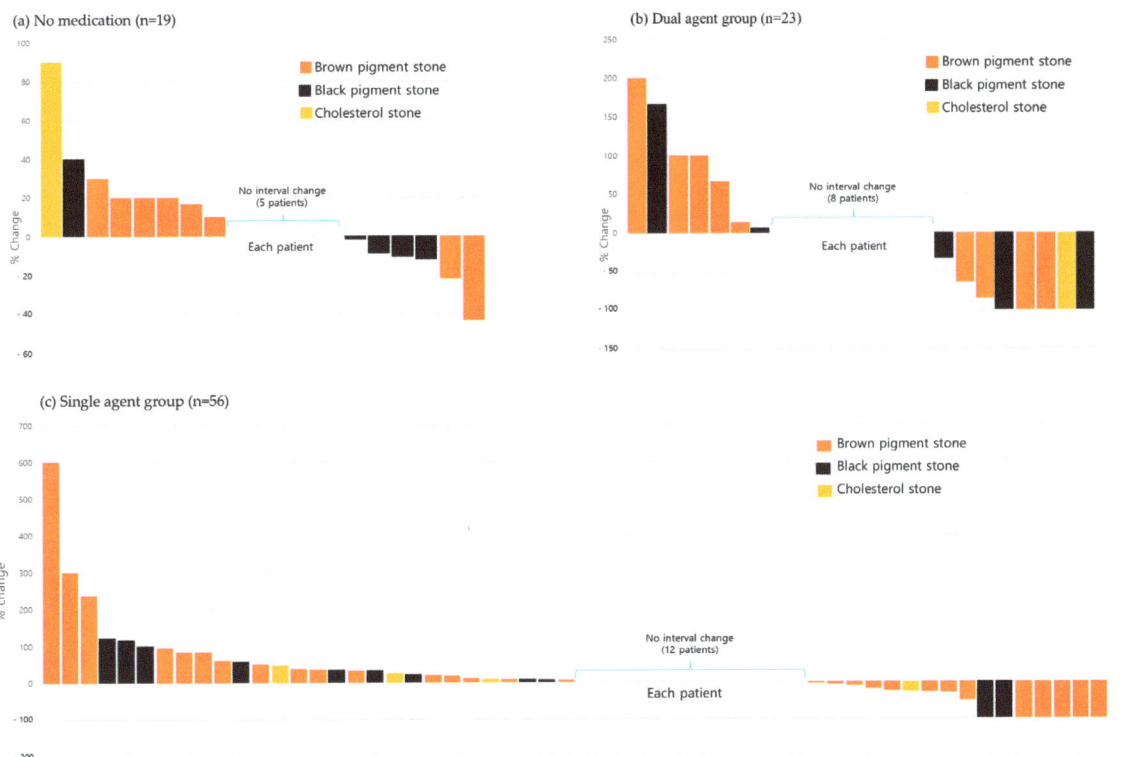

Figure 5. Gallbladder stone resolution by medication group and stone type. Percentage changes in stone size are shown for patients in (a) the no-medication group, (b) the dual-agent group, and (c) the single-agent group. Complete stone resolution was achieved in 7 patients (12.5%) in the single-agent group and 5 patients (21.7%) in the dual-agent group.

4. Discussion

This study shows that stone dissolution medications lowered CBD stone recurrence rates from 41.5% with no medication to 12.7% for single-agent and 9.8% for dual-agent C&U plus terpene therapy treatments. Subgroup analysis revealed that the CBD stone recurrence rate was significantly lower for C&U plus terpene than all other medication regimens combined (5.2% vs. 13.5%). The overall CBD recurrence rate of 17.2% was in line with previously reported recurrence rates of 1–20% [26]. Notably, dual-agent therapy was more effective than single-agent treatment or no medication for GB stone resolution; these treatments achieved > 30% stone reductions in 34.8%, 14.3%, and 5.3% of patients, respectively.

Medication use significantly reduced the risk of CBD stone recurrence, with HRs of 0.122 and 0.109 for single-agent or double-agent treatment, respectively, versus no therapy. In addition, the study showed an age > 70 years (HR, 2.041), bile duct diameter >13 mm (HR, 1.802), EST (HR, 0.445), and EST + EPBD (HR, 2.061) as risk factors of CBD stone recurrence. Previously reported risk factors were age, a large CBD diameter, CBD angle, periampullary diverticulum, EST, mechanical lithotripsy, biliary stenting, and remnant GB [27]. Periampullary diverticulum was not a risk factor via multivariate analysis in the current study, and mechanical lithotripsy was associated with the risk of CBD recurrence via univariate analysis but not multivariate analysis. When we set a cut-off value of 13 mm, according to receiver operating characteristic (ROC) curve analysis (area under the curve [AUC] of 0.610 and highest sensitivity and specificity at a mean bile duct diameter of 12.3 mm), a CBD diameter of >13 mm was also a risk factor for CBD recurrence via univariate but not multivariate analysis. When we set a cut-off value of 145° for the CBD angle based on the findings of another study [28], neither univariate nor multivariate analysis showed an association with CBD stone recurrence, and ROC analysis produced an AUC of 0.557. A large CBD diameter and periampullary diverticulum are associated with cholestatic effects. Furthermore, after ERCP, the possibility of reflux cholangitis increases because of EST, and cholestasis of bile promotes CBD stone recurrence. However, medications such as UDCA or CDCA that enhance bile acid synthesis [29] reduce bile reflux, and thus, stone recurrence.

Combining medications can have additive or synergistic effects on the prevention of CBD stone recurrence. Several studies have demonstrated that UDCA plus CDCA is more effective than either agent alone at dissolving gallstones [21,22,30]. Furthermore, the percentage of cholelitholytic bile acids in bile was nearly 80% for the combination and only ~65% for UDCA alone. Achieving these beneficial changes in bile acid composition is not feasible by administering UDCA or CDCA alone. Specifically, high UDCA doses reduce bile CDCA levels, and thus, reduce cholesterol solubilization into micelles [22]. When CDCA is administered alone, cholesterol does not dissolve in the liquid crystal phase, and bile may remain cholesterol-saturated, even at high CDCA doses, which are poorly tolerated [22]. Terpene alone also has a limited ability to dissolve gallstones, [13] but when combined with CDCA, it provided complete or partial gallstone dissolution in 41% of patients over 6 months [31]. In addition, for patients with CBD stones, three terpene capsules daily resulted in stone dissolution (complete or partial) in 46% of patients after 6 months and 67% of patients after 1 year [32]. Given that combining stone dissolution medications provides effective treatment for established GB or CBD stones, it is likely that combinations are also effective at preventing CBD stone formation.

Several studies have demonstrated gut microbiota dysbiosis after cholecystectomy [33,34] and in patients with GB stones [35], which resulted in studies on the effectiveness of stone dissolution therapy for gut dysbiosis. UDCA treatment restored gut microbiota in patients with non-alcoholic steatohepatitis or primary biliary cholangitis [36,37]. In another study, gut microbiota dysbiosis was partially reversed by C&U treatment in patients with GB stones [35]. Moreover, a recent study that analyzed changes in bile metabolism and composition after UDCA treatment found that UDCA might play a protective role related to gut microbiota in patients with CBD stones [38]. Thus, dissolution therapy may reduce

CBD stone recurrence even after therapy by altering the gut microbiome. Moreover, although the effects of terpene on gut dysbiosis have not been evaluated, it might have similar protective effects.

Biliary stones are classified as cholesterol, black pigment, or brown pigment stones. Pigment stones are more common in East Asia and cholesterol stones are most common in Western countries [39,40], and understanding the mechanisms responsible for their formation is essential for the optimal use of stone-dissolving medicines. Cholesterol stones form mainly when bile concentrations of cholesterol are elevated, and all medications used for biliary stones (UDCA, CDCA, and terpene) reduce bile cholesterol levels by controlling HMG-CoA reductase [27,41]. On the other hand, pigment stones originate from increased unconjugated bilirubin levels when the hepatic glucuronic acid concentration is diminished. Reductions in glucuronic acid have many causes, including bacterial β-glucuronidase activity [11]. Regarding treatments, terpene is metabolized to menthol-glucuronic acid, which can combine with unconjugated bilirubin to reduce pigment stone formation. Recurrent CBD stones after EST are usually brown pigment stones [42]. Terpene is the only medication that can suppress bile glucuronic acid reductions and decrease bile cholesterol saturation. Thus, terpene alone might be considered to be capable of resolving or preventing biliary stones. However, clinical data indicate that terpene monotherapy is inadequate [12,23]. Furthermore, brown pigment stones are associated with bacterial ascending cholangitis, which can be caused by EST after ERCP. The use of UDCA or CDCA to enhance bile acid synthesis would be expected to reduce recurrent brown pigment stone formation by decreasing reflux cholangitis, and UDCA-CDCA combination therapy would be expected to be more effective for biliary stone resolution or prevention than a single therapy treatment with either agent. In a study of CBD stones, the complete dissolution rate was 42% for terpene monotherapy and 73% for terpene plus CDCA or UDCA [12], and in a study of GB stones, the complete resolution rate was 37.5% for UDCA monotherapy and 53% for UDCA plus terpene [23]. It has been reported that terpene is more effective when used in combination therapy, and that CDCA and UDCA function more effectively when combined [43]. In the current study, we found that C&U plus terpene was more effective at preventing CBD recurrence than the other treatments. Numerous studies have shown that UDCA, CDCA, and terpene in various combinations act additively or synergistically, and our results suggest that they provide the best CBD stone prevention when combined.

The duration of medication use required to prevent CBD stone recurrence has not been established, though theoretically, treatment should be continued for life. However, this would be difficult and not cost-effective. After initial complete GB stone resolution, stones recur in around 10% of patients during the year following medication discontinuation and in up to 50% of patients by 5 years [44], and the recurrence rate is even higher in patients who do not achieve complete GB stone resolution. Small stone particles or bile sludge may remain after apparent complete CBD stone removal by ERCP, which highlights the importance of determining the appropriate duration of medication administered to dissolve any remaining stone material. Our results suggest that 6–7 months is appropriate, and ROC curve analysis showed that a cut-off value of 6.4 months had the greatest sensitivity and specificity for preventing CBD stone recurrence (AUC, 0.605; sensitivity, 0.353; specificity, 0.773). Also, after removing CBD stone(s) by ERCP, clinical practice guidelines recommend cholecystectomy when GB stone(s) are confirmed upon imaging. However, in patients with significant co-morbidities or other reasons to avoid surgery, medications could be continued as an alternative treatment. Additionally, CBD dilation after cholecystectomy in young patients may be another risk factor for CBD stones [45].

Our study has several limitations. First, due to its retrospective design, medication duration was not controlled, and some differences in group baseline characteristics were detected. Furthermore, the adverse effects of the medications could not be thoroughly investigated. In particular, medication durations differed markedly between patients, and some patients changed medications during the follow-up period, which introduced potential bias. On the other hand, a large cohort of patients was enrolled to reduce the effects of bias. Second, patients probably stopped taking medications during follow-up, and thus, we could not determine how long medication effects persisted after discontinuation. However, beneficial effects probably persisted due to improvements in gut dysbiosis, especially if microlithiasis was completely removed by medications. Third, the number of patients enrolled in the GB cohort was too small to allow for definitive conclusions. Nonetheless, it can be assumed that medication was effective, and the results obtained provide ample evidence to support the design of future large-scale studies.

5. Conclusions

The combination of CDCA and UDCA plus terpene was more effective at preventing CBD stone recurrence than other medication regimens. Furthermore, terpene-containing dual-agent regimens were more effective at resolving GB stones than no medication or single-agent treatments. Further research is required to confirm our results and improve our understanding of the mechanisms underlying effective CBD stone prevention.

Supplementary Materials: The following supporting information can be downloaded at https://www.mdpi.com/article/10.3390/jcm13237414/s1: Figure S1: Recurrence of the medication subgroups; Figure S2: Time to recurrence of the medication subgroups; Figure S3: Duration of medication use of the medication subgroups; Table S1: Common bile duct stone recurrence results by medication type; Table S2: Baseline characteristics with common bile duct stone recurrence.

Author Contributions: Conceptualization, S.J. and S.I.J.; methodology, S.Y.H.; formal analysis S.Y.H.; investigation, S.Y.H., M.J.S., J.H.L., T.I.K., D.U.K., C.-I.K., S.I.J., J.H.C., J.W.C., J.J.H., J.K.Y., T.H.L., J.L. and S.J.; resources, S.Y.H., M.J.S., J.H.L., T.I.K., D.U.K., C.-I.K., S.I.J., J.H.C., J.W.C., J.J.H., J.K.Y., T.H.L., J.L. and S.J.; software, M.J.S. and S.Y.H.; data curation, S.Y.H.; writing—original draft preparation, S.Y.H. and M.J.S.; writing—review and editing, S.Y.H., M.J.S., S.I.J. and S.J.; visualization S.Y.H., M.J.S. and S.I.J.; validation, M.J.S.; supervision, S.J. and S.I.J.; funding acquisition, S.I.J.; project administration, S.J. and S.I.J. All authors have read and agreed to the published version of the manuscript.

Funding: This study was funded by the 2024 domestic medical device new product association linked user (Medical Institution) multi-institution evaluation support project (S.I.J.); a faculty research grant from the Yonsei University College of Medicine (6-2023-0209) (S.I.J.).

Institutional Review Board Statement: This study was conducted in accordance with the guidelines of the Declaration of Helsinki (revised in 2013), and the study protocol was approved beforehand by our Institutional Review Board (Approval No. 2021-11-011, Approval date: 29 November 2021).

Informed Consent Statement: Patient consent was waived because of the retrospective nature of the study.

Data Availability Statement: The datasets generated and analyzed in the present study are available upon reasonable request to the corresponding author.

Conflicts of Interest: The authors declare no conflicts of interest.

References

1. Buxbaum, J.L.; Fehmi, S.M.A.; Sultan, S.; Fishman, D.S.; Qumseya, B.J.; Cortessis, V.K.; Schilperoort, H.; Kysh, L.; Matsuoka, L.; Yachimski, P.; et al. ASGE guideline on the role of endoscopy in the evaluation and management of choledocholithiasis. *Gastrointest. Endosc.* **2019**, *89*, 1075–1105.e15. [CrossRef] [PubMed]
2. Manes, G.; Paspatis, G.; Aabakken, L.; Anderloni, A.; Arvanitakis, M.; Ah-Soune, P.; Barthet, M.; Domagk, D.; Dumonceau, J.M.; Gigot, J.F.; et al. Endoscopic management of common bile duct stones: European Society of Gastrointestinal Endoscopy (ESGE) guideline. *Endoscopy* **2019**, *51*, 472–491. [CrossRef] [PubMed]
3. Collins, C.; Maguire, D.; Ireland, A.; Fitzgerald, E.; O'Sullivan, G.C. A prospective study of common bile duct calculi in patients undergoing laparoscopic cholecystectomy: Natural history of choledocholithiasis revisited. *Ann. Surg.* **2004**, *239*, 28–33. [CrossRef] [PubMed]
4. Lammert, F.; Gurusamy, K.; Ko, C.W.; Miquel, J.F.; Mendez-Sanchez, N.; Portincasa, P.; van Erpecum, K.J.; van Laarhoven, C.J.; Wang, D.Q. Gallstones. *Nat. Rev. Dis. Primers* **2016**, *2*, 16024. [CrossRef] [PubMed]
5. Kawai, K.; Akasaka, Y.; Murakami, K.; Tada, M.; Koli, Y. Endoscopic sphincterotomy of the ampulla of Vater. *Gastrointest. Endosc.* **1974**, *20*, 148–151. [CrossRef]

6. Staritz, M.; Ewe, K.; Meyer zum Büschenfelde, K.H. Endoscopic papillary dilation (EPD) for the treatment of common bile duct stones and papillary stenosis. *Endoscopy* **1983**, *15* (Suppl 1), 197–198. [CrossRef]
7. McAlister, V.C.; Davenport, E.; Renouf, E. Cholecystectomy deferral in patients with endoscopic sphincterotomy. *Cochrane Database Syst. Rev.* **2007**, *2007*, Cd006233. [CrossRef]
8. Freeman, M.L.; Nelson, D.B.; Sherman, S.; Haber, G.B.; Herman, M.E.; Dorsher, P.J.; Moore, J.P.; Fennerty, M.B.; Ryan, M.E.; Shaw, M.J.; et al. Complications of endoscopic biliary sphincterotomy. *N. Engl. J. Med.* **1996**, *335*, 909–918. [CrossRef]
9. Prat, F.; Malak, N.A.; Pelletier, G.; Buffet, C.; Fritsch, J.; Choury, A.D.; Altman, C.; Liguory, C.; Etienne, J.P. Biliary symptoms and complications more than 8 years after endoscopic sphincterotomy for choledocholithiasis. *Gastroenterology* **1996**, *110*, 894–899. [CrossRef]
10. Hawes, R.H.; Cotton, P.B.; Vallon, A.G. Follow-up 6 to 11 years after duodenoscopic sphincterotomy for stones in patients with prior cholecystectomy. *Gastroenterology* **1990**, *98*, 1008–1012. [CrossRef]
11. Yamamoto, R.; Tazuma, S.; Kanno, K.; Igarashi, Y.; Inui, K.; Ohara, H.; Tsuyuguchi, T.; Ryozawa, S. Ursodeoxycholic acid after bile duct stone removal and risk factors for recurrence: A randomized trial. *J. Hepatobiliary Pancreat. Sci.* **2016**, *23*, 132–136. [CrossRef] [PubMed]
12. Somerville, K.W.; Ellis, W.R.; Whitten, B.H.; Balfour, T.W.; Bell, G.D. Stones in the common bile duct: Experience with medical dissolution therapy. *Postgrad. Med. J.* **1985**, *61*, 313–316. [CrossRef] [PubMed]
13. Han, J.; Moon, J.H.; Koo, H.C.; Kang, J.H.; Choi, J.H.; Jeong, S.; Lee, D.H.; Lee, M.S.; Kim, H.G. Effect of biliary stenting combined with ursodeoxycholic acid and terpene treatment on retained common bile duct stones in elderly patients: A multicenter study. *Am. J. Gastroenterol.* **2009**, *104*, 2418–2421. [CrossRef]
14. Katsinelos, P.; Kountouras, J.; Paroutoglou, G.; Chatzimavroudis, G.; Zavos, C. Combination of endoprostheses and oral ursodeoxycholic acid or placebo in the treatment of difficult to extract common bile duct stones. *Dig. Liver Dis.* **2008**, *40*, 453–459. [CrossRef]
15. Lee, T.H.; Han, J.H.; Kim, H.J.; Park, S.M.; Park, S.H.; Kim, S.J. Is the addition of choleretic agents in multiple double-pigtail biliary stents effective for difficult common bile duct stones in elderly patients? A prospective, multicenter study. *Gastrointest. Endosc.* **2011**, *74*, 96–102. [CrossRef]
16. Song, M.E.; Chung, M.J.; Lee, D.J.; Oh, T.G.; Park, J.Y.; Bang, S.; Park, S.W.; Song, S.Y.; Chung, J.B. Cholecystectomy for Prevention of Recurrence After Endoscopic Clearance of Bile Duct Stones in Korea. *Yonsei Med. J.* **2016**, *57*, 132–137. [CrossRef]
17. Baek, Y.H.; Kim, H.J.; Park, J.H.; Park, D.I.; Cho, Y.K.; Sohn, C.I.; Jeon, W.K.; Kim, B.I. Risk factors for recurrent bile duct stones after endoscopic clearance of common bile duct stones. *Korean J. Gastroenterol.* **2009**, *54*, 36–41. [CrossRef]
18. May, G.R.; Sutherland, L.R.; Shaffer, E.A. Efficacy of bile acid therapy for gallstone dissolution: A meta-analysis of randomized trials. *Aliment. Pharmacol. Ther.* **1993**, *7*, 139–148. [CrossRef] [PubMed]
19. Venneman, N.G.; Besselink, M.G.; Keulemans, Y.C.; Vanberge-Henegouwen, G.P.; Boermeester, M.A.; Broeders, I.A.; Go, P.M.; van Erpecum, K.J. Ursodeoxycholic acid exerts no beneficial effect in patients with symptomatic gallstones awaiting cholecystectomy. *Hepatology* **2006**, *43*, 1276–1283. [CrossRef]
20. European Association for the Study of the Liver. Electronic address, e.e.e. EASL Clinical Practice Guidelines on the prevention, diagnosis and treatment of gallstones. *J. Hepatol.* **2016**, *65*, 146–181. [CrossRef]
21. Rubin, R.A.; Kowalski, T.E.; Khandelwal, M.; Malet, P.F. Ursodiol for hepatobiliary disorders. *Ann. Intern. Med.* **1994**, *121*, 207–218. [CrossRef] [PubMed]
22. Podda, M.; Zuin, M.; Battezzati, P.M.; Ghezzi, C.; de Fazio, C.; Dioguardi, M.L. Efficacy and safety of a combination of chenodeoxycholic acid and ursodeoxycholic acid for gallstone dissolution: A comparison with ursodeoxycholic acid alone. *Gastroenterology* **1989**, *96*, 222–229. [CrossRef] [PubMed]
23. Leuschner, M.; Leuschner, U.; Lazarovici, D.; Kurtz, W.; Hellstern, A. Dissolution of gall stones with an ursodeoxycholic acid menthol preparation: A controlled prospective double blind trial. *Gut* **1988**, *29*, 428–432. [CrossRef]
24. Yoo, E.S.; Yoo, B.M.; Kim, J.H.; Hwang, J.C.; Yang, M.J.; Lee, K.M.; Kim, S.S.; Noh, C.K. Evaluation of risk factors for recurrent primary common bile duct stone in patients with cholecystectomy. *Scand. J. Gastroenterol.* **2018**, *53*, 466–470. [CrossRef] [PubMed]
25. Keizman, D.; Shalom, M.I.; Konikoff, F. An angulated common bile duct predisposes to recurrent symptomatic bile duct stones after endoscopic stone extraction. *Surg. Endosc. Other Interv. Tech.* **2006**, *20*, 1594–1599. [CrossRef]
26. Park, B.K.; Seo, J.H.; Jeon, H.H.; Choi, J.W.; Won, S.Y.; Cho, Y.S.; Lee, C.K.; Park, H.; Kim, D.W. A nationwide population-based study of common bile duct stone recurrence after endoscopic stone removal in Korea. *J. Gastroenterol.* **2018**, *53*, 670–678. [CrossRef]
27. Wu, Y.; Xu, C.J.; Xu, S.F. Advances in risk factors for recurrence of common bile duct stones. *Int. J. Med. Sci.* **2021**, *18*, 1067. [CrossRef]
28. Keizman, D.; Ish Shalom, M.; Konikoff, F.M. Recurrent symptomatic common bile duct stones after endoscopic stone extraction in elderly patients. *Gastrointest. Endosc.* **2006**, *64*, 60–65. [CrossRef]
29. Tint, G.S.; Salen, G.; Shefer, S. Effect of ursodeoxycholic acid and chenodeoxycholic acid on cholesterol and bile acid metabolism. *Gastroenterology* **1986**, *91*, 1007–1018. [CrossRef]
30. Czygan, P.; Stiehl, A.; Raedsch, R.; Seitz, H.; Kommerell, B. *Dissolution of Cholesterol Gallstones by Combination Therapy of Urso/Cheno Versus Urso*; MTP Press Lancaster: Lancaster, UK, 1985; pp. 351–353.
31. Ellis, W.R.; Bell, G.D.; Middleton, B.; White, D.A. Adjunct to bile-acid treatment for gall-stone dissolution: Low-dose chenodeoxycholic acid combined with a terpene preparation. *Br. Med. J.* **1981**, *282*, 611–612. [CrossRef]

32. Ellis, W.R.; Bell, G.D. Treatment of biliary duct stones with a terpene preparation. *Br. Med. J.* **1981**, *282*, 611. [CrossRef] [PubMed]
33. Yoon, W.J.; Kim, H.N.; Park, E.; Ryu, S.; Chang, Y.; Shin, H.; Kim, H.L.; Yi, S.Y. The Impact of Cholecystectomy on the Gut Microbiota: A Case-Control Study. *J. Clin. Med.* **2019**, *8*, 79. [CrossRef] [PubMed]
34. Li, Y.D.; Liu, B.N.; Zhao, S.H.; Zhou, Y.L.; Bai, L.; Liu, E.Q. Changes in gut microbiota composition and diversity associated with post-cholecystectomy diarrhea. *World J. Gastroenterol.* **2021**, *27*, 391–403. [CrossRef]
35. Lee, J.; Lee, S.; Kim, H.; Bae, J.; Park, J.S. Gut Microbial Profile Changes in Patients with Gallbladder Stones after UDCA/CDCA Treatment. *Biomedicines* **2023**, *11*, 777. [CrossRef] [PubMed]
36. Tang, R.; Wei, Y.; Li, Y.; Chen, W.; Chen, H.; Wang, Q.; Yang, F.; Miao, Q.; Xiao, X.; Zhang, H.; et al. Gut microbial profile is altered in primary biliary cholangitis and partially restored after UDCA therapy. *Gut* **2018**, *67*, 534–541. [CrossRef]
37. Li, H.; Wang, Q.; Chen, P.; Zhou, C.; Zhang, X.; Chen, L. Ursodeoxycholic Acid Treatment Restores Gut Microbiota and Alleviates Liver Inflammation in Non-Alcoholic Steatohepatitic Mouse Model. *Front. Pharmacol.* **2021**, *12*, 788558. [CrossRef]
38. Guan, Y.; Xu, F.; Zhang, X.; Fu, X.; Wang, J.; Song, S.; Sun, Y.; Yuan, Q.; Zhu, F. Roles of ursodeoxycholic acid in the bile biochemistry and metabolomics in patients with choledocholithiasis: A prospective study. *Metabolomics* **2022**, *18*, 46. [CrossRef]
39. Kim, J.W.; Oh, H.C.; Do, J.H.; Choi, Y.S.; Lee, S.E. Has the prevalence of cholesterol gallstones increased in K orea? A preliminary single-center experience. *J. Dig. Dis.* **2013**, *14*, 559–563. [CrossRef]
40. Diehl, A.K. Epidemiology and natural history of gallstone disease. *Gastroenterol. Clin. N. Am.* **1991**, *20*, 1–19. [CrossRef]
41. Parker, R.A.; Garcia, R.; Ryan, C.S.; Liu, X.; Shipkova, P.; Livanov, V.; Patel, P.; Ho, S.P. Bile acid and sterol metabolism with combined HMG-CoA reductase and PCSK9 suppression. *J. Lipid Res.* **2013**, *54*, 2400–2409. [CrossRef]
42. Sugiyama, M.; Atomi, Y. Risk factors predictive of late complications after endoscopic sphincterotomy for bile duct stones: Long-term (more than 10 years) follow-up study. *Am. J. Gastroenterol.* **2002**, *97*, 2763–2767. [CrossRef] [PubMed]
43. Hyun, J.J.; Lee, H.S.; Kim, C.D.; Dong, S.H.; Lee, S.-O.; Ryu, J.K.; Lee, D.H.; Jeong, S.; Kim, T.N.; Lee, J. Efficacy of magnesium trihydrate of ursodeoxycholic acid and chenodeoxycholic acid for gallstone dissolution: A prospective multicenter trial. *Gut Liver* **2015**, *9*, 547. [CrossRef] [PubMed]
44. National Institutes of Health (US), Office of Medical Applications of Research. *Gallstones and Laparoscopic Cholecystectomy*; National Institutes of Health (US), Office of Medical Applications of Research: Bethesda, MD, USA, 1992; Volume 10, pp. 1–28.
45. Caddy, G.R.; Kirby, J.; Kirk, S.J.; Allen, M.J.; Moorehead, R.J.; Tham, T.C. Natural history of asymptomatic bile duct stones at time of cholecystectomy. *Ulst. Med. J.* **2005**, *74*, 108–112.

Disclaimer/Publisher's Note: The statements, opinions and data contained in all publications are solely those of the individual author(s) and contributor(s) and not of MDPI and/or the editor(s). MDPI and/or the editor(s) disclaim responsibility for any injury to people or property resulting from any ideas, methods, instructions or products referred to in the content.

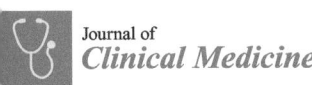

Article

Impact of Interhospital Transfer on Outcomes in Acute Pancreatitis: Implications for Healthcare Quality

Tamara F. Kahan [1], Matthew Antony Manoj [2], Ankit Chhoda [2], Anabel Liyen Cartelle [1], Kelsey Anderson [1], Shaharyar A. Zuberi [1], Steven D. Freedman [2] and Sunil G. Sheth [2,*]

[1] Department of Medicine, Beth Israel Deaconess Medical Center, Boston, MA 02215, USA; tkahan@bidmc.harvard.edu (T.F.K.); aliyenca@bidmc.harvard.edu (A.L.C.); kander17@bidmc.harvard.edu (K.A.); shaharyar.zuberi@nyulangone.org (S.A.Z.)

[2] Division of Gastroenterology, Department of Medicine, Beth Israel Deaconess Medical Center, Harvard Medical School, 330 Brookline Ave., Boston, MA 02215, USA; mmanoj1@bidmc.harvard.edu (M.A.M.); ankitchhoda@gmail.com (A.C.); sfreedma@bidmc.harvard.edu (S.D.F.)

* Correspondence: ssheth@bidmc.harvard.edu

Abstract: Background/Objectives: Effective management of acute pancreatitis (AP) hinges on prompt volume resuscitation and is adversely affected by delays in diagnosis. Given diverse clinical settings (tertiary care vs. community hospitals), further investigation is needed to understand the impact of the initial setting to which patients presented on clinical outcomes and quality of care. This study aimed to compare outcomes and quality indicators between AP patients who first presented to the emergency department (ED) of a tertiary care center and AP patients transferred from community hospitals. **Methods**: This study included AP patients managed at our tertiary care hospital between 2008 and 2018. We compared demographics and outcomes, including length of stay (LOS), intensive care unit (ICU) admission, rates of local and systemic complications, re-admission rates, and one-year mortality in transferred patients and those admitted from the ED. Quality indicators of interest included duration of volume resuscitation, time until advancement to enteral feeding, pain requiring opioid medication [measured in morphine milliequivalent (MME) dosing], and surgical referrals for cholecystectomy. Categorical variables were analyzed by chi-square or Fisher's exact test; continuous variables were compared using Kruskal–Wallis tests. Regression was performed to assess the impact of transfer status on our outcomes of interest. **Results**: Our cohort of 882 AP patients comprised 648 patients admitted from the ED and 234 patients transferred from a community hospital. Transferred patients were older (54.6 vs. 51.0 years old, $p < 0.01$) and had less frequent alcohol use (28% vs. 39%, $p < 0.01$). Transferred patients had a significantly greater frequency of gallstone AP (40% vs. 23%), but a lower frequency of alcohol AP (16% vs. 22%) and idiopathic AP (29% vs. 41%) ($p < 0.001$). Regarding clinical outcomes, transferred patients had significantly higher rates of severe AP (revised Atlanta classification) (10% vs. 2% severe, $p < 0.001$) and ICU admission (8% vs. 2%, $p < 0.001$) and longer median LOS (5 vs. 4 days, $p < 0.001$). Regarding quality indicators, there was no significant difference in the number of days of intravenous fluid administration, or days until advancement to enteral feeding, pain requiring opioid pain medication, or rates of surgical referral for cholecystectomy. **Conclusions**: Though the quality of care was similar in both groups, transferred patients had more severe AP with higher rates of systemic complications and ICU admissions and longer LOS, with no difference in quality indicators between groups.

Keywords: acute pancreatitis; quality of care; tertiary care center; community hospital

Citation: Kahan, T.F.; Manoj, M.A.; Chhoda, A.; Liyen Cartelle, A.; Anderson, K.; Zuberi, S.A.; Freedman, S.D.; Sheth, S.G. Impact of Interhospital Transfer on Outcomes in Acute Pancreatitis: Implications for Healthcare Quality. *J. Clin. Med.* **2024**, *13*, 6817. https://doi.org/10.3390/jcm13226817

Academic Editor: Stanley W. Ashley

Received: 24 October 2024
Revised: 9 November 2024
Accepted: 11 November 2024
Published: 13 November 2024

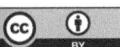

Copyright: © 2024 by the authors. Licensee MDPI, Basel, Switzerland. This article is an open access article distributed under the terms and conditions of the Creative Commons Attribution (CC BY) license (https://creativecommons.org/licenses/by/4.0/).

1. Introduction

Acute pancreatitis (AP) is a severe inflammatory disorder of the pancreas accounting for over 300,000 hospitalizations in the United States each year [1]. The financial burden of AP is substantial, with costs reaching up to $2.6 billion annually [2]. Despite a decline in mortality rates over the past decade, AP continues to present considerable mortality risks particularly in high-risk groups; approximately 25% of patients develop severe AP which has a mortality rate of 20% [3].

As the incidence of AP has increased, recently reported to be at a rate of 2–5% per year, guidelines for early evidence-based interventions for management have been developed to mitigate AP-related mortality [4]. While AP has numerous etiologies that are managed differently, there are consistencies in the management of AP that are recommended regardless of etiology, namely intravenous fluid resuscitation and the prevention of local and systemic complications. Current ACG guidelines based on expert opinion and clinical trials recommend moderately aggressive fluid resuscitation with lactated ringer within the first 24 h of admission [5–7]. In patients with mild AP, oral feeding should be initiated based on patient hunger. The initiation of oral feeding within 24–48 h of presentation is associated with superior outcomes. Randomized controlled trials have demonstrated that there is no indication for the slow advancement of diet from clear liquids to solids [8].

Patients with AP present to community hospitals and tertiary care centers, with community hospitals vastly outnumbering tertiary care centers. Patients who initially present to a community hospital may be transferred to a tertiary care center, often for subspecialty care or prolonged intensive care that cannot be offered at the community hospital. Studies comparing outcomes of transferred patients with AP to patients admitted from the emergency department (ED) are limited and results are difficult to interpret, as higher mortality among transferred patients may reflect their increased illness severity rather than the care delivered at the community hospital or risks associated with discontinuity of care during the transfer process [9–11]. While community hospitals may not have robust advanced endoscopy resources or a team of gastroenterologists with expertise in pancreaticobiliary disease, the key early interventions—fluid resuscitation and nutritional support—can be delivered both in community settings and tertiary care [5].

Studies assessing outcomes for transferred and non-transferred patients with non-pancreatitis acute conditions have yielded mixed results. A multi-center study of 885,392 general adult inpatients found that transferred patients spend more time in intensive care units and have higher inpatient mortality [12]. This trend was corroborated and expanded upon in an analysis using National Inpatient Sample data, which included 1,397,712 transferred patients and 31,692,211 patients admitted from the ED and demonstrated that transferred patients had more frequent in-hospital adverse events and more complex discharge disposition [13]. However, the above analyses were limited by not being disease-specific and thus included transfers that occurred for specialty services or procedural intervention. Furthermore, both studies utilized administrative data and were not able to characterize patients as completely as would have been possible through chart review. While inter-hospital transfer confers risks related to discontinuity of care, results must be interpreted with acknowledgement of the increased severity and complexity of illness in this patient population. Within a nationally representative sample of Medicare claims for acute coronary syndrome, congestive heart failure, arrhythmia, sepsis, and pneumonia, among other conditions, transferred patients had greater resource utilization and variable results for 3-day and 30-day mortality. Patients transferred with acute coronary syndrome, sepsis, stroke, or respiratory disease had lower odds of 3-day and 30-day mortality. Patients transferred with esophageal or gastrointestinal disease, congestive heart failure, or renal failure, among other conditions, had greater odds of 3-day and 30-day mortality [14]. Finally, a study of outcomes of transferred and non-transferred patients with acute non-ST elevation myocardial infarctions in British Columbia found similar 30-day and 1-year mortality rates among both groups of patients.

Our study aimed to compare baseline characteristics and clinical outcomes between patients with AP admitted from the ED of a tertiary care center and patients with AP transferred from community hospitals in the referral network. Specifically, we sought to examine length of stay, in-hospital adverse events, intensive care unit (ICU) admissions, and mortality. We also compared quality indicators of care for AP. We hypothesize that transferred patients may have worse outcomes given the relative lack of resources at community hospitals and the tendency to transfer patients who have clinically worsened over their hospital stay. We aim to elucidate disparities in AP outcomes with the ultimate goal of guiding interventions to reduce these disparities.

2. Methods

2.1. Study Design and Setting

We conducted a retrospective cohort study of patients diagnosed with AP and hospitalized at a tertiary care center in the Boston area between 1 January 2008 and 31 December 2018. This study was approved by our center's Institutional Review Board (Protocol ID: 2016P000158). This study is reported in accordance with the Strengthening the Reporting of Observational Studies in Epidemiology (STROBE) reporting guideline (Supplement S1) [15].

2.2. Patient Population

Adult patients (aged $\geq$ 18 years) were identified through International Classification of Diseases, Ninth and Tenth Revision codes 577.1 and K85.9 [16]. Electronic health records were then manually reviewed to confirm the diagnosis of AP. The diagnosis of AP was based on revised Atlanta classification (two of the following during hospitalization: typical abdominal pain, elevation of serum lipase level three times upper limit of normal, or evidence of pancreatitis on cross-sectional imaging) [17]. Patients who carried a diagnosis of chronic pancreatitis or pancreaticobiliary malignancy were excluded.

2.3. Data Collection

We collected demographic data including age, sex, race, ethnicity, body mass index (BMI), alcohol use, tobacco smoking history, and etiology of AP. Clinical data included comorbidities such as pre-existing DM, kidney disease, pulmonary disease, and cardiovascular disease quantified through the age-adjusted Charlson Comorbidity Index (CCI) and pain at time of presentation [measured through the visual analog scale (VAS)] [18]. The severity of AP at presentation was graded based on the revised Atlanta classification [coded as mild AP (no local or systemic complications), moderately severe AP (transient organ failure, local complications, or exacerbation of co-morbid disease) and severe AP (characterized by persistent organ failure for more than 48 h) [19]. The patients' BISAP score, which predicts in-hospital mortality in AP based on clinical and laboratory variables, was calculated on presentation [20]. Opioid use during the entire hospitalization was quantified and converted into morphine milliequivalent (MME) units.

2.4. Outcomes of Interest

Outcome variables included length of stay, ICU admission, local complications of AP (i.e., pancreatic pseudocysts, peri-pancreatic fluid collections, pancreatic necrosis, and splenic vein thrombosis), systemic complications of AP (i.e., renal failure, acute hypoxemic respiratory failure requiring intubation, and sepsis), extra-pancreatic complications (i.e., alcohol withdrawal, gastrointestinal bleeding, and delirium), re-admissions within thirty days of discharge from index hospitalization, and mortality within one year of index hospitalization. Finally, we assessed quality indicators of care for AP including duration of volume resuscitation, time until advancement to enteral feeding, opioid use during the entire hospitalization [quantified and converted into morphine milliequivalent (MME) units], and surgical referrals for cholecystectomy, with the aforementioned quality indicators chosen based on a review of ACG guidelines and the literature [5,21,22].

2.5. Statistical Analysis

Categorical data are presented as proportions while continuous variables are reported as medians with interquartile ranges. Statistical differences in categorical variables were assessed using chi-square tests or Fisher's exact tests, while continuous variables were analyzed using Kruskal–Wallis tests. Outcome variables (length of stay, ICU admission, local complications, systemic complications, extra-pancreatic complications, readmissions, and one-year mortality) served as dependent variables and were analyzed using univariate linear and logistic regression to identify associations with transferred or non-transferred status. Multivariate regression, controlling for age, sex, BMI, CCI, and AP etiology was planned for variables with $p < 0.1$ on univariate regression. All statistical analysis was performed using STATA software (StataCorp LLC, Version 17.0, College Station, TX, USA) A p-value < 0.05 was considered statistically significant.

3. Results

We identified 882 patients who met our inclusion criteria for AP and who did not carry a diagnosis of chronic pancreatitis or pancreaticobiliary malignancy. The sample included 648 patients admitted from the ED (73.4%) and 234 patients transferred from community hospitals (26.5%).

3.1. Demographics and Clinical Features

Baseline demographics and patient characteristics of the study cohort are summarized in Table 1. The mean age of the full cohort was 51.8 years (SD 21.2); patients admitted from the ED were significantly younger than transferred patients (51.0 vs. 54.6, $p < 0.01$). The cohort was 49% female and 73% Caucasian; median BMI was 26.3 (7.1) kg/m². There were no statistically significant differences in distribution of sex, race, or BMI between the two groups. We observed a substantial psychosocial burden within our study sample, with 310 patients (36%) reporting active alcohol use and 241 patients (27%) reporting active smoking at time of admission. Notably, active alcohol use was significantly more prevalent in patients admitted from the ED compared to transferred patients (39% vs. 28%, $p < 0.01$). The median CCI of patients was 1; there was no difference in CCI when comparing transferred patients to patients admitted from the ED.

3.2. Pancreatitis Etiology and Severity

The etiology of AP varied between groups, with transferred patients having significantly higher rates of gallstone pancreatitis (40% vs. 23%) and post-ERCP pancreatitis (4% vs. 2%), and lower rates of alcoholic pancreatitis (16% vs. 22%) and idiopathic pancreatitis (29% vs. 41%) compared to patients admitted from the ED ($p < 0.01$). On presentation, out of the full sample of 882 patients, 642 patients (76%) met criteria for mild pancreatitis, 172 patients (20%) met criteria for moderate pancreatitis, and 34 patients (4%) met criteria for severe pancreatitis by revised Atlanta classification. Transferred patients had significantly higher rates of moderate (32% vs. 16%) and severe (10% vs. 2%) pancreatitis ($p < 0.01$). Median BISAP score was 1 among both patients admitted from the ED and transferred patients.

3.3. Clinical Outcomes

3.3.1. Length of Stay and Intensive Care Unit Admission

Transferred patients had a significantly longer median length of stay (5 vs. 4 days, $p < 0.001$) and were more likely to be transferred to the ICU (8% vs. 2%, $p < 0.001$) compared to patients admitted from the ED (Table 2). These associations were statistically significant on regression analysis (Table 3). When controlling for age, sex, BMI, CCI, and AP etiology, transferred patients had significantly longer lengths of stay (OR 3.09; 95%CI 2.08–4.10) and were significantly more likely to be transferred to the ICU compared to patients admitted from the ED (OR 7.05; 95%CI 3.22–15.44) (Table 4).

Table 1. Demographic and clinical characteristics of patients admitted from the ED and transferred patients with acute pancreatitis.

	Demographics			
	Total (N = 882)	Patients Admitted from ED (N = 648)	Transferred Patients (N = 234)	p-Value
Age [mean (SD)]	51.8 (21.2)	51.0 (20.6)	54.6 (21.8)	<0.01
Body Mass Index [M (IQR)]	26.3 (8.3)	26.0 (8.7)	26.7 (7.1)	0.54
Sex [Female n (%)]	431 (49%)	310 (48%)	121 (52%)	0.31
Race [Caucasian n (%)]	633 (73%)	460 (72%)	173 (78%)	0.1
Active Alcohol use [n (%)]	310 (36%)	246 (39%)	64 (28%)	<0.01
Active Tobacco Use [n (%)]	241 (27%)	187 (29%)	54 (23%)	0.08
Revised Atlanta Classification [mild/moderate/severe: n (%)]	642 (76%)	518 (82%)	124 (57%)	<0.001
	172 (20%)	102 (16%)	70 (32%)	
	34 (4%)	12 (2%)	22 (10%)	
Etiology of AP [n (%)]				
Gallstone	237 (27%)	145 (23%)	92 (40%)	<0.001
Alcohol	179 (20%)	143 (22%)	36 (16%)	
Post-ERCP	24 (3%)	14 (2%)	10 (4%)	
Other [1]	102 (13%)	81 (12%)	28 (11.5%)	
Idiopathic	327 (37%)	261 (41%)	66 (29%)	
Charlson Comorbidity Index [M (IQR)]	1 (1)	0 (1)	1 (2)	0.3
BISAP [M (IQR)]	1 (0)	1 (0)	1 (1)	<0.001

[1] Includes hypertriglyceridemia, medication-induced, autoimmune pancreatitis, pancreatic mass, and acute on chronic acute pancreatitis.

3.3.2. Local and Systemic Complications

We compared the frequency of local complications of AP, including pancreatic pseudocysts, peri-pancreatic fluid collections, pancreatic necrosis, and splenic vein thrombosis, between transferred patients and patients admitted from the ED. There was no difference in the rates of any of these local complications between groups. We also assessed systemic complications of AP, including renal failure, acute hypoxemic respiratory failure requiring intubation, and sepsis. Transferred patients had significantly higher rates of systemic complications overall (29% vs. 7%, $p < 0.001$), and higher rates of each complication when analyzed individually ($p < 0.001$). On multivariate regression, transferred patients were significantly more likely to have systemic complications of AP (OR 4.22; 95% CI 2.61–6.84) (Table 4). Regarding extra-pancreatic complications, there was no difference between patients admitted from the ED and transferred patients when considering all extra-pancreatic complications (i.e., alcohol withdrawal, gastrointestinal bleeding, and delirium) in aggregate though when considered individually, patients admitted from the ED had higher rates of alcohol withdrawal (5.7% vs. 1%, $p < 0.01$) and lower rates of delirium (1.5% vs. 6%, $p < 0.01$) compared to transferred patients.

3.3.3. Thirty-Day Re-Admissions and One-Year Mortality

Overall, 166 (19%) patients were re-admitted within 30-days of discharge; re-admission rates did not vary between transferred patients and patients admitted from the ED. One-year mortality in the sample was 2.5%; one-year mortality was not significantly different when comparing transferred patients and patients admitted from the ED.

Table 2. Clinical outcomes and quality of care measures of patients admitted from the ED and transferred patients with acute pancreatitis.

	Clinical Outcomes			
	Total (N = 882)	Patients Admitted from ED (N = 648)	Transferred Patients (N = 234)	p-Value
Length of Stay (days) [M (IQR)]	4 (3.6)	4 (4)	5 (5.8)	<0.001
ICU transfer [n (%)]	29 (3%)	10 (2%)	19 (8%)	<0.001
Local complications (defined as one or more of the following: pseudocysts, peri-pancreatic fluid collections, pancreatic necrosis, and splenic vein thrombosis) [n (%)]	128 (15%)	89 (14%)	39 (17%)	0.28
Systemic complications (defined as one or more of the following: renal failure, acute hypoxemic respiratory failure requiring intubation, and sepsis) [n (%)]	112 (13%)	43 (7%)	69 (29%)	<0.001
Renal failure	52 (6%)	22 (3%)	30 (13%)	<0.001
Acute hypoxemic respiratory failure requiring intubation	18 (2%)	4 (0.6%)	14 (6%)	<0.001
Sepsis	41 (5%)	16 (2%)	25 (11%)	<0.001
Extra-pancreatic complications (including alcohol withdrawal, gastrointestinal bleeding, and delirium) [n (%)]	83 (9%)	61 (9%)	22 (9%)	0.99
Alcohol withdrawal [n (%)]	39 (4%)	37 (6%)	2 (1%)	<0.01
Delirium [n (%)]	24 (3%)	10 (2%)	14 (6%)	<0.01
Re-admitted within 30-days of discharge [n (%)]	166 (19%)	131 (20%)	35 (11%)	0.08
One-year mortality [n (%)]	22 (3%)	13 (3%)	9 (5%)	0.15
	Quality of Care Measures			
	Total (N = 882)	Patients Admitted from ED (N = 648)	Transferred Patients (N = 234)	p-Value
Days of IV fluid resuscitation [M (IQR)]	3 (2)	3 (2)	3 (3)	0.69
Initial pain assessment through visual analog scale (VAS) [M (IQR)]	7 (4)	7 (4)	7 (4)	0.38
MME within first 24 hours of admission [M (IQR)]	8.5 (14)	8.5 (16)	8.5 (10)	0.79
Total MME over admission [M (IQR)]	14 (44.6)	12 (41)	16 (59.8)	0.36
Time to PO nutrition (days) [M (IQR)]	2 (2)	2 (2)	2 (3)	0.44
Received IV fluids within 4 hours of admission [n (%)]	554 (81%)	413 (82%)	141 (78%)	0.32
Surgical referral for cholecystectomy [n (%)]	169 (19%)	104 (16%)	65 (28%)	0.57

Table 3. Univariate linear and logistic regression analysis assessing the association of transfer status with various outcomes of AP (n = 882).

Parameter	Odds Ratio	p-Value
Length of stay	3.09 (95%CI: 2.08–4.10)	<0.001
ICU admission	7.05 (95%CI: 3.22–15.44)	<0.001
Local complications	1.14 (95%CI: 0.74–1.75)	0.57
Systemic complications	4.22 (95%CI: 2.61–6.84)	<0.001
Extra-pancreatic complications	1.05 (95%CI: 0.61–1.80)	0.86
Re-admission within 30 days	0.86 (95%CI: 0.57–1.29)	0.46
One-year mortality	1.55 (95%CI: 0.47–5.11)	0.56

Table 4. Multivariate regression analysis assessing the association of transfer status with various outcomes of AP, controlling for age, gender, BMI, CCI, and etiology of AP (n = 882).

Parameter	Odds Ratio	p-Value
Length of stay	3.16 (95%CI: 1.99–4.33)	<0.001
ICU admission	8.23 (95%CI: 3.26–20.72)	<0.001
Systemic complications	3.75 (95%CI: 2.01–5.89)	<0.001

3.4. Quality of Care Measures

An initial pain assessment score using VAS demonstrated a median score of seven (IQR: 4). Regarding pain management with opioids, patients received a median of 8.5 MME within the first 24 h of admission and 14 MME over the course of admission. Regarding IV fluid resuscitation, 554 patients (62.8%) of patients received IV fluids within four hours of presentation and patients received a median of 3 days (IQR: 2) of IV fluids. Diet was advanced to oral nutrition in a median of 2 days (IQR: 2). On discharge, 169 patients (19.1%) received a surgical referral for cholecystectomy. There was no significant difference in any of the above measures when comparing transferred patients to patients admitted from the ED.

4. Discussion

We found numerous differences in baseline characteristics and outcomes for patients with AP when comparing those transferred from community hospitals to those who presented to the ED of our tertiary care center. We found that transferred patients had a higher incidence of moderate and severe AP and higher rates of gallstone-related and post-ERCP pancreatitis. Patients who presented to the ED had a higher baseline rate of active alcohol use and higher rates of alcohol-related pancreatitis. Transferred patients had longer lengths of stay, higher rates of admission to the ICU, and higher rates of systemic complications of pancreatitis compared to patients admitted from the ED.

There are numerous possible explanations for the above findings. The higher incidence of moderate and severe pancreatitis, longer lengths of stay, higher rates of admission to the ICU, and higher rates of systemic complications of transferred patients may represent greater illness severity among transferred patients or suboptimal initial management at community hospitals; however, there were no differences in the quality of care between groups. Reassuringly, mortality rates were not significantly different between transferred patients and patients admitted from the ED, reflecting uniform high-quality care delivered at our tertiary care pancreas center. Unfortunately, we did not have access to data on fluid resuscitation delivered at community hospitals, with fluid resuscitation being one of the cornerstones of management in AP. Inadequate fluid resuscitation is associated with the development of necrotizing pancreatitis and consequent multi-organ failure [23,24]. Data support that delayed presentation for acute pancreatitis is associated with greater pancreatitis severity at the time of presentation, higher rates of organ failure, and greater likelihood of requiring procedural intervention [25].

Our study has a number of strengths. This study is strengthened by rigorous clinical follow-up, detailed clinical history, and meticulous work-up for each AP patient in a large sample of over 800 patients with AP. Manual chart review ensures a high degree of accuracy [26]. The retrospective design of the study mitigates the "Hawthorne effect", providing a more accurate reflection of real-time practices. We have included a wide range of outcome variables including systemic and extra-pancreatic complications of AP, which are responsible for a substantial mortality and morbidity burden.

Despite these strengths, there are a number of limitations which should be noted. First, these findings stem from the population of a large single-center tertiary referral center, and thus may not be generalizable to all other hospital systems. Second, our current sample size limits the ability to detect small differences between groups. Third, our results may reflect referral bias, with transfer patients having more severe AP at the time of transfer. Last, as a retrospective study, although many clinical and demographic variables were captured, the likelihood of unmeasured confounding always exists.

In conclusion, we found that relative to patients admitted from the ED of a tertiary care center, transferred patients had longer lengths of stay, higher rates of admission to the ICU, and higher rates of systemic complications though readmissions within 30-days of discharge and one-year mortality was not significantly different between groups, indicating that high quality care delivered by our pancreas center serves to mitigate possible greater illness severity or suboptimal management of transferred patients prior to their transfer. Further prospective studies are needed to identify reasons for disparities in outcomes between the two groups of AP patients.

Supplementary Materials: The following supporting information can be downloaded at: https://www.mdpi.com/article/10.3390/jcm13226817/s1, Supplement S1: Strengthening the Reporting of Observational Studies in Epidemiology (STROBE) Statement.

Author Contributions: Conceptualization, T.F.K., A.C., S.D.F. and S.G.S.; Methodology, T.F.K., A.C., A.L.C., K.A., S.A.Z. and S.G.S.; Formal analysis, T.F.K., M.A.M. and A.C.; Investigation, T.F.K. and A.C.; Data curation, T.F.K., A.L.C., K.A. and S.A.Z.; Writing—original draft, T.F.K., M.A.M. and A.C.; Writing—review & editing, A.L.C., K.A., S.A.Z., S.D.F. and S.G.S.; Supervision, S.D.F. and S.G.S.; Project administration, S.D.F. and S.G.S. All authors have read and agreed to the published version of the manuscript.

Funding: This research received no external funding.

Institutional Review Board Statement: The study was approved by the Institutional Review Board (or Ethics Committee) of the Beth Israel Deaconess Medical Center (Protocol ID: 2016P000158) on the date of November 2016 for studies involving humans.

Informed Consent Statement: Patient consent was waived due to the investigation posing no more than minimal risk to human subjects.

Data Availability Statement: The original contributions presented in the study are included in the article/Supplementary Materials, further inquiries can be directed to the corresponding author.

Acknowledgments: This article is a revised and expanded version of an abstract entitled "Outcomes and Quality of Care of Transferred and Non-Transferred Patients with Acute Pancreatitis", which was presented at Digestive Disease Week, Washington, DC, USA, 18–21 May 2024.

Conflicts of Interest: The authors declare no conflicts of interest.

References

1. Peery, A.F.; Crockett, S.D.; Murphy, C.C.; Jensen, E.T.; Kim, H.P.; Egberg, M.D.; Lund, J.L.; Moon, A.M.; Pate, V.; Barnes, E.L. Burden and cost of gastrointestinal, liver, and pancreatic diseases in the United States: Update 2021. *Gastroenterology* **2022**, *162*, 621–644. [CrossRef] [PubMed]
2. Li, C.; Jiang, M.; Pan, C.; Li, J.; Xu, L. The global, regional, and national burden of acute pancreatitis in 204 countries and territories, 1990–2019. *BMC Gastroenterol.* **2021**, *21*, 332. [CrossRef] [PubMed]

1. Di, M.-Y.; Liu, H.; Yang, Z.-Y.; Bonis, P.A.L.; Tang, J.-L.; Lau, J. Prediction Models of Mortality in Acute Pancreatitis in Adults: A Systematic Review. *Ann. Intern. Med.* **2016**, *165*, 482. [CrossRef] [PubMed]
2. Xiao, A.Y.; Tan, M.L.Y.; Wu, L.M.; Asrani, V.M.; Windsor, J.A.; Yadav, D.; Petrov, M.S. Global incidence and mortality of pancreatic diseases: A systematic review, meta-analysis, and meta-regression of population-based cohort studies. *Lancet Gastroenterol. Hepatol.* **2016**, *1*, 45–55. [CrossRef]
3. Tenner, S.; Vege, S.S.; Sheth, S.G.; Sauer, B.; Yang, A.; Conwell, D.L.; Yadlapati, R.H.; Gardner, T.B. American College of Gastroenterology Guidelines: Management of Acute Pancreatitis. *Off. J. Am. Coll. Gastroenterol. | ACG* **2024**, *119*, 419. [CrossRef]
4. Gardner, T.B. Fluid Resuscitation in Acute Pancreatitis—Going over the WATERFALL. *N. Engl. J. Med.* **2022**, *387*, 1038–1039. [CrossRef]
5. Garg, P.K.; Mahapatra, S.J. Optimum Fluid Therapy in Acute Pancreatitis Needs an Alchemist. *Gastroenterology* **2021**, *160*, 655–659. [CrossRef]
6. Yao, Q.; Liu, P.; Peng, S.; Xu, X.; Wu, Y. Effects of immediate or early oral feeding on acute pancreatitis: A systematic review and meta-analysis. *Pancreatology* **2022**, *22*, 175–184. [CrossRef]
7. Mueller, S.K.; Zheng, J.; Orav, E.J.; Schnipper, J.L. Rates, Predictors and Variability of Interhospital Transfers: A National Evaluation. *J. Hosp. Med.* **2017**, *12*, 435–442. [CrossRef]
8. Cohen, M.D.; Hilligoss, P.B. The published literature on handoffs in hospitals: Deficiencies identified in an extensive review. *BMJ Qual. Saf.* **2010**, *19*, 493–497. [CrossRef]
9. Mueller, S.K.; Shannon, E.; Dalal, A.; Schnipper, J.L.; Dykes, P. Patient and Physician Experience with Interhospital Transfer: A Qualitative Study. *J. Patient Saf.* **2021**, *17*, e752. [CrossRef] [PubMed]
10. Sokol-Hessner, L.; White, A.A.; Davis, K.F.; Herzig, S.J.; Hohmann, S.F. Interhospital transfer patients discharged by academic hospitalists and general internists: Characteristics and outcomes. *J. Hosp. Med.* **2016**, *11*, 245–250. [CrossRef] [PubMed]
11. Hernandez-Boussard, T.; Davies, S.; McDonald, K.; Wang, N.E. Interhospital facility transfers in the United States: A nationwide outcomes study. *J. Patient Saf.* **2017**, *13*, 187–191. [CrossRef] [PubMed]
12. Mueller, S.; Zheng, J.; Orav, E.J.; Schnipper, J.L. Inter-hospital transfer and patient outcomes: A retrospective cohort study. *BMJ Qual. Saf.* **2019**, *28*, e1. [CrossRef] [PubMed]
13. Von Elm, E.; Altman, D.G.; Egger, M.; Pocock, S.J.; Gøtzsche, P.C.; Vandenbroucke, J.P. The Strengthening the Reporting of Observational Studies in Epidemiology (STROBE) statement: Guidelines for reporting observational studies. *Lancet* **2007**, *370*, 1453–1457. [CrossRef]
14. CDC. *International Classification of Diseases, Tenth Revision, Clinical Modification (ICD-10-CM)*; CDC: Atlanta, GA, USA, 2023. Available online: https://www.cdc.gov/nchs/icd/icd-10-cm/index.html (accessed on 21 October 2024).
15. Banks, P.A.; Bollen, T.L.; Dervenis, C.; Gooszen, H.G.; Johnson, C.D.; Sarr, M.G.; Tsiotos, G.G.; Vege, S.S. Classification of acute pancreatitis—2012: Revision of the Atlanta classification and definitions by international consensus. *Gut* **2013**, *62*, 102–111. [CrossRef]
16. Charlson, M.E.; Pompei, P.; Ales, K.L.; MacKenzie, C.R. A new method of classifying prognostic comorbidity in longitudinal studies: Development and validation. *J. Chronic Dis.* **1987**, *40*, 373–383. [CrossRef]
17. Wu, B.U.; Johannes, R.S.; Sun, X.; Tabak, Y.; Conwell, D.L.; Banks, P.A. The early prediction of mortality in acute pancreatitis: A large population-based study. *Gut* **2008**, *57*, 1698–1703. [CrossRef]
18. Gao, W.; Yang, H.-X.; Ma, C.-E. The value of BISAP score for predicting mortality and severity in acute pancreatitis: A systematic review and meta-analysis. *PLoS ONE* **2015**, *10*, e0130412. [CrossRef]
19. Ketwaroo, G.; Sealock, R.J.; Freedman, S.; Hart, P.A.; Othman, M.; Wassef, W.; Banks, P.; Vege, S.S.; Gardner, T.; Yadav, D.; et al. Quality of Care Indicators in Patients with Acute Pancreatitis. *Dig. Dis. Sci.* **2019**, *64*, 2514–2526. [CrossRef]
20. Sheth, S.G.; Maratt, J.K.; Newberry, C.; Hung, K.W.; Henry, Z.; Leiman, D.A. AGA Institute Quality Indicator Development and Uses. *Clin. Gastroenterol. Hepatol.* **2023**, *21*, 1399–1402. [CrossRef] [PubMed]
21. Brown, A.; Baillargeon, J.-D.; Hughes, M.D.; Banks, P.A. Can fluid resuscitation prevent pancreatic necrosis in severe acute pancreatitis? *Pancreatology* **2002**, *2*, 104–107. [CrossRef] [PubMed]
22. Brown, A.; Orav, J.; Banks, P.A. Hemoconcentration is an early marker for organ failure and necrotizing pancreatitis. *Pancreas* **2000**, *20*, 367–372. [CrossRef] [PubMed]
23. Mallick, B.; Dhaka, N.; Sharma, V.; Malik, S.; Sinha, S.K.; Dutta, U.; Gupta, P.; Gulati, A.; Yadav, T.D.; Gupta, V. Impact of timing of presentation of acute pancreatitis to a tertiary care centre on the outcome. *Pancreatology* **2019**, *19*, 143–148. [CrossRef]
24. Kahn, M.G.; Eliason, B.B.; Bathurst, J. Quantifying clinical data quality using relative gold standards. *AMIA Annu. Symp. Proc.* **2010**, *2010*, 356–360. Available online: https://www.ncbi.nlm.nih.gov/pmc/articles/PMC3041459/ (accessed on 21 October 2024).

Disclaimer/Publisher's Note: The statements, opinions and data contained in all publications are solely those of the individual author(s) and contributor(s) and not of MDPI and/or the editor(s). MDPI and/or the editor(s) disclaim responsibility for any injury to people or property resulting from any ideas, methods, instructions or products referred to in the content.

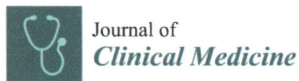

Article

Pericholecystic Fat Stranding as a Predictive Factor of Length of Stays of Patients with Acute Cholecystitis: A Novel Scoring Model

Suh-Won Lee [1,†], Cheng-Han Tsai [1,†], Hui-An Lin [1,2,3], Yu Chen [1], Sen-Kuang Hou [1,2,*] and Sheng-Feng Lin [1,3,4,5,*]

1. Department of Emergency Medicine, Taipei Medical University Hospital, Taipei 110, Taiwan; 173122@h.tmu.edu.tw (S.-W.L.); b101101122@h.tmu.edu.tw (C.-H.T.); 133005@h.tmu.edu.tw (H.-A.L.); b101102093@tmu.edu.tw (Y.C.)
2. Department of Emergency Medicine, School of Medicine, College of Medicine, Taipei Medical University, Taipei 110, Taiwan
3. School of Public Health, College of Public Health, Taipei Medical University, Taipei 110, Taiwan
4. Department of Public Health, School of Medicine, College of Medicine, Taipei Medical University, Taipei 110, Taiwan
5. Department of Evidence-Based Medicine, Taipei Medical University Hospital, Taipei 110, Taiwan
* Correspondence: 992001@h.tmu.edu.tw (S.-K.H.); linshengfeng@tmu.edu.tw (S.-F.L.); Tel.: +886-2-27372181 (ext. 8107) (S.-K.H. & S.-F.L.)
† These authors contributed equally to this work.

Abstract: Background: The 2018 Tokyo Guidelines (TG18) are used to classify the severity of acute cholecystitis (AC) but insufficient to predict the length of hospital stay (LOS). **Methods:** For patients with AC, clinical factors and computed tomography features, including our proposed grading system of pericholecystic fat stranding were used for predicting an LOS of ≥ 7 days in the logistic regression models. **Results:** Our multivariable model showed age ≥ 65 years (OR: 2.56, $p < 0.001$), C-reactive protein (CRP) ≥ 2 mg/dL (OR: 1.97, $p = 0.013$), gamma-glutamyltransferase levels (OR: 2.460, $p = 0.001$), TG18 grade (OR: 2.89 per grade, $p < 0.001$), and moderate to severe pericholecystic fat stranding (OR: 2.14, $p = 0.012$) exhibited prolonged LOS ≥ 7 days. **Conclusions:** We developed a scoring model, including TG18 grades (score of 1–3 per grade), our grading system of fat stranding (score of 1), CRP (score of 1), and gamma-glutamyltransferase (score of 1), and a cutoff of >3 had highest diagnostic performance.

Keywords: acute cholecystitis; length of stays; Tokyo guidelines; pericholecystic fat stranding; computed tomography

Citation: Lee, S.-W.; Tsai, C.-H.; Lin, H.-A.; Chen, Y.; Hou, S.-K.; Lin, S.-F. Pericholecystic Fat Stranding as a Predictive Factor of Length of Stays of Patients with Acute Cholecystitis: A Novel Scoring Model. *J. Clin. Med.* **2024**, *13*, 5734. https://doi.org/ 10.3390/jcm13195734

Academic Editors: Antonio M. Caballero-Mateos and Emmanuel Andrès

Received: 28 August 2024
Revised: 14 September 2024
Accepted: 23 September 2024
Published: 26 September 2024

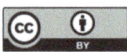

Copyright: © 2024 by the authors. Licensee MDPI, Basel, Switzerland. This article is an open access article distributed under the terms and conditions of the Creative Commons Attribution (CC BY) license (https:// creativecommons.org/licenses/by/ 4.0/).

1. Introduction

Acute cholecystitis (AC) is a common diagnosis for patients presenting in the emergency department with abdominal pain. In general, history taking, physical examination, and abdominal sonography are adequate for making a clinical diagnosis of AC [1]. However, distinguishing between complicated and uncomplicated AC generally requires multislice computed tomography (MSCT). Abdominal MSCT has high sensitivity (85% to 94%) for the detection of AC [2,3]. MSCT plays an essential role in evaluating the severity of AC [4].

The 2018 Tokyo Guidelines (TG18) regarding the diagnostic and severity grading criteria for AC are widely used to classify AC severity. The severity of AC is classified as grade I (mild), grade II (moderate), and grade III (severe) [5]. Patients with signs of cardiovascular, neurological, hematological, respiratory, renal, or hepatic system organ dysfunction are categorized as having grade III (severe) AC. Patients with an elevated white blood cell count (>18,000/mm^3), a palpable tender mass in the right upper abdominal quadrant, onset > 72 h, or marked local inflammation are categorized as having grade II (moderate) AC. Patients with uncomplicated AC who do not meet the criteria for grades II and III are categorized as having grade I (mild) AC. Patients with grade I or II AC can be treated surgically, whereas those with grade III AC are generally treated using percutaneous transhepatic gallbladder drainage [5,6]. MSCT information is not included in the TG18 diagnostic criteria for AC.

Remarkable MSCT features, such as gallbladder distension, wall thickening, and pericholecystic fat stranding, are valuable for their role in diagnosis [7]. The present study proposes that fat stranding may be associated with AC severity. In addition, other MSCT features may assist in distinguishing between complicated and uncomplicated AC. To our knowledge, few studies have evaluated the use of fat stranding signs to assess AC severity [8].

The present study determined whether fat stranding signs were associated with an increased length of hospital stay (LOS) and developed a simple and accessible scoring system that can be implemented in emergency departments.

2. Materials and Methods

2.1. Participants and Design

This single-center retrospective study was conducted between 1 January 2018 and 31 December 2020 in the emergency department of Taipei Medical University Hospital, Taipei, Taiwan. This hospital is a tertiary care center. The emergency department of this hospital is run by certified emergency physicians and has approximately 60,000 patient visits per year. Study participants were treated in the usual manner. We used the disease codes of the International Statistical Classification of Diseases, Tenth Revision, Clinical Modification (Supplementary Table S1) to enroll eligible patients. Patients who were aged ≥ 18 years, who presented to our emergency department with a confirmed diagnosis of cholecystitis (including both calculus and acalculous cholecystitis), and who were admitted to a ward for subsequent care were enrolled. Furthermore, the management of AC was by the consensus of the emergency physician and the general surgeon (laparoscopic cholecystectomy, percutaneous transhepatic gallbladder drainage [PTGBD], and endoscopic retrograde cholangiopancreatography [ERCP]). Patients were excluded if their MSCT images were not taken at the emergency department, if they were discharged directly from the emergency department, including if they were discharged against medical advice, or if their final diagnosis was not compatible with cholecystitis. The medical charts of the patients were reviewed by Suh-Won Lee, Cheng-Han Tsai, and Yu Chen. This study was approved by the Joint Institutional Review Board (reference number: N202303059).

2.2. Data Collection

Patient information relating to age, sex, vital signs, Glasgow Coma Scale score, and a history of hypertension, diabetes mellitus, chronic kidney disease, liver cirrhosis, or malignant disease was obtained upon the arrival of each patient to the emergency department. Blood samples for laboratory tests, including a complete blood cell count and differential count, C-reactive protein (CRP, normal range < 0.5 mg/dL), total bilirubin, and gamma-glutamyl transpeptidase (normal range 5–40 U/L) levels, were obtained within 2 h of the arrival of each patient to the emergency department. TG18 and fat stranding grades were analyzed by reviewing the patients' data after their discharge. The LOS was considered to be the total number of days spent in the hospital, including the days of the patient's emergency department stay. The patients were categorized into groups of LOS < 7 and LOS ≥ 7 days.

2.3. MSCT Imaging

Abdominal MSCT images were obtained by using the 128-slice SOMATOM Perspective MSCT scanner (Siemens Healthineers Inc., Forchheim, Germany). Scans were obtained from the top of the liver to the pubic symphysis in the pelvic cavity with a 0.625 mm slice thickness. All patients were administered 95 mL of Optiray 350 (Mallinckrodt Medical

Inc., Pointe Claire, QC, Canada) contrast medium intravenously. The initial interpretation of the MSCT images was performed by the on-duty emergency physician. All original MSCT images were reviewed by Suh-Won Lee, Cheng-Han Tsai, and Yu Chen to ensure the accuracy of the data.

2.4. Classification of Fat Stranding

The gallbladder fat stranding signs were categorized into four grades (Figure 1). Grade 0 was defined as definitely no sign of fat stranding. Grade 1 was considered to be gallbladder wall thickening > 0.3 cm without obvious fat stranding. Grade 2 was considered to be linear fat stranding of the fat adjacent to the gallbladder. Grade 3 was considered to be severe fat stranding extending outside the gallbladder with or without pericholecystic abscess or a gangrene change in the gallbladder wall.

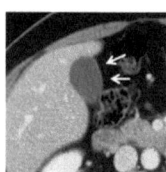
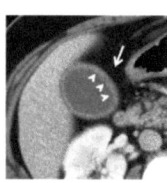
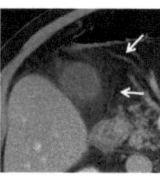
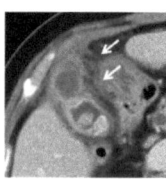

(a) Grade 0
No pericholecystic fat stranding (arrow) or gallbladder wall thickening

(b) Grade 1
Gallbladder wall thickening > 0.3 cm (arrowhead) without pericholecystic fat stranding (arrow)

(c) Grade 2
Linear pericholecystic fat stranding (arrow)

(d) Grade 3
Prominent pericholecystic reticular dirty fat (arrow)

Figure 1. Categorization of fat stranding signs. (**a**) Grade 0: no pericholecystic fat stranding or gallbladder wall thickening. (**b**) Grade 1: gallbladder wall thickening > 0.3 cm without pericholecystic fat stranding. (**c**) Grade 2: linear pericholecystic fat stranding. (**d**) Grade 3: prominent pericholecystic reticular dirty fat.

2.5. Statistical Analysis

Tests of normality for continuous variables, including the Kolmogorov–Smirnov and the Shapiro–Wilk tests, were performed (Supplementary Table S2). Continuous variables with non-Gaussian distribution were presented as median and interquartile range and were compared using the Mann–Whitney U tests. Categorical variables were presented as proportions and were analyzed using Pearson's chi-square test or Fisher's exact test. The cutoff values for age [9–11], CRP levels [12], gamma-glutamyltransferase levels, fat stranding TG18 [13,14], and LOS [15–17] were determined with reference to the relevant literature.

Univariable and multivariable logistic regression models were used to obtain the odds ratios (ORs) and corresponding 95% confidence intervals (CIs) for predicting an LOS of ≥ 7 days. To identify suitable predictors or variables for our multivariable logistic regression models, we used univariable logistic regression analysis and determined which factors were statistically significant (indicated by $p < 0.05$). All significant factors were incorporated into the multivariable logistic regression model. To construct our scoring system, we assigned point values to different potential predictors on the basis of their ORs. The diagnostic performance of each model was obtained by calculating the areas under the curve (AUCs) of the receiver operating characteristics curves. The Youden index was used to determine the optimal cutoff values (the point with the maximum value of sensitivity + specificity $-$ 1) for our developed scoring system. A p value < 0.05 was considered statistically significant. All statistical analyses were performed using SPSS version 20 (IBM, Armonk, NY, USA).

3. Results

A total of 390 patients with AC were included in this study. There were 324 of 390 (83.1%) patients who had the first episode of cholecystitis; the remaining 66 patients had recurrent cholecystitis. The patients were categorized into groups of LOS $\geq$ 7 and LOS < 7. The patient characteristics are presented in Table 1. The mean age was significantly higher in the LOS $\geq$ 7 group (70.0 [IQR, 58.0–80.3] years) than in the LOS < 7 group (54.5 [IQR, 43.3–66.8] years; p < 0.001). Gallbladder length was greater in the LOS $\geq$ 7 group (7.3 [IQR, 5.6–9.0] cm) than in the LOS < 7 group (6.9 [IQR, 5.2–8.1] cm; p = 0.0079). Gallbladder width was greater in the LOS $\geq$ 7 group (4.1 [IQR, 3.5–4.7] cm) than in the LOS < 7 group (3.9 [IQR, 3.2–4.4] cm; p = 0.0083). Gallbladder size was greater in the LOS $\geq$ 7 group (30.4 [IQR, 21.3–41.3] cm^2) than in the LOS < 7 group (26.0 [IQR, 18.0–33.9] cm^2, p = 0.0020). A total of 138 patients in the LOS < 7 days group (58.5%) underwent laparoscopic cholecystectomy. By contrast, only 34 patients (22.1%) in the LOS $\geq$ 7 days group underwent laparoscopic cholecystectomy. In total, 1 of 172 patients (0.6%) had conversion from laparoscopic cholecystectomy to open surgery. Percutaneous transhepatic gallbladder drainage was more common in the LOS $\geq$ 7 days group than in the LOS < 7 days group (44.2% vs. 14.0%, respectively; p < 0.0001). Endoscopic retrograde cholangiopancreatography was more common in the LOS $\geq$ 7 days group than in the LOS < 7 days group (27.3% vs. 12.7%, respectively; p = 0.0003). The TG18 grades were higher in the LOS $\geq$ 7 days group (Grade II, III 75.3%) than in the LOS < 7 days group (Grade II, III 50.4%).

Table 1. Population characteristics (N = 390).

Characteristics	LOS < 7 Days	LOS $\geq$ 7 Days	p Value
Number (N)	236 (60.5%)	154 (39.5%)	
Age (years)	54.5 (43.3–66.8)	70.0 (58.0–80.3)	<0.0001 *
Age subgroups			<0.0001 *
20–29 years (N)	10/236 (4.2%)	1/154 (0.7%)	
30–39 years (N)	28/236 (11.9%)	5/154 (3.3%)	
40–49 years (N)	55/236 (23.3%)	15/154 (9.7%)	
50–59 years (N)	51/236 (21.6%)	24/154 (15.6%)	
60–69 years (N)	43/236 (18.2%)	30/154 (19.5%)	
70–79 years (N)	32/236 (13.6%)	40/154 (26.0%)	
$\geq$80 years (N)	17/236 (7.2%)	39/154 (25.3%)	
Body mass index (kg/m^2)	24.6 (22.6–27.3)	24.9 (22.0–27.6)	0.7548
Onset of symptoms to ED (days)	1.0 (1.0–3.0)	1.0 (1.0–3.0)	0.8720
Onset of symptoms to ED > 72 h	30/236 (12.7%)	27/154 (17.5%)	0.1877
ICU admission	8/236 (3.4%)	35/154 (22.7%)	<0.0001
Procedures			
Laparoscopic cholecystectomy	138/236 (58.5%)	34/154 (22.1%)	<0.0001 *
PTGBD	33/236 (14.0%)	68/154 (44.2%)	<0.0001 *
ERCP	30/236 (12.7%)	42/154 (27.3%)	0.0003 *
Imaging findings			
Gallbladder length (cm)	6.9 (5.2–8.1)	7.3 (5.6–9.0)	0.0079 *
Gallbladder width (cm)	3.9 (3.2–4.4)	4.1 (3.5–4.7)	0.0083 *
Gallbladder size (cm^2)	26.0 (18.0–33.9)	30.4 (21.3–41.3)	0.0020 *
Gallbladder volume (mL)	186.4 (129.9–269.3)	209.1 (135.5–305.0)	0.0863
Gallbladder wall thickness	0.4 (0.3–0.7)	0.5 (0.3–0.7)	0.3118
Calculus cholecystitis	133/236 (56.4%)	82/154 (53.2%)	0.5467
Multiple Gallbladder stone (N)	75/236 (31.8%)	52/154 (33.8%)	0.6824
Abscess (N)	8/236 (3.4%)	10/154 (6.5%)	0.1533
Grades of pericholecystic fat stranding			0.0518
Grade 0	55/236 (23.3%)	32/154 (20.8%)	
Grade 1	94/236 (39.8%)	45/154 (29.2%)	
Grade 2	44/236 (18.6%)	34/154 (22.1%)	
Grade 3	43/236 (18.2%)	43/154 (27.9%)	
Tokyo guideline grading			<0.0001 *
Grade I	117/236 (49.6%)	38/154 (24.7%)	
Grade II	94/236 (39.8%)	47/154 (30.5%)	
Grade III	25/236 (10.6%)	69/154 (44.8%)	

Continuous variables were expressed as median (interquartile range). Abbreviations: ED, emergency department; ERCP, endoscopic retrograde cholangiopancreatography; PTGBD, percutaneous transhepatic gallbladder drainage. * Statistical significance at p value < 0.05.

3.1. Univariate Analysis

Univariate analysis was used to investigate the factors significantly associated with LOS $\geq$ 7 days. Age, gallbladder width, size, and volume, common bile duct diameter, fat stranding, TG18 grade, and the laboratory markers of CRP and gamma-glutamyltransferase levels were associated with LOS $\geq$ 7 days (Table 2).

Table 2. Univariate analysis of LOS < 7 days and LOS $\geq$ 7 days.

Characteristics	Univariate Analysis		
	OR (95% CI)	p Value	AUC
Age	1.05 (1.04–1.07)	<0.001 *	0.716
Gallbladder width	1.38 (1.10–1.72)	0.005 *	0.581
Gallbladder size	1.03 (1.01–1.04)	0.001 *	0.596
Gallbladder volume	1.00 (1.00–1.00)	0.034 *	0.555
Gallbladder stone	0.88 (0.59–1.33)	0.546	0.482
Gallbladder wall	1.15 (0.66–2.00)	0.628	0.532
Gallbladder wall HU	1.01 (1.00–1.02)	0.064	0.544
CBD diameter	2.47 (1.26–4.88)	0.009 *	0.589
TG18 grade	2.79 (2.09–3.73)	<0.001 *	0.695
Fat stranding	1.25 (1.03–1.52)	0.022 *	0.563
Fat stranding (0 vs. 1–3)	1.16 (0.71–1.90)	0.558	0.512
Fat stranding (0–1 vs. 2–3)	1.71 (1.13–2.59)	0.010 *	0.563
Fat stranding (0–2 vs. 3)	1.74 (1.07–2.82)	0.025 *	0.549
Abscess	1.98 (0.76–5.13)	0.160	0.516
Gangrene change	1.45 (0.96–2.19)	0.077	0.546
Symptom duration (0–7 and >7)	1.04 (0.92–1.16)	0.561	0.507
Symptom duration (0–7 vs. >7)	0.65 (0.17–2.55)	0.537	0.495
Symptom duration (0–3 vs. >3)	1.46 (0.83–2.57)	0.189	0.524
CRP (normal range <0.5 mg/dL)	1.05 (1.02–1.07)	<0.001 *	0.631
CRP $\geq$ 0.5 mg/dL	2.26 (1.48–3.46)	<0.001 *	0.598
CRP $\geq$ 0.8 mg/dL	2.41 (1.59–3.66)	<0.001 *	0.608
CRP $\geq$ 2 mg/dL	2.46 (1.62–3.74)	<0.001 *	0.608
g-GT (normal range 5–40 U/L)	1.00 (1.00–1.00)	0.007 *	0.556
g-GT $\geq$ 60 U/L	2.53 (1.53–4.18)	<0.001 *	0.575
g-GT $\geq$ 40 U/L	2.57 (1.60–4.14)	<0.001 *	0.585

Abbreviations: HU, Hounsfield unit; CBD, common bile duct; CRP, C-reactive protein; g-GT, gamma-glutamyltransferase. * Statistical significance at p value < 0.05.

3.2. Multivariable Analysis

Multivariate logistic regression analysis revealed that a high TG18 grade (OR: 2.89 per grade, p < 0.001), a fat stranding grade > 2 (OR: 2.14, p = 0.012), CRP level $\geq$ 2 mg/dL (OR: 1.97, p = 0.013), gamma-glutamyltransferase level $\geq$ 40 U/L (OR: 2.460, p = 0.001), and age $\geq$ 65 years (OR: 2.56, p < 0.001) were independent predictors of LOS $\geq$ 7 days (Table 3)

Table 3. Multivariate Analysis of LOS < 7 Days and LOS $\geq$ 7 Days.

Characteristics	OR (95% CI)	p Value	Score
TG18 grade (per grade)	2.89 (2.04–4.10)	<0.001 *	1–3 †
Fat stranding grade > 2	2.14 (1.18–3.86)	0.012 *	1
CRP level $\geq$ 2 mg/dL	1.97 (1.15–3.35)	0.013 *	1
g-GT level $\geq$ 40 U/L	2.46 (1.44–4.22)	0.001 *	1
Age $\geq$ 65 years	2.56 (1.59–4.12)	<0.001 *	1

Abbreviations: CRP, C-reactive protein; g-GT, gamma-glutamyltransferase. * Statistical significance at p < 0.05.
† 1–3 According to TG18, Grade I (mild) = 1, Grade II (moderate) = 2, Grade III (severe) = 3.

3.3. Area under the Receiver Operating Characteristics Curve Analysis

In a univariate receiver operating characteristics curve analysis (Figure 2), age $\geq$ 65 years (AUC: 0.657, 95% CI, 0.601–0.713), gamma-glutamyltransferase $\geq$ 40 U/L (AUC: 0.587, 95% CI, 0.528–0.646), TG18 grade (AUC: 0.698, 95% CI, 0.643–0.752), fat stranding grade > 2 (AUC: 0.566, 95% CI, 0.507–0.624), and CRP level $\geq$ 2 mg/dL (AUC: 0.608, 95% CI, 0.551–0.666) were comparable for predicting LOS $\geq$ 7 days. In the multivariable model including the five significant predictors, the diagnostic performance for predicting LOS $\geq$ 7 days reached a moderate-to-high level (AUC: 0.769, 95% CI, 0.720–0.817). After exclusion of TG18 grade, the multivariable model exhibited a moderate diagnostic performance (AUC: 0.714, 95% CI, 0.662–0.767).

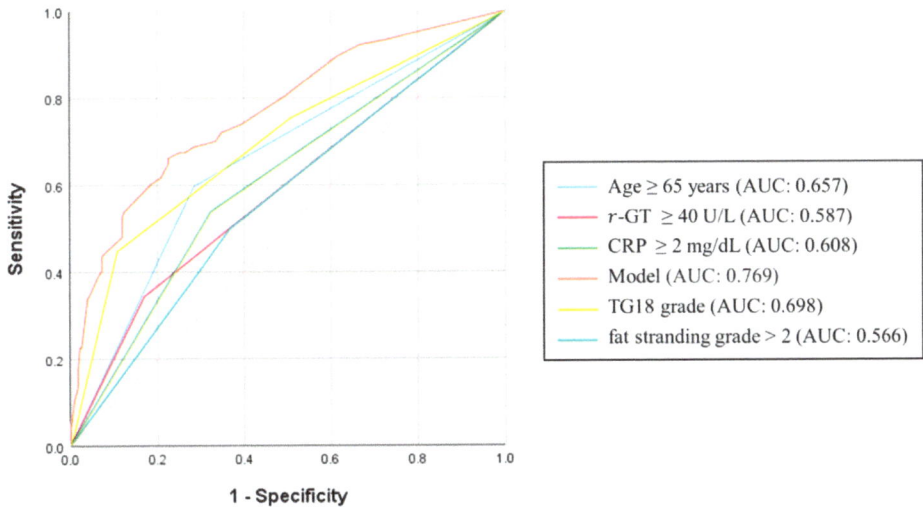

Figure 2. Receiver of operating characteristic curve of the multivariable model.

3.4. Development of New Scoring System Model

In our model, TG18 grades I, II, and III were assigned 1, 2, and 3 points, respectively. In addition, fat stranding grade > 2, CRP level ≥ 2 mg/dL, gamma-glutamyltransferase level ≥ 40 U/L, and age ≥ 65 years were assigned 1 point each (Table 3). After the Youden index was applied (Figure 3), a cutoff value of 2 exhibited a sensitivity of 79.9%, a specificity of 48.7%, and a Youden index value of 28.6%. A cutoff value of 3 exhibited a sensitivity of 66.2%, a specificity of 66.5%, and a Youden index value of 32.7%. By contrast, a cutoff value of 4 exhibited a sensitivity of 46.1%, a specificity of 87.3%, and a Youden index value of 33.4%. On the basis of the Youden index results, an optimal cutoff value of >3 was determined.

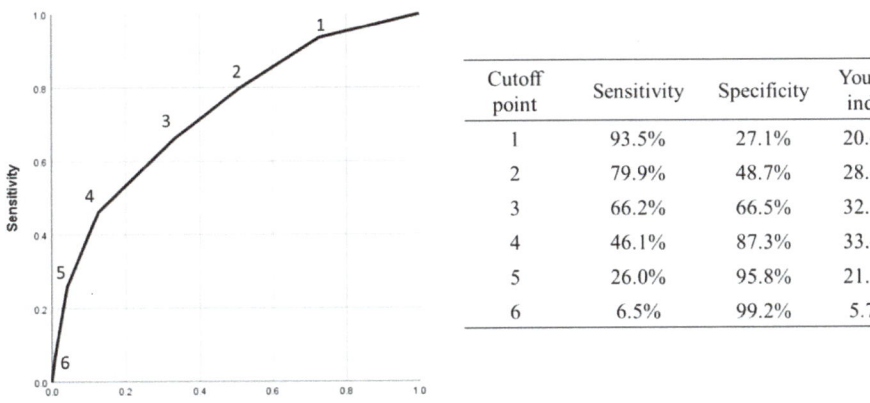

Cutoff point	Sensitivity	Specificity	Youden index
1	93.5%	27.1%	20.6%
2	79.9%	48.7%	28.6%
3	66.2%	66.5%	32.7%
4	46.1%	87.3%	33.4%
5	26.0%	95.8%	21.8%
6	6.5%	99.2%	5.7%

Figure 3. Receiver of operating characteristic curve of the scoring system model.

4. Discussion

Our study revealed that older age, elevated inflammatory marker levels, and more pronounced fat stranding signs were associated with a prolonged hospital stay. In our multivariate analysis, age, CRP levels, gamma-glutamyltransferase levels, TG18 grade, and fat stranding were significant predictors for a prolonged hospital stay.

A distinctive feature of our study is the inclusion of fat stranding signs. Our study model's diagnostic performance was comparable to that of an earlier model that employed ten variables, namely age, sex, body mass index, white blood cell count, neutrophil fraction, platelet count, alanine transaminase levels, admission from the emergency department, gallbladder wall thickening, and pericholecystic fluid levels [18]. In general, severe inflammation of the gallbladder leads to more pronounced fat stranding signs [19,20]. Notably, a novel feature of our study is the proposal of the four grades of fat stranding into a predictive model. Fat stranding is caused by increased congestion and engorgement of lymphatics [21]. Disproportionate fat stranding observed on MSCT is used to evaluate the severity of intra-abdominal inflammation such as acute appendicitis, diverticulitis, and cholecystitis [22]. In case of worsening acute cholecystitis, the gallbladder wall becomes venously engorged and leads to reduced atrial blood flow and subtle ischemic changes. As inflammation progresses, fat stranding becomes more apparent. In addition to fat stranding, our selection of other variables was well justified. The cutoff values we used for LOS, age, CRP levels, and gamma-glutamyltransferase levels were determined based on the relevant literature. First, AC severity is positively correlated with LOS [16], and in most studies, the median LOS was 7 days [15]. Accordingly, LOS $\geq$ 7 days was defined as a poor outcome (prolonged LOS), while LOS < 7 days was considered a more favorable outcome [16,17]. Second, age was a major risk factor for gallbladder stone formation [23] and increased mortality [24]. Numerous studies have defined age $\geq$ 65 years as old age [9–11]. Third, CRP is considered a strong predictor of complicated AC [13], and a cutoff value of $\geq$2 mg/dL was reported to exhibit a sensitivity of 71.9% and a specificity of 69.6% [12]. Fourth, gamma-glutamyltransferase levels are elevated in patients with AC, and we selected the upper normal limit value of $\geq$40 U/L as the cutoff value in our model. Last, TG18 grades are widely used for grading AC severity [14,25]. We assigned scores of 1 to 3 for TG18 grades I to III, respectively, in our model.

In our univariate analysis, the TG18 grades solely had poor-to-moderate diagnostic performance for predicting LOS (AUC: 0.698); however, the multivariable model including age, CRP levels, gamma-glutamyltransferase levels, fat stranding, and the TG18 grades had improved diagnostic performance (AUC: 0.769). To facilitate clinical practice, we constructed a scoring model with a total score of 7. The score was named the FACTT score based on its components: fat stranding, age, CRP levels, TG18, and gamma-glutamyltransferase. Points were allocated based on the OR of each variable. We determined the optimal cutoff value to be a score of 3. Although a score of 4 exhibited the highest Youden index value, it exhibited relatively low sensitivity (46.1%). In contrast, a score of 3 exhibited a sensitivity of 66.2% and a specificity of 66.5%.

Overall, our study's results are consistent with previous research. Several studies have examined the LOS in patients with AC. For example, patients who received PTGBD before cholecystectomy had a longer LOS [26]. Similarly, another study showed patients receiving PTGBD alone rather than cholecystectomy experienced a longer hospital stay [27]. Our study also found that patients in the LOS > 7 days group were more likely to receive PTGBD (14.0% vs. 44.2%). The duration of symptoms before ED presentation did not significantly affect LOS [28]. Our study similarly found no statistically significant differences in LOS related to the onset time of symptoms before presenting to the ED. The previous literature has shown that increased pericholecystic fat stranding is significantly associated with the severity of AC [29]. In our study, using LOS as a measure of severity for AC, we confirmed that fat stranding is associated with a longer LOS.

Higher grades of TG18, specifically moderate and severe AC, are associated with an increased complication rate and may necessitate additional imaging studies before surgery for outcome evaluation [5]. MSCT has become the standard imaging modality in most modern EDs. Although sonography is available at the bedside for AC evaluation, it is operator dependent and lacks standardized imaging assessment criteria. In contrast, MSCT benefits from standardized procedures and well-defined imaging protocols, which contribute to more reliable and consistent interpretations of results. This standardization reduces variability and enhances the clarity of diagnostic images, making MSCT a more dependable tool for evaluating the severity of AC. Our model incorporates the novel classification of a pericholecystic fat-stranding sign to address the limitations of TG18.

Our study has several limitations. First, this was a single-center retrospective study. Unmeasured confounding factors remained. Second, patients were of Han Chinese ethnicity; however, we do not believe the clinical course of AC for patients of Han Chinese ethnicity differs to that for patients of other ethnicities.

5. Conclusions

Fat stranding, C-reactive protein levels, gamma-glutamyltransferase levels, and age are predictors of length of stays in addition to the 2018 Tokyo Guidelines grade among patients with acute cholecystitis. An increased severity of these factors is associated with more severe acute cholecystitis and longer length of stays. Our simple scoring system is currently being used for the primary evaluation of acute cholecystitis in our emergency department.

Supplementary Materials: The following supporting information can be downloaded at: https://www.mdpi.com/article/10.3390/jcm13195734/s1, Table S1: The List of the International Statistical Classification of Diseases, Tenth Revision, Clinical Modification (ICD-10-CM) of screening all eligible patients aged $\geq$ 18 years presenting to this ED with confirmed cholecystitis; Table S2. Normality tests of the Kolmogorov-Smirnova and the Shapiro-Wilk's statistics.

Author Contributions: Conceptualization, S.-W.L., C.-H.T., H.-A.L., Y.C., S.-K.H. and S.-F.L.; methodology, S.-W.L., C.-H.T. and S.-F.L.; software, S.-W.L., C.-H.T. and S.-F.L.; validation, S.-K.H. and S.-F.L.; formal analysis, S.-W.L. and C.-H.T.; investigation, S.-W.L. and C.-H.T.; data curation, S.-W.L., C.-H.T., and Y.C.; writing—original draft preparation, S.-W.L. and C.-H.T.; writing—review and editing, S.-F.L.; visualization, C.-H.T.; supervision, H.-A.L., S.-K.H. and S.-F.L.; funding acquisition, S.-K.H. All authors have read and agreed to the published version of the manuscript.

Funding: This research was funded by Taipei Medical University, Taipei, Taiwan, grant number TMU112-AE1-B25; the National Science and Technology Council, Taipei Taiwan, grant number 113-2314-B-038-051.

Institutional Review Board Statement: This study was conducted in accordance with the Declaration of Helsinki and approved by the Joint Institutional Review Board of Taipei Medical University, Taipei, Taiwan (reference number: N202303059, 28 March 2023).

Informed Consent Statement: Patient consent was waived due to retrospective study design and the de-identified and de-linked data were used.

Data Availability Statement: Due to the "Personal Data Protection Act," the personal health data were not publicly available. Request of the data needs the formal proposal to the Joint Institutional Review Board of Taipei Medical University and the Office of Human Research of Taipei Medical University, Taipei, Taiwan (ohr@tmu.edu.tw).

Acknowledgments: This study was supported by staff of the Department of Emergency Medicine, Taipei Medical University Hospital, Taipei, Taiwan.

Conflicts of Interest: The authors declare no conflicts of interest.

References

1. Shea, J.A.; Berlin, J.A.; Escarce, J.J.; Clarke, J.R.; Kinosian, B.P.; Cabana, M.D.; Tsai, W.W.; Horangic, N.; Malet, P.F.; Schwartz, J.S.; et al. Revised estimates of diagnostic test sensitivity and specificity in suspected biliary tract disease. *Arch. Intern. Med.* **1994**, *154*, 2573–2581. [CrossRef]
2. Kiewiet, J.J.; Leeuwenburgh, M.M.; Bipat, S.; Bossuyt, P.M.; Stoker, J.; Boermeester, M.A. A systematic review and meta-analysis of diagnostic performance of imaging in acute cholecystitis. *Radiology* **2012**, *264*, 708–720. [CrossRef]
3. Wertz, J.R.; Lopez, J.M.; Olson, D.; Thompson, W.M. Comparing the Diagnostic Accuracy of Ultrasound and CT in Evaluating Acute Cholecystitis. *AJR Am. J. Roentgenol.* **2018**, *211*, W92–W97. [CrossRef] [PubMed]
4. Sandomenico, F.; Sanduzzi, L.; La Verde, E.; Vicenzo, E.; Pirolo, L.; Maione, S.; Setola, F.R.; Macchia, V.; Dello Iacono, U.; Barbato, D.; et al. Multidetector Computed Tomography (MDCT) Findings of Complications of Acute Cholecystitis. A Pictorial Essay. *Tomography* **2022**, *8*, 1159–1171. [CrossRef] [PubMed]

5. Yokoe, M.; Hata, J.; Takada, T.; Strasberg, S.M.; Asbun, H.J.; Wakabayashi, G.; Kozaka, K.; Endo, I.; Deziel, D.J.; Miura, F.; et al Tokyo Guidelines 2018: Diagnostic criteria and severity grading of acute cholecystitis (with videos). *J. Hepatobiliary Pancreat. Sci* **2018**, *25*, 41–54. [CrossRef] [PubMed]
6. Yokoe, M.; Takada, T.; Strasberg, S.M.; Solomkin, J.S.; Mayumi, T.; Gomi, H.; Pitt, H.A.; Gouma, D.J.; Garden, O.J.; Büchler, M.W. et al. New diagnostic criteria and severity assessment of acute cholecystitis in revised Tokyo Guidelines. *J. Hepatobiliary Pancreat. Sci.* **2012**, *19*, 578–585. [CrossRef]
7. Shakespear, J.S.; Shaaban, A.M.; Rezvani, M. CT findings of acute cholecystitis and its complications. *AJR Am. J. Roentgenol.* **2010**, *194*, 1523–1529. [CrossRef]
8. Charalel, R.A.; Jeffrey, R.B.; Shin, L.K. Complicated cholecystitis: The complementary roles of sonography and computed tomography. *Ultrasound Q.* **2011**, *27*, 161–170. [CrossRef]
9. Asiltürk Lülleci, Z.; Başyiğit, S.; Pirinçci Sapmaz, F.; Uzman, M.; Kefeli, A.; Yeniova, A.; Nazlıgül, Y. Comparison of ultrasonographic and laboratory findings of acute cholecystitis between elderly and nonelderly patients. *Turk. J. Med. Sci.* **2016**, *46*, 1428–1433. [CrossRef]
10. McGillicuddy, E.A.; Schuster, K.M.; Brown, E.; Maxfield, M.W.; Davis, K.A.; Longo, W.E. Acute cholecystitis in the elderly: Use of computed tomography and correlation with ultrasonography. *Am. J. Surg.* **2011**, *202*, 524–527. [CrossRef]
11. Riall, T.S.; Zhang, D.; Townsend, C.M., Jr.; Kuo, Y.F.; Goodwin, J.S. Failure to perform cholecystectomy for acute cholecystitis in elderly patients is associated with increased morbidity, mortality, and cost. *J. Am. Coll. Surg.* **2010**, *210*, 668–677. [CrossRef] [PubMed]
12. Yuzbasioglu, Y.; Ucoz, D.; Icme, F.; Haydar, G.; Uzunosmanoglu, H.; Pekcici, R. The role of C-reactive protein in the evaluation of the severity of acute cholecystitis. *Acta Medica Mediterr.* **2020**, *2017*, 475. [CrossRef]
13. Kabul Gurbulak, E.; Gurbulak, B.; Akgun, I.E.; Duzkoylu, Y.; Battal, M.; Celayir, M.F.; Demir, U. Prediction of the grade of acute cholecystitis by plasma level of C-reactive protein. *Iran. Red. Crescent Med. J.* **2015**, *17*, e28091. [CrossRef] [PubMed]
14. Lin, Y.N.; Wu, Y.T.; Fu, C.Y.; Liao, C.H.; Cheng, C.T.; Wang, S.Y.; Lin, B.C.; Hsu, Y.P.; Kang, S.C.; Liu, E.H.; et al. Evaluating the advantages of treating acute cholecystitis by following the Tokyo Guidelines 2018 (TG18): A study emphasizing clinical outcomes and medical expenditures. *Surg. Endosc.* **2021**, *35*, 6623–6632. [CrossRef] [PubMed]
15. Paul Wright, G.; Stilwell, K.; Johnson, J.; Hefty, M.T.; Chung, M.H. Predicting length of stay and conversion to open cholecystectomy for acute cholecystitis using the 2013 Tokyo Guidelines in a US population. *J. Hepatobiliary Pancreat. Sci.* **2015**, *22*, 795–801 [CrossRef] [PubMed]
16. Sert, İ.; İpekci, F.; Engin, Ö.; Karaoğlan, M.; Çetindağ, Ö. Outcomes of early cholecystectomy (within 7 days of admission) for acute cholecystitis according to diagnosis and severity grading by Tokyo 2013 Guideline. *Turk. J. Surg.* **2017**, *33*, 80–86. [CrossRef]
17. Yuksekdag, S.; Bas, G.; Okan, I.; Karakelleoglu, A.; Alimoglu, O.; Akcakaya, A.; Sahin, M. Timing of laparoscopic cholecystectomy in acute cholecystitis. *Niger. J. Clin. Pract.* **2021**, *24*, 156–160. [CrossRef]
18. Kim, K.H.; Kim, S.J.; Lee, S.C.; Lee, S.K. Risk assessment scales and predictors for simple versus severe cholecystitis in performing laparoscopic cholecystectomy. *Asian J. Surg.* **2017**, *40*, 367–374. [CrossRef]
19. Chawla, A.; Bosco, J.I.; Lim, T.C.; Srinivasan, S.; Teh, H.S.; Shenoy, J.N. Imaging of acute cholecystitis and cholecystitis-associated complications in the emergency setting. *Singap. Med. J.* **2015**, *56*, 438–443, quiz 444. [CrossRef]
20. Woo, S.H.; Lee, W.J.; Seol, S.H.; Kim, D.H.; Choi, S.P. The accuracies of abdominal computed tomography and the neutrophil-to-lymphocyte ratio used to predict the development of clinically severe acute cholecystitis in elderly patients visiting an emergency department. *Niger. J. Clin. Pract.* **2018**, *21*, 645–652. [CrossRef] [PubMed]
21. Thornton, E.; Mendiratta-Lala, M.; Siewert, B.; Eisenberg, R.L. Patterns of fat stranding. *AJR Am. J. Roentgenol.* **2011**, *197*, W1–W14. [CrossRef] [PubMed]
22. Pereira, J.M.; Sirlin, C.B.; Pinto, P.S.; Jeffrey, R.B.; Stella, D.L.; Casola, G. Disproportionate fat stranding: A helpful CT sign in patients with acute abdominal pain. *Radiographics* **2004**, *24*, 703–715. [CrossRef]
23. Pak, M.; Lindseth, G. Risk Factors for Cholelithiasis. *Gastroenterol. Nurs.* **2016**, *39*, 297–309. [CrossRef] [PubMed]
24. Lee, S.O.; Yim, S.K. Management of Acute Cholecystitis. *Korean J. Gastroenterol.* **2018**, *71*, 264–268. [CrossRef] [PubMed]
25. Rice, C.P.; Vaishnavi, K.B.; Chao, C.; Jupiter, D.; Schaeffer, A.B.; Jenson, W.R.; Griffin, L.W.; Mileski, W.J. Operative complications and economic outcomes of cholecystectomy for acute cholecystitis. *World J. Gastroenterol.* **2019**, *25*, 6916–6927. [CrossRef]
26. Choi, J.W.; Park, S.H.; Choi, S.Y.; Kim, H.S.; Kim, T.H. Comparison of clinical result between early laparoscopic cholecystectomy and delayed laparoscopic cholecystectomy after percutaneous transhepatic gallbladder drainage for patients with complicated acute cholecystitis. *Korean J. Hepatobiliary Pancreat. Surg.* **2012**, *16*, 147–153. [CrossRef]
27. Loozen, C.S.; van Santvoort, H.C.; van Duijvendijk, P.; Besselink, M.G.; Gouma, D.J.; Nieuwenhuijzen, G.A.; Kelder, J.C.; Donkervoort, S.C.; van Geloven, A.A.; Kruyt, P.M.; et al. Laparoscopic cholecystectomy versus percutaneous catheter drainage for acute cholecystitis in high risk patients (CHOCOLATE): Multicentre randomised clinical trial. *Bmj* **2018**, *363*, k3965. [CrossRef]
28. Tur-Martínez, J.; Escartín, A.; Muriel, P.; González, M.; Cuello, E.; Pinillos, A.; Salvador, H.; Olsina, J.J. Days of symptoms and days of hospital admission before surgery do not influence the results of cholecystectomy in moderate acute calculous cholecystitis-Cholecystectomy remains the best treatment. *Rev. Esp. Enferm. Dig.* **2022**, *114*, 213–218. [CrossRef]
29. Prakash, G.; Hasan, M. The Accuracy of Neutrophil-to-Lymphocyte Ratio and Abdominal Computed Tomography to Predict the Severity of Acute Cholecystitis. *Cureus* **2022**, *14*, e32243. [CrossRef]

Disclaimer/Publisher's Note: The statements, opinions and data contained in all publications are solely those of the individual author(s) and contributor(s) and not of MDPI and/or the editor(s). MDPI and/or the editor(s) disclaim responsibility for any injury to people or property resulting from any ideas, methods, instructions or products referred to in the content.

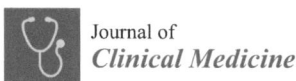 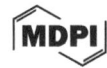

Article

The Experience of a Tertiary Referral Center with Endoscopic Management and Combining Percutaneous Intervention for the Treatment of Walled-Off Necrosis: A Stepwise Approach

Ali Atay [1,*] and Ilhami Yuksel [1,2]

[1] Department of Gastroenterology, Ankara Bilkent City Hospital, Ankara 06800, Turkey; yukselilhami@hotmail.com
[2] Department of Gastroenterology, School of Medicine, Ankara Yildirim Beyazit University, Ankara 06800, Turkey
* Correspondence: draliatay@hotmail.com; Tel.: +90-(505)-520-67-67

Abstract: Background: This study aimed to assess the effectiveness and safety of endoscopic management in patients with walled-off necrosis and additionally explore the results of a stepwise approach for combining percutaneous intervention in cases where endoscopic management was inadequate. **Methods:** We included cases of endoscopic management for walled-off necrosis between February 2019 and December 2023. **Results:** Endoscopic management was performed in 11 patients. The median largest dimension was 150 mm. Multiple cavities were present in four patients. Technical success was 90.9%, while clinical success with only endoscopic management was 36.3%. Clinical success could not be achieved with only endoscopic management in patients with a large diameter (≥ 125 mm) or multi-lobulated walled-off necrosis. Combining percutaneous intervention resulted in success for all patients. Two patients experienced major complications: one suffered from major bleeding, while the other experienced perforation, necessitating surgical intervention. The patient with perforation died due to multi-organ failure. **Conclusions:** Endoscopic management is recommended as the primary treatment method for walled-off necrosis due to its less invasive and higher safety profile. In cases involving large or multi-lobulated walled-off necrosis where clinical success cannot be achieved, combining percutaneous intervention is highly successful and safe. Ultimately, this approach can minimize the need for more invasive surgery.

Keywords: walled-off necrosis; endoscopic cystogastrostomy; lumen-apposing metallic stent; percutaneous intervention

Citation: Atay, A.; Yuksel, I. The Experience of a Tertiary Referral Center with Endoscopic Management and Combining Percutaneous Intervention for the Treatment of Walled-Off Necrosis: A Stepwise Approach. *J. Clin. Med.* **2024**, *13*, 4916. https://doi.org/10.3390/jcm13164916

Academic Editor: Jun Kato

Received: 29 July 2024
Revised: 11 August 2024
Accepted: 17 August 2024
Published: 20 August 2024

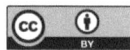

Copyright: © 2024 by the authors. Licensee MDPI, Basel, Switzerland. This article is an open access article distributed under the terms and conditions of the Creative Commons Attribution (CC BY) license (https://creativecommons.org/licenses/by/4.0/).

1. Introduction

Walled-off necrosis (WON) is a late complication of acute necrotizing pancreatitis that can lead to permanent organ failure and even death [1,2]. Necrosis in the pancreas develops in approximately 15–20% of all acute pancreatitis (AP) cases, and about 40% of these cases progress to infected or complicated WON [3–8]. In the historical process, WON was often managed with surgical methods. However, minimally invasive procedures involving endoscopic interventions, video-assisted retroperitoneal debridement, and percutaneous drainage have become preferred modalities due to their lower morbidity, mortality, cost, and complication rates, as well as providing a better quality of life. Among minimally invasive approaches, endoscopic interventions are the preferred initial method [1,9,10]. In cases of sterile pancreatic necrosis presenting with symptoms such as abdominal pain, nausea, vomiting, and nutritional insufficiency, or in patients with associated complications such as biliary obstruction, recurrent acute pancreatitis, fistulas, or persistent systemic inflammatory response syndrome, drainage may be necessary [11]. If drainage proves inadequate, necrosectomy is advised [12,13].

This study was conducted to evaluate the effectiveness and safety of endoscopic treatment in the management of WON and to assess combining percutaneous intervention in cases where endoscopic management was inadequate in a tertiary care center.

2. Materials and Methods

2.1. Patients and Pre-Procedure Evaluation

In the retrospective analysis of our prospective database, consecutive cases of endoscopic cystogastrostomy for WON between February 2019 and December 2023 were included in the study. All patients underwent preprocedural endoscopic evaluation. Additionally, the presence of vascular structures between the cavity and the lumen was assessed using computed tomography (CT) imaging. If vascular structures were observed or could not be clearly evaluated, the assessment was conducted using an echoendoscope (EUS) (Olympus GF-UE160 echoendoscope, Olympus, Tokyo, Japan). Patients without capsule integrity of the cavity, those with a distance of more than 10 mm between the lumen and the cavity, and individuals with visible vessels at the site where the cavity contacted the lumen were excluded.

Data collected from patients included demographic information, etiology, clinical manifestations, and results of imaging studies prior to the procedure. Furthermore, we documented the findings, results, and complications of our approach.

2.2. Definition

Walled-off necrosis was defined according to the revised Atlanta Classification [2]. Technical success was defined as the cannulation of the cavity, successful placement of a lumen-apposing metallic stent (LAMS) (Micro-Tech Co., Ltd., Nanjing, China) in the cavity, and successful necrosectomy if necessary. Clinical success was defined as the complete normalization of disease-related findings in clinical, laboratory, and CT imaging, or a reduction in WON size to 2 cm or a decrease in size by 25%. Recurrence was defined as the reappearance of fluid collection or necrosis after resolution. Complications such as bleeding, perforation, multi-organ failure, stent blockage, infection, and migration were documented. Complications were graded according to the AGREE classification [14].

2.3. Procedure

All endoscopic procedures were performed using carbon dioxide insufflation by an experienced endoscopist under moderate sedation. Broad-spectrum antibiotics were administered to all patients before and after the procedure. A nasogastric tube was placed into the gastric lumen before the procedure, and fluid aspiration post-dilation was performed to prevent respiratory aspiration. In cases of luminal compression, the therapeutic duodenoscope (Fujinon ED-530XT Flexible Video Duodenoscope, Fujifilm Medical Co., Saitama, Japan) was utilized to identify the area of maximum pressure. Subsequently, the identified area was punctured with a needle knife sphincterotome as a conventional transmural drainage method. In patients without significant luminal compression, a 19-gauge fine needle aspiration needle was used to puncture the area determined as the safest location with an EUS. Afterward, the guidewire was advanced into the cavity. Cystogastrostomy tract dilation with a 6 or 8 mm dilatation balloon was performed to facilitate stent placement at the discretion of the endoscopist. This decision was based on factors such as the thickness of the collection wall and the density of the contents to be drained. After dilatation, a LAMS was deployed into the cavity under endoscopic and fluoroscopic guidance. To prevent LAMS migration, a double pigtail plastic stent (DPPS) was inserted through the LAMS (Figure 1). Patients with disconnected pancreatic duct syndrome (DPDS) identified during the imaging method were additionally subjected to pancreatic duct cannulation for transpapillary drainage. A pancreatic sphincterotomy was performed, and a pancreatic stent was placed to extend to the closest localization of duct disruption.

After the procedure, all patients followed up as inpatients and underwent clinical and laboratory examinations. If necessary, CT scans were performed, and the timing of follow-up procedures was decided on an individual basis. The decision of direct endoscopic necrosectomy (DEN) was made at the discretion of the physician based on insufficient resolution of necrosis. Necrosectomy was performed using a balloon, basket catheter, irrigation with sterile saline, and cytology brush (Figure 2). As a step-by-step approach, a percutaneous drainage catheter was placed in patients where clinical success could not be achieved after at least three successful endoscopic interventions (Figure 3). To expedite the resolution of necrosis and prevent stent and drain blockage, lavage was performed at least four times a day during subsequent follow-ups.

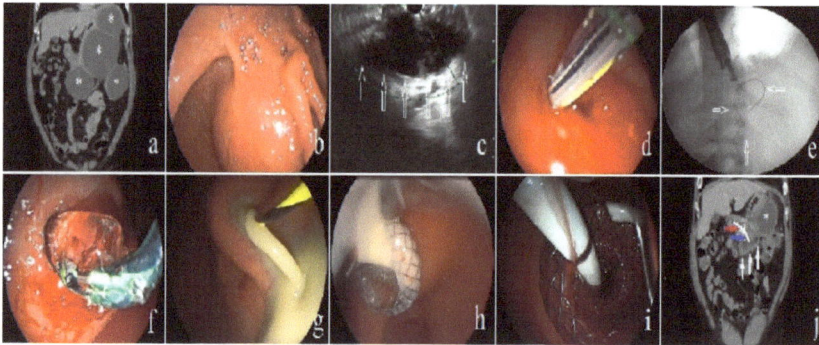

Figure 1. Placement of lumen-apposing metallic stent (LAMS) in the walled-off necrosis (WON) cavity. (**a**) CT demonstrating multi-lobulated WON cavities (asterisk). (**b**) Endoscopy demonstrating bulging of the gastric lumen. (**c**) Determining the WON cavity and selecting an appropriate drainage site with echoendoscope in a patient exhibiting no signs of bulging on the intestinal lumen (arrow). (**d**) Cavity puncture was performed with a needle knife sphincterotome. (**e**) Subsequently, a guidewire was carefully introduced into the cavity to facilitate further procedures (arrow). (**f**) Balloon dilatation was performed on the cystogastrostomy tract. (**g**) Purulent fluid was seen flowing into the lumen. (**h**) LAMS was placed to extend into the WON cavity. (**i**) To prevent migration, a double pigtail stent was positioned through the LAMS, extending into the cavity. (**j**) Three days post-procedure, the CT demonstrated the LAMS (red arrow), double pigtail stent (blue arrow), a visibly reduced volume of the drained WON cavity (white arrow), and another WON cavity (asterixis) that remained unaffected by endoscopic drainage.

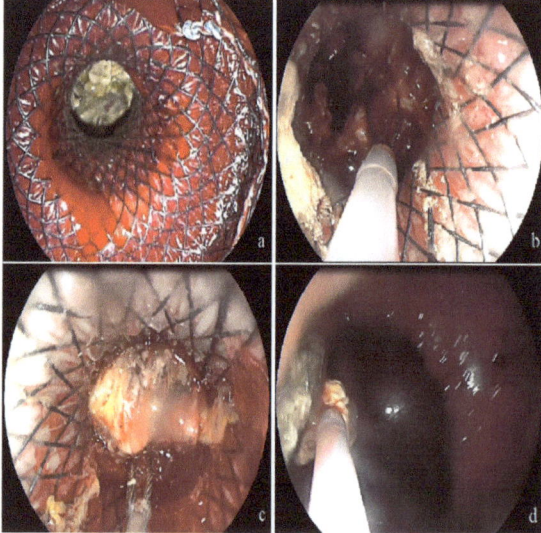

Figure 2. Direct endoscopic necrosectomy procedure. (**a**) Necrotic tissue in the walled-off necrosis cavity was seen through the lumen-apposing metallic stent (LAMS) with the endoscope. (**b**) The necrotic tissue was captured with a basket catheter. (**c**) The necrotic tissue was pulled through the LAMS into the gastric lumen. (**d**) Subsequently, the necrotic tissue was released into the gastric lumen.

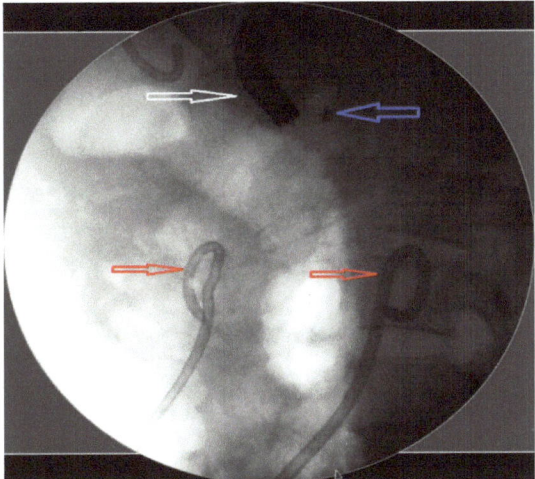

Figure 3. Image of a double pigtail stent with a lumen-apposing metallic stent and percutaneous drainage catheters on fluoroscopy. Figure 3 Fluoroscopy demonstrating the presence of the lumen-apposing metallic stent (white arrow) in the cystogastrostomy tract, along with the double pigtail stent (blue arrow) and two percutaneous drainage catheters (red arrows).

2.4. Post-Procedure Follow-Up

The stents were removed upon achieving clinical success, and patients were monitored with clinical, laboratory, and ultrasound examinations every three months for the first year. For patients with recurrent symptoms or documented recurrence of collections, CT imaging was repeated. In patients with clinical success, the total number of procedures was determined by including the last session in which the stent was removed.

2.5. Statistics

Statistical analysis was conducted using the 21st version of the Statistical Package for the Social Sciences (SPSS, IBM, Armonk, NY, USA). Continuous variables are presented as the median and interquartile range (IQR), while categorical data are presented as numbers and percentages. Due to the non-normal distribution of the data, outcomes between groups were compared using the Mann–Whitney U test for variance. The receiver operating characteristic (ROC) curve was utilized to calculate the area under the curve (AUC) for assessing the diagnostic value and accuracy of different parameters, with the best sensitivity and specificity determined by given cut-off values.

3. Results
3.1. Characteristics of Patients

A total of 11 patients (63.6% male, median age 48 years) with infected or complicated WON who underwent endoscopic intervention were included in this study. The causes underlying AP in these patients were gallstone (45.4%), alcohol (18.1%), acute-on-chronic pancreatitis (18.1%), and hypertriglyceridemia (9.0%). The cause of AP could not be determined in one (9.0%) patient. The median time interval between the diagnosis of AP attack and the diagnosis of WON was 54 days (IQR, 30 to 240 days). Abdominal pain was present in all patients, abdominal distension in 54.5%, early satiety in 54.5%, vomiting in 18.1%, and fever in 9.0% of cases. In laboratory examinations, white blood cell counts were above the upper limit of normal (ULN) in two (18%) patients, and amylase and/or lipase levels were above the ULN in eight (73%). Carcinoembryonic antigen and CA 19-9 levels were within normal limits in all patients. Diagnosis of WON was confirmed in all patients through abdominal CT scans. The median largest dimension of the WON was

150 mm (IQR, 92 to 238 mm). Single WON cavities were present in seven (63.6%) patients, while multiple cavities in four (36.3%) patients. Among these patients, the main location of WON involved the body and tail in six (54.5%) patients, the entire pancreas in two (18.1%), the body alone in one (9.0%), and the tail alone in one (9.0%). Additionally, in one (9.0%) patient, the cavity was located outside the pancreas. DPDS was detected in five (45.4%) patients, and gastric lumen bulging was observed in six (54.5%) patients during imaging examinations (Table 1).

Table 1. Characteristics of patients with walled-off necrosis who underwent endoscopic management.

	Total n (%)
Age (median years)	48 (24–61)
Sex	
Male	7 (63.6)
Female	4 (36.3)
Cause of pancreatitis	
Alcohol	2 (18.1)
Gallstone	5 (45.4)
Acute or chronic pancreatitis	2 (18.1)
Hypertriglyceridemia	1 (9.0)
Idiopathic	1 (9.0)
Diagnosis time from pancreatitis to WON (median days)	54 (30–240)
Clinical presentation	
Abdominal pain	11 (100)
Vomiting	2 (18.1)
Fever	1 (9.0)
Abdominal distention	6 (54.5)
Early satiety	6 (54.5)
Laboratory investigation	
Elevated WBC	2 (18.1)
Elevated amylase and lipase	8 (72.7)
Normal CEA and Ca 19-9	11 (100)
Diagnosis by imaging	
Abdominal CT or MRI	11 (100)
Largest dimension of WON cavity (mm)	150 (92–238)
No. of WON cavities	
Single	7 (63.6)
Multiple	4 (36.3)
Main location of WON	
Body	1 (9.0)
Tail	1 (9.0)
Body and tail	6 (54.5)
Entire pancreas	2 (18.1)
Extrapancreatic location	1 (9.0)
Presence of DPD	5 (45.4)
Presence of bulging into the stomach	6 (54.5)
Intra-cavity echogenicity	
Anechogenic	11 (100)

Data are presented as median (IQR) or frequency (%). WON, walled-off necrosis. DPD, disconnected pancreatic duct. WBC, white blood cell. CEA, carcinoembryonic antigen. CT, computed tomography. MRI, magnetic resonance imaging.

3.2. Initial Outcomes of Endoscopic Intervention

Out of the 11 patients who underwent endoscopic intervention, 6 (54.5%) did so due to gastric outlet obstruction, 5 (45.4%) due to intractable pain, and 1 (9.0%) due to suspected infection. The conventional transmural drainage method was employed in six (54.5%) patients, while EUS-guided drainage was utilized in five (45.4%) patients. Successful cannulation of the cavity was achieved in all patients with the first puncture attempt. The cystogastrostomy tract was dilated in nine (81.8%) patients. LAMS with DPPS was placed into the WON in all patients. DEN was performed in seven (63.6%) patients. Additionally, transpapillary drainage was performed in five (45.4%) patients for DPDS. Surgical treatment was required in one (9.0%) patient due to perforation that occurred during the initial procedure. Technical success was 90.9%, while clinical success with only endoscopic treatment methods was 36.3% (Table 2).

Table 2. Procedural details and outcomes of a step-up approach in patients with walled-off necrosis.

	Total n (%)
Indication of intervention	
Suspected infection	1 (9.0)
Intractable pain	5 (45.4)
Gastric outlet obstruction	6 (54.5)
Preprocedural intravenous antibiotics	11 (100)
Drainage method	
CTD	6 (54.5)
EUS	5 (45.4)
Additional transpapillary drainage	5 (45.4)
Route	
Transgastric	11 (100)
Transduodenal	0 (0)
Insufflation during the procedure	
Room air	0 (0)
CO_2 gas	11 (100)
Cavity cannulation success at first attempt	11 (100)
Tract dilatation	9 (81.8)
Types of stents	
LAMS with DPPS	11 (100)
Size of LAMS	
16 × 15 mm	5 (45.4)
16 × 20 mm	6 (54.5)
Direct endoscopic necrosectomy needed	7 (63.6)
Additional percutaneous intervention	6 (54.5)
Surgery treatment needed	1 (9.0)
Technical success	10 (90.9)
Clinical success with only endoscopic management	4 (36.3)
Largest dimension of WON cavity (mm)	100–110 (92–120)
Single WON cavity	4 (100)
Multiple WON cavities	0 (0)
Clinical success with a combination of percutaneous and endoscopic management	6 (54.5)
Largest dimension of WON cavity (mm)	200 (130–238)
Single WON cavity	2 (33.3)
Multiple WON cavities	4 (66.6)
Clinical failure	1 (9.0)

Data are presented as median (IQR) or frequency (%). CTD, conventional transmural drainage. EUS, endoscopic ultrasonography. CO_2, carbon dioxide. LAMS, lumen-apposing metallic stent. DPPS, double pigtail plastic stent.

3.3. The Addition of Percutaneous Intervention as a Step-Up Approach

In six (54.5%) patients, clinical success could not be achieved with three sessions of endoscopic management alone. Consequently, a step-up approach was adopted by inserting a percutaneous drainage catheter into the WON cavity. Both technical and clinical success were attained in all patients with a combination of percutaneous and endoscopic management (Table 2).

Patients who achieved clinical success with only endoscopic management had a median cavity diameter of 100–110 mm (IQR, 92 to 120 mm), whereas those who succeeded with a combined treatment method had a median cavity diameter of 200 mm (IQR, 130 to 238 mm) ($p = 0.034$). The cut-off value for endoscopic treatment success based on cavity diameter was 125 mm (AUC = 1.00; 95% CI: 1.00–1.00; p = 0.011). Additionally, all patients who achieved clinical success with endoscopic management alone had a single cavity whereas among those successfully treated with a combination treatment method, four had two or more cavities (Table 2).

3.4. Outcomes of Complications, Recurrence, and Follow-Up

A total of 53 procedures were performed, with a median of five procedures (IQR, one to nine). Among the patients, two (18.2%) experienced major complications, with one (9.0%) encountering perforation and the other (9.0%) suffering from major bleeding necessitating replacement. In perforated patients, EUS-guided cannulation of the WON cavity was followed by balloon dilatation of the cystogastrostomy tract; however, despite the placement of LAMS, surgical treatment was ultimately necessary. The patient died due to multi-organ failure during the post-operative follow-up. Additionally, minor complications were observed in six patients, including LAMS migration and minor bleeding in two patients, LAMS migration and procedure-related infection in one patient, LAMS migration and blockage in one patient, and LAMS migration in two patients. LAMS migration was observed in those who were considered sufficiently drained with only LAMS without the need for DPPS during subsequent procedures. Out of the six patients, LAMS migration occurred into the gastric lumen in four patients, while it migrated into the cavity in two patients. In the two cases where LAMS migrated into the cavity, it was retrieved endoscopically through the cystogastrostomy tract, captured with a snare, removed, and then replaced. In two out of the four patients in whom LAMS migrated into the stomach lumen, the size of the WON cavity had significantly reduced, indicating no remaining necrosis. In these cases, only a DPPS extending into the cavity was placed through the cystogastrostomy tract. In the other two patients, no additional procedure was necessary as clinical success had already been achieved. Additionally, no complications related to stent infection or acute pancreatitis were detected after drainage or at the 1-month follow-up.

No major complications, such as organ perforation or major bleeding, related to the placement of percutaneous drainage catheter occurred in any of the patients. However, minor complications occurred in three (50%) patients. All of these were related to catheter occlusion, requiring either drain replacement or the use of a guide to clear the blockage.

The median length of hospital stay was 32 (IQR, 14 to 58) days, with a median follow-up time of 94 (IQR, 22 to 1105) days. Among the 10 patients who achieved clinical remission with a step-up treatment approach, recurrence occurred in only 1 patient during follow-up (Table 3).

Table 3. Outcomes of complications, recurrence, and follow-up.

	Total n (%)
No. of procedures	5 (1–9)
Complications of endoscopic management	
Major complications	2 (18.1)
Major bleeding	1 (9.0)
Perforation	1 (9.0)
Minor complications	6 (54.5)
Minor bleeding	2 (18.1)
LAMS blockage	1 (9.0)
Procedure-related infection	1 (9.0)
LAMS migration into the lumen	4 (36.3)
LAMS migration into the cavity	2 (18.1)
Complications of percutaneous intervention	
Blockage	3 (50)
Recurrence	1 (9.0)
Mortality	1 (9.0)
Hospital stay (median days)	32 (14–58)
Total follow-up (median days)	123 (55–1125)

Data are presented as median (IQR) or frequency (%). LAMS, lumen-apposing metallic stent.

4. Discussion

The incidence of acute necrotizing pancreatitis is increasing, and it can be a disease associated with a mortality rate ranging from 20% to 80%, attributed to septic complications and multiple organ failure [15]. Endoscopic treatment methods have been reported to achieve high success rates with low morbidity and mortality rates, along with offering lower total costs and improved quality of life [4,16,17]. Additionally, the choice of stent for transmural drainage in endoscopic management is a current area of debate. A recent review highlighted the use of LAMS in patients with WON, reporting a resolution rate of 87.7% with transmural drainage using LAMS. Complications included stent occlusion (7.5%), bleeding (6.2%), perforation (3.8%), migration (7.8%), and occlusion (11.7%) [18]. Consequently, while surgery has traditionally been the predominant approach, minimally invasive methods, particularly endoscopic treatments, are increasingly favored as the initial step [19–21].

We included 11 consecutive patients with infected or complicated WON who were referred to our tertiary referral center over a 4-year period. Technical success was achieved in 90.9% despite the development of retroperitoneal perforation in one patient, while clinical success with endoscopic treatment alone was 36.3%. An additional percutaneous drainage catheter was placed in patients where an adequate response could not be achieved. Clinical success was attained in all patients who underwent this combination treatment method. During a total of 53 procedures, major complications occurred in 18.1% of patients, while minor complications occurred in 6% of patients. Among all complications, LAMS migration (54.5%) was the most common, and all of these occurred after the decision not to place DPPS in the follow-up procedures. Our clinical success and major complication results were comparable to previous studies (20–25).

In our study, the clinical success achieved through endoscopic management alone was relatively low (36.3%), despite achieving high technical success rates, transpapillary drainage in all patients with DPDS, the placement of LAMS in all patients to facilitate drainage, and DEN in indicated cases. We attribute this low success rate of endoscopic treatment alone compared to previous studies to several factors, including the significantly large average cavity diameter, the presence of multiple unrelated cavities in four patients, and the complexity of cases typically referred to our center as a tertiary referral center. Out of our patient cohort, only one individual encountered a procedure-related perforation, which occurred during cannulation utilizing the EUS-guided method. The absence of perforations in patients undergoing cavity cannulation via conventional transmural drainage in our study can be attributed to several factors. These include thorough preprocedural evaluation of patients radiologically and endoscopically, the performance of cystogastrostomy tract dilation in deemed necessary cases (the fluidity of the drainage fluid was the main factor), the use of LAMS in all patients, and the fact that an experienced endoscopist conducted all procedures. The recent systematic review and meta-analysis by Bang et al. evaluated the use of LAMS and plastic stent, reporting no significant difference in clinical outcomes except for procedure duration [22]. Since our study did not include a patient group with only plastic stent placement for the drainage of WON, we could not make a comparison. However, we believe that there are additional benefits to using LAMS. The most significant of these is the closure of gaps without causing a clinical outcome in minor perforation cases that we cannot detect during the procedure. Another benefit is facilitating entry into the cavity during necrosectomy procedures. In cases where adequate necrosis resolution could not be achieved, additional procedures were required for cavity washing. In patients with an additional percutaneous drainage catheter, providing drainage to the intestinal lumen through external washing with a low risk of blockage is also a valuable contribution. Additionally, washing could be easily performed within the day without the need for repeated procedures. Mohan et al. reported a migration rate of 5.1% for LAMS [23]. Our migration rate for LAMS was 11.3% in a total of 53 procedures. All migrations occurred in follow-up procedures after procedures where DPPS was not placed. It is clear that placing DPPS in every session where LAMS will be left in place will reduce migration rates. Additionally, re-cavity cannulation after migration was quite easy in our patients in whom LAMS was placed before, and this can be considered an additional advantage of using LAMS.

We achieved clinical success with the combination of endoscopic and percutaneous treatment, as a step-up therapeutic approach, in all six patients for whom clinical success could not be achieved with three sessions of endoscopic management alone. We believe there are several main reasons for this high success rate. Firstly, the addition of percutaneous drainage to the treatment allows for the drainage of cavities that cannot be drained endoscopically. Secondly, the reduction in the size of large cavities through endoscopic drainage may lead to the development of collapsed regions within the cavity, impeding effective drainage by endoscopic modalities alone. The addition of percutaneous drainage enables the drainage of regions distant from the cystogastrostomy tract, which may be difficult to access solely through endoscopic means. Additionally, frequent cavity washouts within the day help to maintain optimal drainage and promote the resolution of necrotic tissue, contributing to improved patient outcomes. In our study, we conducted a comparative analysis between patients who achieved successful outcomes with endoscopic management alone and those who required a combined treatment approach for success. The findings suggest that in instances involving multiple cavities or cavities of significant size (≥ 125 mm), relying solely on endoscopic management may prove insufficient. In such cases, a combined treatment approach emerges as an effective strategy.

According to the recent results of 117 patients with WON treated with a percutaneous drainage catheter reported by Mallick et al., complications included external pancreatic fistula in 34.2% of patients, drain blockage in 14.5%, drain slippage in 11.1%, and bleeding in 5.1%. Among those with an external pancreatic fistula, 80% required the placement of a pancreatic stent. Additionally, 12% of patients required surgery, and mortality occurred in 13.7% [24]. None of our patients experienced major complications such as organ perforation or significant bleeding during the percutaneous interventions. A total of 50% of our patients with combining percutaneous modalities experienced drain obstruction. No instances of external pancreatic fistula, drain slippage, or bleeding were observed. None of the patients required surgery due to percutaneous intervention, and there was no mortality. We believe that the placement of a pancreatic stent before percutaneous intervention in patients with pre-existing DPDS, along with meticulous follow-up to prevent drain slippage, was effective.

The strength of this study lies in its inclusion of patients treated with a pre-defined step-up strategy and the performance of all procedures by an experienced endoscopist. However, our study has several limitations. Firstly, it is retrospective in design; however, we believe that this limitation is largely overcome by the pre-defined treatment strategy and the retrospective analysis of our prospective database. Secondly, another limitation is the number of included patients. This can be attributed to the fact that our clinic is a tertiary referral center. Therefore, severe cases that cannot be adequately managed in other healthcare institutions are often referred to our hospital. We anticipate that addressing this issue in future multi-center studies or meta-analyses may provide a more comprehensive perspective. Another limitation is that EUS-guided interventions were not performed in all patients. However, no major complications occurred in patients where we utilized the conventional transmural drainage method for interventions. Therefore, we are confident that this limitation did not significantly impact our results.

In conclusion, endoscopic management is recommended as the primary treatment method for WON due to its less invasive nature and higher safety profile. However, in cases where there are large (≥ 125 mm) or multi-lobulated WON cavities and clinical success cannot be achieved with three interventions, the inclusion of percutaneous drainage in the treatment is highly successful and safe. Ultimately, it can minimize the need for surgery, which is a more invasive treatment modality.

Author Contributions: A.A.: investigation, data collection, writing—original draft preparation, statistics, reviewing and editing, visualization. I.Y.: conceptualization, methodology, investigation, supervision, writing—reviewing and editing. All authors have read and agreed to the published version of the manuscript.

Funding: The authors declared that this study has received no financial support.

Institutional Review Board Statement: This study was conducted in accordance with the ethical guidelines of the institutional research committee, the 1964 Declaration of Helsinki and its subsequent amendments, or comparable ethical standards. The Ankara Bilkent City Hospital Scientific Research and Ethics Committee accepted the project on 27 December 2023 with approval No: E1-23-4492.

Informed Consent Statement: Written informed consent has been obtained from the patients to publish this paper.

Data Availability Statement: The data used and analyzed in the current study are available from the corresponding author upon reasonable request.

Conflicts of Interest: The authors declare that they have no conflicts of interest.

References

1. Hyun, J.J.; Sahar, N.; Singla, A.; Ross, A.S.; Irani, S.S.; Gan, S.I.; Larsen, M.C.; Kozarek, R.A.; Gluck, M. Outcomes of Infected versus Symptomatic Sterile Walled-Off Pancreatic Necrosis Treated with a Minimally Invasive Therapy. *Gut Liver* **2019**, *13*, 215–222. [CrossRef]
2. Banks, P.A.; Bollen, T.L.; Dervenis, C.; Gooszen, H.G.; Johnson, C.D.; Sarr, M.G.; Tsiotos, G.G.; Vege, S.S.; Acute Pancreatitis Classification Working Group. Classification of acute pancreatitis—2012: Revision of the Atlanta classification and definitions by international consensus. *Gut* **2013**, *62*, 102–111. [CrossRef]
3. Perez, A.; Whang, E.E.; Brooks, D.C.; Moore, F.D., Jr.; Hughes, M.D.; Sica, G.T.; Zinner, M.J.; Ashley, S.W.; Banks, P.A. Is severity of necrotizing pancreatitis increased in extended necrosis and infected necrosis? *Pancreas* **2002**, *25*, 229–233. [CrossRef]
4. van Santvoort, H.C.; Bakker, O.J.; Bollen, T.L.; Besselink, M.G.; Ali, U.A.; Schrijver, A.M.; Boermeester, M.A.; van Goor, H.; Dejong, C.H.; van Eijck, C.H.; et al. A conservative and minimally invasive approach to necrotizing pancreatitis improves outcome. *Gastroenterology* **2011**, *141*, 1254–1263. [CrossRef] [PubMed]
5. Shahid, H. Endoscopic management of pancreatic fluid collections. *Transl. Gastroenterol. Hepatol.* **2019**, *4*, 15. [CrossRef]
6. Seifert, H.; Wehrmann, T.; Schmitt, T.; Zeuzem, S.; Caspary, W.F. Retroperitoneal endoscopic debridement for infected peripancreatic necrosis. *Lancet* **2000**, *356*, 653–655. [CrossRef] [PubMed]
7. Banks, P.A.; Freeman, M.L. Practice Guidelines in Acute Pancreatitis. *Am. J. Gastroenterol.* **2006**, *101*, 2379–2400. [CrossRef] [PubMed]
8. Zhao, K.; Adam, S.Z.; Keswani, R.N.; Horowitz, J.M.; Miller, F.H. Acute Pancreatitis: Revised Atlanta Classification and the Role of Cross-Sectional Imaging. *Am. J. Roentgenol.* **2015**, *205*, W32–W41. [CrossRef]
9. Braden, B.; Koutsoumpas, A.; Silva, M.A.; Soonawalla, Z.; Dietrich, C.F. Endoscopic ultrasound-guided drainage of pancreatic walled-off necrosis using self-expanding metal stents without fluoroscopy. *World J. Gastrointest. Endosc.* **2018**, *10*, 93–98. [CrossRef]
10. Kim, Y.S.; Cho, J.H.; Cho, D.H.; Park, S.W.; Moon, S.H.; Park, J.S.; Lee, Y.N.; Lee, S.S. Long-Term Outcomes of Direct Endoscopic Necrosectomy for Com-Plicated or Symptomatic Walled-Off Necrosis: A Korean Multicenter Study. *Gut Liver* **2021**, *15*, 930–939. [CrossRef]
11. Baron, T.H.; DiMaio, C.J.; Wang, A.Y.; Morgan, K.A. American Gastroenterological Association Clinical Practice Update: Management of Pancreatic Necrosis. *Gastroenterology* **2020**, *158*, 67–75.e1. [CrossRef]
12. Dutch Pancreatitis Study Group; van Grinsven, J.; van Santvoort, H.C.; Boermeester, M.A.; Dejong, C.H.; van Eijck, C.H.; Fockens, P.; Besselink, M.G. Timing of catheter drainage in infected necrotizing pancreatitis. *Nat. Rev. Gastroenterol. Hepatol.* **2016**, *13*, 306–312. [CrossRef]
13. Freeman, M.L.; Werner, J.; Van Santvoort, H.C.; Baron, T.H.; Besselink, M.G.; Windsor, J.A.; Horvath, K.D.; Bollen, T.L.; Vege, S.S. Interventions for necrotizing pancreatitis: Summary of a multidisciplinary consensus conference. *Pancreas* **2012**, *41*, 1176–1194. [CrossRef]
14. Nass, K.J.; Zwager, L.W.; van der Vlugt, M.; Dekker, E.; Bossuyt, P.M.; Ravindran, S.; Thomas-Gibson, S.; Fockens, P. Novel classification for adverse events in GI endos-copy: The AGREE classification. *Gastrointest. Endosc.* **2022**, *95*, 1078–1085.e8. [CrossRef]
15. Yasuda, I.; Nakashima, M.; Iwai, T.; Isayama, H.; Itoi, T.; Hisai, H.; Inoue, H.; Kato, H.; Kanno, A.; Kubota, K.; et al. Japanese multicenter experience of endoscopic necrosectomy for infected walled-off pancreatic necrosis: The JENIPaN study. *Endoscopy* **2013**, *45*, 627–634. [CrossRef] [PubMed]
16. Wronski, M.; Cebulski, W.; Karkocha, D.; Slodkowski, M.; Wysocki, L.; Jankowski, M. Ultrasound-guided percutaneous drainage of infected pancreatic necrosis. *Surg. Endosc.* **2013**, *27*, 2841–2848. [CrossRef]
17. Yasuda, I.; Takahashi, K. Endoscopic management of walled-off pancreatic necrosis. *Dig. Endosc.* **2021**, *33*, 335–341. [CrossRef]

18. Bazerbachi, F.; Sawas, T.; Vargas, E.J.; Prokop, L.J.; Chari, S.T.; Gleeson, F.C.; Levy, M.J.; Martin, J.; Petersen, B.T.; Pearson R.K.; et al. Metal stents versus plastic stents for the management of pancreatic walled-off necrosis: A systematic review and meta-analysis. *Gastrointest. Endosc.* **2018**, *87*, 30–42.e15. [CrossRef] [PubMed]
19. Bang, J.Y.; Holt, B.A.; Hawes, R.H.; Hasan, M.K.; Arnoletti, J.P.; Christein, J.D.; Wilcox, C.M.; Varadarajulu, S. Outcomes after implementing a tailored endoscopic step-up approach to walled-off necrosis in acute pancreatitis. *Br. J. Surg.* **2014**, *101*, 1729–1738 [CrossRef]
20. Kumar, N.; Conwell, D.L.; Thompson, C.C. Direct endoscopic necrosectomy versus step-up approach for walled-off pancreatic necrosis: Comparison of clinical outcome and health care utilization. *Pancreas* **2014**, *43*, 1334–1339. [CrossRef] [PubMed]
21. Gardner, T.B.; Chahal, P.; Papachristou, G.I.; Vege, S.S.; Petersen, B.T.; Gostout, C.J.; Topazian, M.D.; Takahashi, N.; Sarr, M.G.; Baron, T.H. A comparison of direct endoscopic necrosectomy with transmural endoscopic drainage for the treatment of walled-off pancreatic necrosis. *Gastrointest. Endosc.* **2009**, *69*, 1085–1094. [CrossRef] [PubMed]
22. Bang, J.Y.; Wilcox, C.M.; Navaneethan, U.; Hawes, R.H.; Varadarajulu, S. Treatment of walled-off necrosis using lumen-apposing metal stents versus plastic stents: A systematic review and meta-analysis of data from randomized trials. *Endoscopy* **2023**, *56*, 184–195. [CrossRef] [PubMed]
23. Mohan, B.P.; Jayaraj, M.; Asokkumar, R.; Shakhatreh, M.; Pahal, P.; Ponnada, S.; Navaneethan, U.; Adler, D.G. Lumen apposing metal stents in drainage of pancreatic walled-off necrosis, are they any better than plastic stents? A systematic review and meta-analysis of studies published since the revised Atlanta classification of pancreatic fluid collections. *Endosc. Ultrasound* **2019**, *8*, 82–90. [PubMed]
24. Mallick, B.; Dhaka, N.; Gupta, P.; Gulati, A.; Malik, S.; Sinha, S.K.; Yadav, T.D.; Gupta, V.; Kochhar, R. An audit of percutaneous drainage for acute necrotic collections and walled off necrosis in patients with acute pancreatitis. *Pancreatology* **2018**, *18*, 727–733 [CrossRef]

Disclaimer/Publisher's Note: The statements, opinions and data contained in all publications are solely those of the individual author(s) and contributor(s) and not of MDPI and/or the editor(s). MDPI and/or the editor(s) disclaim responsibility for any injury to people or property resulting from any ideas, methods, instructions or products referred to in the content.

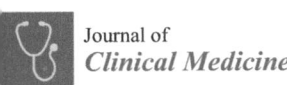

Article

β1600 Q.Clear Digital Reconstruction of [⁶⁸Ga]Ga-DOTANOC PET/CT Improves Image Quality in NET Patients

Martina Di Franco [1,*,†], Emilia Fortunati [2,*,†], Lucia Zanoni [2], Norma Bonazzi [1], Cristina Mosconi [3,4], Claudio Malizia [2], Simona Civollani [2], Davide Campana [3,5], Elisa Andrini [3,5], Giuseppe Lamberti [3,5], Vincenzo Allegri [2], Stefano Fanti [1,2] and Valentina Ambrosini [1,2]

1. Nuclear Medicine, Alma Mater Studiorum, University of Bologna, 40126 Bologna, Italy; norma.bonazzi@studio.unibo.it (N.B.); stefano.fanti@aosp.bo.it (S.F.); valentina.ambrosini@unibo.it (V.A.)
2. Nuclear Medicine, IRCCS, Azienda Ospedaliero-Universitaria di Bologna, 40138 Bologna, Italy; lucia.zanoni@aosp.bo.it (L.Z.); claudio.malizia@aosp.bo.it (C.M.); simona.civollani@aosp.bo.it (S.C.); vincenzo.allegri@aosp.bo.it (V.A.)
3. Department of Medical and Surgical Sciences (DIMEC), Alma Mater Studiorum, University of Bologna, 40138 Bologna, Italy; cristina.mosconi@aosp.bo.it (C.M.); davide.campana@unibo.it (D.C.); elisa.andrini3@unibo.it (E.A.); giuseppe.lamberti8@unibo.it (G.L.)
4. Department of Radiology, IRCCS, Azienda Ospedaliero-Universitaria di Bologna, 40138 Bologna, Italy
5. Medical Oncology, IRCCS, Azienda Ospedaliero-Universitaria di Bologna, 40138 Bologna, Italy
* Correspondence: martina.difranco2@studio.unibo.it (M.D.F.); emilia.fortunati@studio.unibo.it (E.F.)
† These authors contributed equally to this work.

Abstract: Background: Image reconstruction is crucial for improving overall image quality and diagnostic accuracy. Q.Clear is a novel reconstruction algorithm that reduces image noise. The aim of the present study is to assess the preferred Q.Clear β-level for digital [⁶⁸Ga]Ga-DOTANOC PET/CT reconstruction vs. standard reconstruction (STD) for both overall scan and single-lesion visualization. **Methods:** Inclusion criteria: (1) patients with/suspected neuroendocrine tumors included in a prospective observational monocentric study between September 2019 and January 2022; (2) [⁶⁸Ga]Ga-DOTANOC digital PET/CT and contrast-enhanced-CT (ceCT) performed at our center at the same time. Images were reconstructed with STD and with Q.Clear β-levels 800, 1000, and 1600. Scans were blindly reviewed by three nuclear-medicine experts: the preferred β-level reconstruction was independently chosen for the visual quality of both the overall scan and the most avid target lesion < 1 cm (t) and >1 cm (T). PET/CT results were compared to ceCT. Semiquantitative analysis was performed (STD vs. β1600) in T and t concordant at both PET/CT and ceCT. Subgroup analysis was also performed in patients presenting discordant t. **Results:** Overall, 52 patients were included. β1600 reconstruction was considered superior over the others for both overall scan quality and single-lesion detection in all cases. The only significantly different ($p < 0.001$) parameters between β1600 and STD were signal-to-noise liver ratio and standard deviation of the liver background. Lesion-dependent parameters were not significantly different in concordant T ($n = 37$) and t ($n = 10$). Among 26 discordant t, when PET was positive, all findings were confirmed as malignant. **Conclusions:** β1600 Q.Clear reconstruction for [⁶⁸Ga]Ga-DOTANOC imaging is feasible and improves image quality for both overall and small-lesion assessment.

Keywords: Q.Clear; PET/CT; [⁶⁸Ga]Ga-DOTANOC; neuroendocrine neoplasms; neuroendocrine tumors; NET

1. Introduction

Technical improvements to Positron Emission Tomography with Computed Tomography (PET/CT) have focused on obtaining better image quality through the improvement of image contrast and the minimization of noise level. Image reconstruction is crucial for improving overall image quality and diagnostic accuracy [1].

A widely used image reconstruction algorithm, OSEM, is based on the repetition of a convergence algorithm that translates PET coincidence data into an image. Iterating the function, a new image is produced. This reconstruction model is affected by increased noise when the convergence is full; therefore, it is stopped after 2–4 iterations. Scarce iterations can lower OSEM quantitative accuracy and misrepresent small lesions.

A Bayesian penalized-likelihood image reconstruction algorithm, named Q.Clear, has recently been implemented for digital PET/CT tomographs (GE Healthcare) to improve quantification accuracy and image quality [2]. Q.Clear reconstruction incorporates a noise-suppression term called "relative difference penalty", for which the formula is available at: https://www.gehealthcare.com (accessed on 18 June 2024). Through regularization, the algorithm reaches full convergence without the need to stop iterations, resulting in preserving the edges and lowering the background at every voxel. The strength of the regularizing term is controlled by a "β" variable. The selection of the best optimal penalization factor (β-level) regulates the penalty term in the reconstruction algorithm with a consecutive variability in signal recovery and background. Lower β-levels are generally associated with higher noise and sharp contrast, while higher β-levels suppress image noise with the possibility of excessive smoothing [3].

It is well known that Q.Clear reconstruction improves overall image quality in comparison to other reconstruction algorithms by improving contrast recovery and noise suppression, therefore resulting in better lesion detectability [4–9].

Small-lesion detection is both a challenging and clinically relevant issue: Q.Clear is expected to improve small-lesion detectability by reducing image noise [10,11]. However, this setting has not been extensively studied, and there is no consensus on the best β-level to employ.

To date, most literature data has investigated the utility of Q.Clear on [^{18}F]F-FDG (Fluorodeoxyglucose) images. Some analyses conducted on phantoms have shown that Q.Clear reconstruction seems to detect sub-centimetric findings better than OSEM reconstruction [12,13].

Regarding the particular setting of small lesions and their characterization, neuroendocrine neoplasms (NEN) could benefit from Q.Clear reconstruction. [^{68}Ga]Ga-DOTA-peptide PET/CT is the gold standard for imaging well-differentiated neuroendocrine tumors (NET, with high expression of somatostatin receptors—SST), mainly for staging, assessing SST status, selecting patients for Peptide Receptor Radionuclide Therapy (PRRT), and monitoring the response to therapy [14–16].

[^{68}Ga]Ga-DOTA-peptide PET/CT shows high sensitivity and specificity for the diagnosis of NET [17–21]. The most common site of NET metastases is the liver (up to 85% of patients), and its involvement is associated with reduced survival. However, the physiological moderate-to-intense and often heterogeneous [^{68}Ga]Ga-DOTA-peptide uptake at the liver level limits the detection of metastases [17,18]. For extra-hepatic metastasis detection (e.g., bone [19] and node [20]), [^{68}Ga]Ga-DOTA-peptide PET/CT resulted in more accuracy than contrast-enhanced diagnostic CT (ceCT).

Q.Clear reconstruction may be crucial for detecting small lesions at both liver and extra-liver levels, with potential impact on patient management.

The literature about Q.Clear utility in NET patients is still very limited, and no definitive β-levels have been reported.

The aim of the present study was to assess the preferred Q.Clear β-level for digital [^{68}Ga]Ga-DOTANOC PET/CT reconstruction vs. standard reconstruction (STD) for both overall scan quality and single-lesion visualization (for the most avid finding < 1 cm and >1 cm, respectively).

2. Materials and Methods

Among the patients with NET or suspected NET who underwent [^{68}Ga]Ga-DOTANOC PET/CT at our center and were included in a prospective monocentric CE-approved electronic archive (131/2017/O/Oss), those meeting the following criteria were included in the analysis: (1) [^{68}Ga]Ga-DOTANOC PET/CT performed on a digital tomograph (GE MI) between September 2019 and January 2022 and ceCT performed at our center at the same time; (2) no significant radiotracer extravasation.

[^{68}Ga]Ga-DOTANOC PET/CT was acquired on a digital tomograph according to standard practice and following EANM guidelines (100–200 MBq, uptake time 60 min, 3 min per bed position) [14,15]. Overall, 52 patients were included. Areas of increased uptake outside the tracer's biodistribution were interpreted as positive (excluding areas of clearly benign/inflammatory findings). Images were reconstructed with standard OSEM (8 subsets, 4 iterations, 6 mm filter) + time of flight (STD) and Q.Clear algorithms with three different βlevels (800, 1000, and 1600) [22].

Scans were reviewed by three expert nuclear-medicine readers, unaware of the clinical data, who independently chose the preferred reconstruction (STD vs. β800 vs. β1000 vs. β1600) for the visual quality of both overall scan and single lesions (for the most avid target finding < 1 cm and >1 cm, respectively). Agreement among readers was assessed to define the best β-level reconstruction, as previously published. PET/CT results were compared to ceCT and revised by one expert radiologist.

Semiquantitative analysis (GE software AW server) of the most avid lesion < 1 cm (t) and > 1 cm (T) concordant at both PET/CT and ceCT was performed both on STD and the best β-level reconstruction: SUVmax, SUVmean, and standard deviation (SD) of, respectively, the most avid target lesion (T and t) and liver background (L); SUVmax-T/SUVmean-L; SUVmax-t/SUVmean-L; signal-to-noise liver ratio (SNR-L = SUVmean /SD); contrast-to-noise ratio (CNR = SUVmean (T or t)-SUVmeanSurroundingBackground/SDBackground). Note that a 5-centimeter-diameter ROI on disease-free liver parenchyma was used to measure liver background uptake.

A subgroup analysis was also performed in patients presenting small-sized discordant lesions on PET/CT and ceCT.

3. Statistical Analysis

All collected data were analyzed using R software version 4.1.0, with a significance level set at 0.05. The Friedman test was applied to semiquantitative parameters. In the case of significant results, post hoc analysis was performed using pair-by-pair Wilcoxon signed-rank tests.

4. Results

Overall, 52 patients with NET or suspected NET were included (M:F = 31:21; age: mean = 60.3 yo, median = 62.5 [52.7–73.0] yo). NET primary tumor sites were ileum (15/52, 29%), pancreas (11/52, 21%), other gastrointestinal (6/52, 11%), lung (4/52, 8%), and unknown (4/52,8%). A total of 12 of 52 (23%) were patients with suspected NET.

Indications to [^{68}Ga]Ga-DOTANOC PET/CT were pre-treatment staging (7/52, 14%), post-surgical staging (6/52, 11%), evaluation of PRRT eligibility (2/52, 4%), suspected relapse (4/52, 8%), assessment during treatment (8/52, 15%), restaging after therapy (10/52, 19%), follow-up (2/52, 4%), localization of unknown primary (2/52, 4%) and for suspected NET (11/52, 21%) [Table 1].

Overall, [^{68}Ga]Ga-DOTANOC PET/CT was positive in 37/52 patients (71%) and negative in 15/52 (29%), while ceCT was positive in 45/52 (87%) and negative in 7/52 (13%) patients.

Visual image quality of PET β-1600 reconstruction was considered superior over the others (STD; β-800; β-1000) for both overall scan quality and single-lesion detection in all cases (52/52, 100%), with full agreement between the three readers (100%) (Figures 1 and 2).

Table 1. Patient epidemiological characteristics.

		Median	Range
Age		62.5	52.7–73.0
Gender		n	%
	Male	31	60
	Female	21	40
Primary tumor site			
	Ileum	15	29
	Pancreas	11	21
	Other GEP	6	11
	Lung	4	8
	CUP	4	8
Suspected NET		12	23
Indication of PET imaging			
	Pre-treatment staging	7	14
	Post-surgical staging	6	11
	Evaluation of PRRT eligibility	2	4
	Suspected relapse	4	8
	Assessment during treatment	8	15
	Restaging after therapy	10	19
	Follow-up	2	4
	Localization of unknown primary	2	4
	Suspected NET	11	21

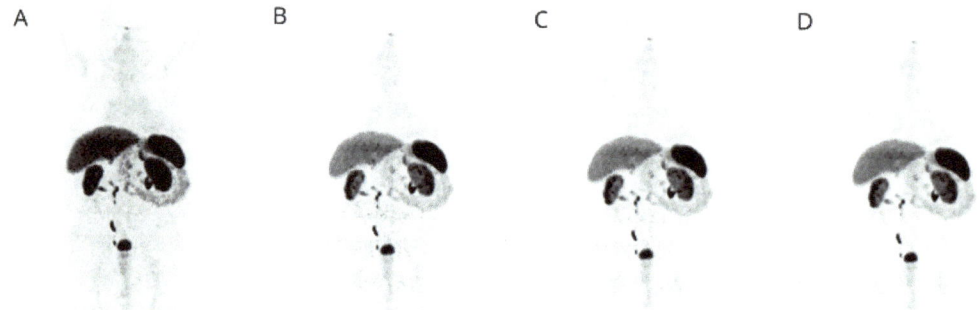

Figure 1. MIP images corresponding to STD (**A**), β-level 800 (**B**), β-level 1000 (**C**), and β-level 1600 (**D**) are displayed: lower image noise is evident in D, confirming the preferred image quality with β-level 1600.

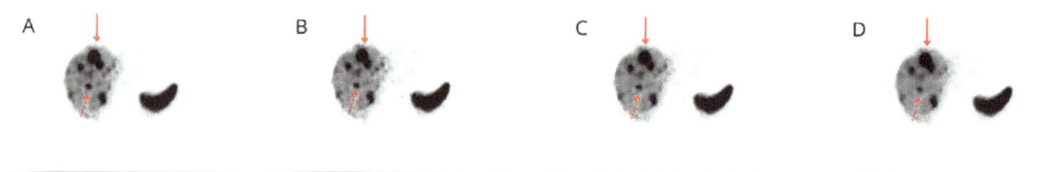

Figure 2. Transaxial PET images corresponding to STD (**A**), β-level 800 (**B**), β-level 1000 (**C**), and β-level 1600 (**D**) are displayed: both T (red arrow) and t (dashed arrow) are better appreciated on the D image corresponding to β-level 1600.

The only significantly different ($p < 0.001$) parameters between β1600 and STD ($p < 0.001$) were signal-to noise liver ratio (SNR-L) (β1600 vs. STD: mean = 9.9 vs. 7.3; median = 9.9 vs. 7.1; range: 4.7–15.7 vs. 4.6–14.0) and standard deviation of the liver background (β1600 vs. STD: mean = 0.5 vs. 0.7; median =0.5 vs. 0.7; range: 0.2–1.1 vs. 0.3–1.3) (Figure 3).

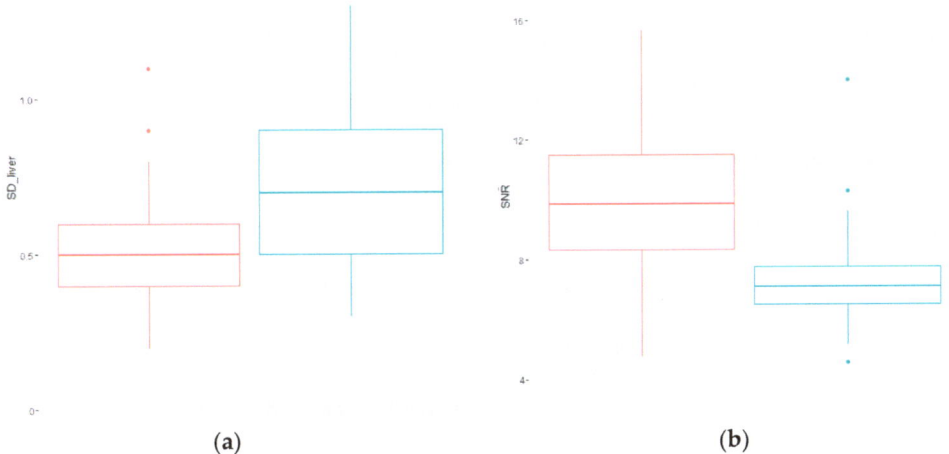

Figure 3. (**a**) Standard deviation of the liver background of β1600 (red) and STD (blue) are significantly different $p < 0.001$; (**b**) Signal-to-noise liver ratio of β1600 (red) and STD (blue) are significantly different at $p < 0.001$.

When lesion-dependent parameters (SUVmax, SUVmean, and CNR) were measured in the most avid lesion (>1 cm, T; n = 37), there were no statistically significant differences between β1600 and STD. This was also confirmed when lesion-dependent parameters were measured in the most avid concordant small lesion (<1 cm, t; n = 10) (Table 2).

Table 2. Lesion-dependent parameters.

	n	β1600			STD			p
		Mean	Median	Range	Mean	Median	Range	
Most avid lesion > 1 cm (T)	37							
SUVmax		26.7	22.7	4–82.7	26.9	24.3	3.4–79.3	0.867
SUVmean		16.9	14.1	2.3–54.5	16.6	15.1	2.1–51.7	1000
CNR		45.6	38.3	2.3–188	35.5	34.8	2.7–125.5	0.165
Most avid lesion < 1 cm	23							
concordant	10							
SUVmax		10.4	7.5	4.7–24	11.7	8.7	5.1–24.3	0.364
SUVmean		6.5	4.6	3–15.6	7.0	5.3	3.3–15.1	0.427
CNR		15.6	5.0	−0.6–60	15.4	5.7	−0.6–49.5	0.734
discordant	13							
SUVmax		14.8	13.4	7.3–18.4	15.1	11.8	7.8–20.4	0.96
SUVmean		9.3	8	4.3–11.3	9.7	7.4	4.6–12.5	0.98
CNR		27.8	18.5	9–32.8	29.6	23.7	10.9–30.7	0.572

In the subgroup of patients presenting small-sized (<1 cm) discordant lesions (n = 26) between PET/CT and ceCT, PET was negative in 13 cases and positive in the remaining half of the cases (13/26).

Among patients with PET-negative small discordant lesions (n = 13/26), in 4 cases, ceCT detected millimetric findings compatible with secondary NET lesions (liver lesions in 3 patients and nodes in 1 patient); in 9 patients, small-sized findings (at lung, nodes, liver, and pancreatic level) were reported as indeterminate on ceCT (4/9 remained stable following imaging).

Among the 13 PET-positive targeted small findings (all true positive), 6/13 cases presented ceCT-negative small lesions (at bone level in 4/6 patients and node level in 2/6 cases) (Figure 4), 2/13 showed both small-sized PET-positive lesions (false negative on ceCT) and additional small-sized lesions reported as indeterminate on ceCT that were not detectable on PET/CT. There was also a small group of only 5/13 patients presenting both concordant and discordant PET-positive findings: each case presented a target PET-positive small finding confirmed by ceCT (concordant true positive) and a small finding clearly avid on PET images (2 pancreatic, 2 nodal and 1 at soft tissue level), known as malignant at ceCT only after expert radiological revision, aware of the PET result.

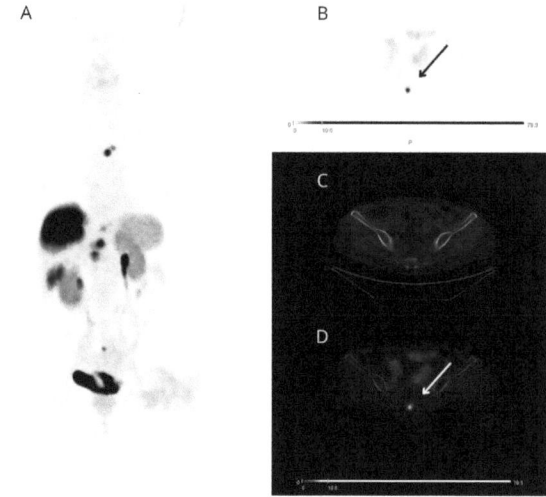

Figure 4. Maximum intensity projection (MIP) (**A**), PET (**B**), CT (**C**), and fused PET/CT (**D**) transaxial images of a patient studied for restaging of metastatic G3 NET, likely of pancreatic origin. [^{68}Ga]Ga-DOTANOC PET shows high and focal uptake at the coccyx (arrows). The uptake area does not correspond to clear morphologic alterations on low-dose CT.

5. Discussion

PET images are generated using image reconstruction algorithms to improve image quality. Q.Clear was developed to enhance image quality through the improvement of CNR, and it is deemed to increase quantitative accuracy [2]. The superiority of Q.Clear over OSEM was documented in phantom and clinical studies, mostly using [^{18}F]F-FDG reconstructed with various β-levels, often between 300 and 400 [4,5,7–9,23–25]. The optimal β-level in the non-FDG setting was only preliminarily explored in different clinical scenarios. In a study conducted using [^{18}F]F-PSMA-1007 PET/CT, the optimal β-level was 700 [26]. In two studies on [^{18}F]-NaF, the preferred levels were, respectively, 400 and 600 (the latter for overweight patients) [27,28]. For [^{89}Zr]-immunoPET tracers, the best value found was 3600 [29].

Few studies regard Gallium-68 tracers. Santoro et al. analyzed OSEM and Q.Clear reconstructed images of NEMA phantoms filled with Gallium-68 to find the optimal β-level according to lesion size and phantom type (mimicking normal or overweight patients). Optimal β-levels ranged from 250 to 800 [3]. A β-level of 600 was suggested for [^{68}Ga]Ga-PSMA PET/CT by Rijnsdrop et al. [30]. Lysvik et al. applied different β-levels to dynamic

[^{18}F]F-PSMA-1007 PET imaging performed in two patients with recurrent glioblastoma, reporting a 25.5% increase of K_i with increased β-levels (from 300 to 1000) [31].

Besides identifying the best reconstruction in terms of overall visual image quality, we conducted additional analysis of ceCT/PET discordant small lesions, expecting improved small-lesion detectability with Q.Clear reconstruction. An improvement in small-lesion detectability in Q.Clear images was previously reported by Macnab et al. In their study, three independent readers blindly compared the visual image quality of active and non-active small objects in OSEM and Q.Clear reconstructions (with a penalization coefficient of 400), finding significant visual-detection improvement in Q.Clear images of active small lesions over OSEM. No significant differences were found for non-active (true-negative) lesions [13]. Miwa et al. recently analyzed the impact on small lesions of another factor of Q.Clear reconstruction, named gamma, whose value of 2 enabled the detection of lesions <6.2 mm in phantoms [32]. Overall, the preferred β-level varies considerably among published studies, also depending on the chosen scan time per bed position. Moreover, semiquantitative measurements are influenced by uptake times and data entries like patient weight, decay-corrected injected dose, and cross-calibration [15].

A potential limitation of this new technology is the occurrence of significant alterations of lesions' semiquantitative parameters that may hamper the direct comparison of their value across different tomographs and time-points: higher SUV values over OSEM were previously reported for Q.Clear image reconstructions performed using [^{68}Ga]Ga-DOTATATE [33], [^{18}F]F-FDG [1,7,34], and [^{18}F]F-PSMA [35]. Devriese et al. reported statistically significant and clinically relevant differences between Q.Clear (β-factor of 400) and OSEM images in terms of SUVmax and SUVpeak in 64 [^{18}F]F-FDG PET/CT examinations [34]. Similarly, Wyrzykowski et al. reported significant discordant clinical assessments (change in Deauville Score) between the two reconstructions in 11 cases (15.7%) of 70 interim [^{18}F]F-FDG PET scans and in 11 cases of 70 end-of-treatment PET scans among a total of 280 patients with lymphoma (β-level of 350) [9].

Published studies investigating Q.Clear of patients with neuroendocrine neoplasms undergoing [^{68}Ga]Ga-DOTANOC PET/CT are limited. We previously analyzed Q.Clear reconstruction in the subgroup of overweight patients with NEN. In these patients, image quality suffers from low-coincidence events and poor attenuation. Applying the Bayesian penalized-likelihood reconstruction with high β-levels (β1600), the perceived image quality was enhanced, followed by significantly increased CNR, SNR-T, and LSNR [21]. The issue of comparability was also addressed by Krokos et al., who performed PET scans with ^{68}Gallium-labelled tracers in 14 patients, reconstructing the images with or without the Q.Clear algorithm. They found that only β-factors of 800–1000 made the two reconstructions comparable in terms of semiquantitative parameters [36].

The present study shows that Q.Clear β1600 reconstruction outperformed STD and β800/β1000 reconstructions. In fact, all readers unanimously agreed that β1600 reconstruction provided the best image quality. When lesion-dependent parameters were analyzed, there were no significant differences between β1600 and STD (regardless of lesion size), confirming that β1600 can be employed in routine clinical practice (allowing the direct comparison of lesions' semiquantitative parameters even when previous images were acquired using different tomographs). Moreover, the β1600 images present significant differences in SNR liver, resulting in better visualization of lesions at the liver level, the most frequent site of metastatic spread. Limitations of the present study include the small-sized cohort and, in particular, the small subgroup with discordant small lesions. However, it is important to note that the setting of small-lesion detection is challenging with all imaging modalities (ceCT and PET), in particular in the setting of NET, which is characterized by a low growth rate over time. Our data show that all clearly PET-positive target findings <1 cm corresponded to true malignant lesions. In particular, the most frequent sites of small PET-positive/ceCT-negative findings were at the bone level and node level. In the case of a lack of significant uptake on PET corresponding to indeterminate small ceCT findings, clinical and radiological surveillance is recommended.

6. Conclusions

Despite the previously mentioned limitations, our data show that when a digital PET/CT is available, β1600 Q.Clear reconstruction for [^{68}Ga]Ga-DOTANOC imaging is feasible and improves image quality for both overall and small-lesion assessment. Further studies are needed to validate these findings in a larger population and to assess the impact on patient management derived from the Q.Clear improved image quality.

Author Contributions: Conceptualization, V.A. (Valentina Ambrosini), L.Z. and S.F.; methodology M.D.F., E.F., L.Z., C.M. (Cristina Mosconi), V.A. (Vincenzo Allegri), C.M. (Claudio Malizia), S.C., S.F. and V.A. (Valentina Ambrosini); formal analysis: C.M. (Claudio Malizia); data curation; M.D.F., E.F. and N.B.; writing—original draft preparation M.D.F. and E.F.; writing—review and editing, M.D.F. E.F., L.Z., N.B., C.M. (Cristina Mosconi), C.M. (Claudio Malizia), S.C., D.C., E.A., G.L., V.A. (Vincenzo Allegri), S.F. and V.A. (Valentina Ambrosini); supervision, V.A. (Valentina Ambrosini), L.Z. and S.F. All authors have read and agreed to the published version of the manuscript.

Funding: This research received no external funding.

Institutional Review Board Statement: This study was conducted in accordance with the Declaration of Helsinki and approved by the Ethics Committee of the "Azienda Ospedaliero-Universitaria di Bologna" (protocol code 131/2017/O/Oss, 22 June 2017).

Informed Consent Statement: Informed consent was obtained from all subjects involved in the study. Written informed consent was obtained from the patients for publication.

Data Availability Statement: Access to the anonymous electronic archive is regulated by the local ethics committee.

Conflicts of Interest: Martina Di Franco, Emilia Fortunati, Norma Bonazzi, Cristina Mosconi, Claudio Malizia, Simona Civollani, Davide Campana, Elisa Andrini, Giuseppe Lamberti and Vincenzo Allegri declare no conflicts of interest. Valentina Ambrosini reports personal fees from EANM, ESMIT, ESMO, Elma Academy, AAA, and Cineca outside the submitted work. Stefano Fanti reports, outside the submitted work, personal honoraria from Novartis and personal fees from AAA, Amgen, Astellas, Bayer, Debio, GE Healthcare, Immedica, Janssen, Sofie, and Telix. Lucia Zanoni reports, outside the submitted work, personal fees from Springer (as a book editor).

References

1. Naghavi-Behzad, M.; Vogsen, M.; Gerke, O.; Dahlsgaard-Wallenius, S.E.; Nissen, H.J.; Jakobsen, N.M.; Braad, P.-E.; Vilstrup, M.H.; Deak, P.; Hildebrandt, M.G.; et al. Comparison of Image Quality and Quantification Parameters between Q.Clear and OSEM Reconstruction Methods on FDG-PET/CT Images in Patients with Metastatic Breast Cancer. *J. Imaging* **2023**, *9*, 65. [CrossRef]
2. In GE Healthcare. Available online: https://www.gehealthcare.com (accessed on 16 May 2024).
3. Santoro, M.; Della Gala, G.; Paolani, G.; Zagni, F.; Civollani, S.; Strolin, S.; Strigari, L. A novel figure of merit to investigate ^{68}Ga PET/CT image quality based on patient weight and lesion size using Q.Clear reconstruction algorithm: A phantom study. *Phys. Medica* **2023**, *106*, 102523. [CrossRef] [PubMed]
4. Ribeiro, D.; Hallett, W.; Tavares, A.A.S. Performance evaluation of the Q.Clear reconstruction framework versus conventional reconstruction algorithms for quantitative brain PET-MR studies. *EJNMMI Phys.* **2021**, *8*, 41. [CrossRef] [PubMed]
5. Te Riet, J.; Rijnsdorp, S.; Roef, M.J.; Arends, A.J. Evaluation of a Bayesian penalized likelihood reconstruction algorithm for low-count clinical 18F-FDG PET/CT. *EJNMMI Phys.* **2019**, *6*, 32. [CrossRef] [PubMed]
6. Teoh, E.J.; McGowan, D.R.; Schuster, D.M.; Tsakok, M.T.; Gleeson, F.V.; Bradley, K.M. Bayesian penalised likelihood reconstruction (Q.Clear) of ^{18}F-fluciclovine PET for imaging of recurrent prostate cancer: Semi-quantitative and clinical evaluation. *Br. J. Radiol.* **2018**, *91*, 20170727. [CrossRef] [PubMed]
7. Parvizi, N.; Franklin, J.M.; McGowan, D.R.; Teoh, E.J.; Bradley, K.M.; Gleeson, F.V. Does a novel penalized likelihood reconstruction of 18F-FDG PET-CT improve signal-to-background in colorectal liver metastases? *Eur. J. Radiol.* **2015**, *84*, 1873–1878. [CrossRef] [PubMed]
8. Teoh, E.J.; McGowan, D.R.; Bradley, K.M.; Belcher, E.; Black, E.; Moore, A.; Sykes, A.; Gleeson, F.V. 18F-FDG PET/CT assessment of histopathologically confirmed mediastinal lymph nodes in non-small cell lung cancer using a penalised likelihood reconstruction. *Eur. Radiol.* **2016**, *26*, 4098–4106. [CrossRef] [PubMed]
9. Wyrzykowski, M.; Siminiak, N.; Kaźmierczak, M.; Ruchała, M.; Czepczyński, R. Impact of the Q.Clear reconstruction algorithm on the interpretation of PET/CT images in patients with lymphoma. *EJNMMI Res.* **2020**, *10*, 99. [CrossRef] [PubMed]

10. Genc, M.; Yildirim, N.; Coskun, N.; Ozdemir, E.; Turkolmez, S. The variation of quantitative parameters and Deauville scores with different reconstruction algorithms in FDG PET/CT imaging of lymphoma patients. *Rev. Espanola Med. Nucl. E Imagen Mol.* **2023**, *42*, 388–392. [CrossRef] [PubMed]
11. Sadeghi, F.; Sheikhzadeh, P.; Farzanehfar, S.; Ghafarian, P.; Moafpurian, Y.; Ay, M. The effects of various penalty parameter values in Q.Clear algorithm for rectal cancer detection on ^{18}F-FDG images using a BGO-based PET/CT scanner: A phantom and clinical study. *EJNMMI Phys.* **2023**, *10*, 63. [CrossRef] [PubMed]
12. Miwa, K.; Wagatsuma, K.; Nemoto, R.; Masubuchi, M.; Kamitaka, Y.; Yamao, T.; Hiratsuka, S.; Yamaguchi, M.; Yoshii, T.; Kobayashi, R.; et al. Detection of sub-centimeter lesions using digital TOF-PET/CT system combined with Bayesian penalized likelihood reconstruction algorithm. *Ann. Nucl. Med.* **2020**, *34*, 762–771. [CrossRef] [PubMed]
13. Macnab, M.R.F.; Biggans, T.J.; Mckiddie, F.I.; Pether, M.I.; Straiton, J.B.; Staff, R.T. Detectability of small objects in PET/computed tomography phantom images with Bayesian penalised likelihood reconstruction. *Nucl. Med. Commun.* **2020**, *41*, 666–673. [CrossRef] [PubMed]
14. Virgolini, I.; Ambrosini, V.; Bomanji, J.B.; Baum, R.P.; Fanti, S.; Gabriel, M.; Papathanasiou, N.D.; Pepe, G.; Oyen, W.; De Cristoforo, C.; et al. Procedure guidelines for PET/CT tumour imaging with ^{68}Ga-DOTA-conjugated peptides: ^{68}Ga-DOTA-TOC, ^{68}Ga-DOTA-NOC, ^{68}Ga-DOTA-TATE. *Eur. J. Nucl. Med. Mol. Imaging* **2010**, *37*, 2004–2010. [CrossRef] [PubMed]
15. Bozkurt, M.F.; Virgolini, I.; Balogova, S.; Beheshti, M.; Rubello, D.; Decristoforo, C.; Ambrosini, V.; Kjaer, A.; Delgado-Bolton, R.; Kunikowska, J.; et al. Guideline for PET/CT imaging of neuroendocrine neoplasms with ^{68}Ga-DOTA-conjugated somatostatin receptor targeting peptides and ^{18}F-DOPA. *Eur. J. Nucl. Med. Mol. Imaging* **2017**, *44*, 1588–1601. [CrossRef] [PubMed]
16. Hope, T.A.; Bodei, L.; Chan, J.A.; El-Haddad, G.; Fidelman, N.; Kunz, P.L.; Mailman, J.; Menda, Y.; Metz, D.C.; Mittra, E.S.; et al. NANETS/SNMMI Consensus Statement on Patient Selection and Appropriate Use of ^{177}Lu-DOTATATE Peptide Receptor Radionuclide Therapy. *J. Nucl. Med. Off. Publ. Soc. Nucl. Med.* **2020**, *61*, 222–227. [CrossRef] [PubMed]
17. Hofman, M.S.; Lau, W.F.E.; Hicks, R.J. Somatostatin receptor imaging with ^{68}Ga DOTATATE PET/CT: Clinical utility, normal patterns, pearls, and pitfalls in interpretation. *Radiogr. Rev. Publ. Radiol. Soc. N. Am. Inc* **2015**, *35*, 500–516.
18. Choi, S.J.; Choi, S.H.; Lee, D.Y.; Lee, J.S.; Kim, D.W.; Jang, J.K. Diagnostic value of [^{68}Ga]Ga-DOTA-labeled-somatostatin analogue PET/MRI for detecting liver metastasis in patients with neuroendocrine tumors: A systematic review and meta-analysis. *Eur. Radiol.* **2022**, *32*, 4628–4637. [CrossRef] [PubMed]
19. Ambrosini, V.; Nanni, C.; Zompatori, M.; Campana, D.; Tomassetti, P.; Castellucci, P.; Allegri, V.; Rubello, D.; Montini, G.; Franchi, R.; et al. ^{68}Ga-DOTA-NOC PET/CT in comparison with CT for the detection of bone metastasis in patients with neuroendocrine tumours. *Eur. J. Nucl. Med. Mol. Imaging* **2010**, *37*, 722–727. [CrossRef] [PubMed]
20. Albanus, D.; Apitzsch, J.; Erdem, Z.; Erdem, O.; Verburg, F.; Behrendt, F.; Mottaghy, F.; Heinzel, A. Clinical value of ^{68}Ga-DOTATATE-PET/CT compared to stand-alone contrast enhanced CT for the detection of extra-hepatic metastases in patients with neuroendocrine tumours (NET). *Eur. J. Radiol.* **2015**, *84*, 1866–1872. [CrossRef] [PubMed]
21. Zanoni, L.; Calabrò, D.; Fortunati, E.; Argalia, G.; Malizia, C.; Allegri, V.; Civollani, S.; Fanti, S.; Ambrosini, V. Two birds with one stone: Can [^{68}Ga]Ga-DOTANOC PET/CT image quality be improved through BMI-adjusted injected activity without increasing acquisition times? *Br. J. Radiol.* **2022**, *95*, 20211152. [CrossRef]
22. Tian, D.; Yang, H.; Li, Y.; Cui, B.; Lu, J. The effect of Q.Clear reconstruction on quantification and spatial resolution of ^{18}F-FDG PET in simultaneous PET/MR. *EJNMMI Phys.* **2022**, *9*, 1. [CrossRef] [PubMed]
23. Caribé, P.R.R.V.; Koole, M.; D'Asseler, Y.; Van Den Broeck, B.; Vandenberghe, S. Noise reduction using a Bayesian penalized-likelihood reconstruction algorithm on a time-of-flight PET-CT scanner. *EJNMMI Phys.* **2019**, *6*, 22. [CrossRef] [PubMed]
24. Rogasch, J.M.; Suleiman, S.; Hofheinz, F.; Bluemel, S.; Lukas, M.; Amthauer, H.; Furth, C. Reconstructed spatial resolution and contrast recovery with Bayesian penalized likelihood reconstruction (Q.Clear) for FDG-PET compared to time-of-flight (TOF) with point spread function (PSF). *EJNMMI Phys.* **2020**, *7*, 2. [CrossRef] [PubMed]
25. Trägårdh, E.; Minarik, D.; Brolin, G.; Bitzén, U.; Olsson, B.; Oddstig, J. Optimization of [^{18}F]PSMA-1007 PET-CT using regularized reconstruction in patients with prostate cancer. *EJNMMI Phys.* **2020**, *7*, 31. [CrossRef] [PubMed]
26. Yoshii, T.; Miwa, K.; Yamaguchi, M.; Shimada, K.; Wagatsuma, K.; Yamao, T.; Kamitaka, Y.; Hiratsuka, S.; Kobayashi, R.; Ichikawa, H.; et al. Optimization of a Bayesian penalized likelihood algorithm (Q.Clear) for ^{18}F-NaF bone PET/CT images acquired over shorter durations using a custom-designed phantom. *EJNMMI Phys.* **2020**, *7*, 56. [CrossRef] [PubMed]
27. Usmani, S.; Ahmed, N.; Gnanasegaran, G.; Rasheed, R.; Marafi, F.; Alnaaimi, M.; Omar, M.; Musbah, A.; al Kandari, F.; De Schepper, S.; et al. The clinical effectiveness of reconstructing ^{18}F-sodium fluoride PET/CT bone using Bayesian penalized likelihood algorithm for evaluation of metastatic bone disease in obese patients. *Br. J. Radiol.* **2021**, *94*, 20210043. [CrossRef] [PubMed]
28. Kirchner, J.; O'Donoghue, J.A.; Becker, A.S.; Ulaner, G.A. Improved image reconstruction of ^{89}Zr-immunoPET studies using a Bayesian penalized likelihood reconstruction algorithm. *EJNMMI Phys.* **2021**, *8*, 6. [CrossRef]
29. Rijnsdorp, S.; Roef, M.J.; Arends, A.J. Impact of the Noise Penalty Factor on Quantification in Bayesian Penalized Likelihood (Q.Clear) Reconstructions of ^{68}Ga-PSMA PET/CT Scans. *Diagnostics* **2021**, *11*, 847. [CrossRef] [PubMed]
30. Lysvik, E.K.; Mikalsen, L.T.G.; Rootwelt-Revheim, M.E.; Emblem, K.E.; Hjørnevik, T. Optimization of Q.Clear reconstruction for dynamic ^{18}F PET imaging. *EJNMMI Phys.* **2023**, *10*, 65. [CrossRef] [PubMed]

31. Miwa, K.; Yoshii, T.; Wagatsuma, K.; Nezu, S.; Kamitaka, Y.; Yamao, T.; Kobayashi, R.; Fukuda, S.; Yakushiji, Y.; Miyaji, N.; et al Impact of γ factor in the penalty function of Bayesian penalized likelihood reconstruction (Q.Clear) to achieve high-resolution PET images. *EJNMMI Phys.* **2023**, *10*, 4. [CrossRef] [PubMed]
32. Chicheportiche, A.; Goshen, E.; Godefroy, J.; Grozinsky-Glasberg, S.; Oleinikov, K.; Meirovitz, A.; Gross, D.J.; Ben-Haim, S. Can a penalized-likelihood estimation algorithm be used to reduce the injected dose or the acquisition time in ^{68}Ga-DOTATATE PET/CT studies? *EJNMMI Phys.* **2021**, *8*, 13. [CrossRef] [PubMed]
33. Devriese, J.; Beels, L.; Maes, A.; Van de Wiele, C.; Pottel, H. Impact of PET reconstruction protocols on quantification of lesions that fulfil the PERCIST lesion inclusion criteria. *EJNMMI Phys.* **2018**, *5*, 35. [CrossRef] [PubMed]
34. Witkowska-Patena, E.; Budzyńska, A.; Giżewska, A.; Dziuk, M.; Walęcka-Mazur, A. Ordered subset expectation maximisation vs Bayesian penalised likelihood reconstruction algorithm in ^{18}F-PSMA-1007 PET/CT. *Ann. Nucl. Med.* **2020**, *34*, 192–199. [CrossRef] [PubMed]
35. Zanoni, L.; Argalia, G.; Fortunati, E.; Malizia, C.; Allegri, V.; Calabrò, D.; Civollani, S.; Campana, D.; Fanti, S.; Ambrosini, V. Can Q.Clear reconstruction be used to improve [^{68}Ga]Ga-DOTANOC PET/CT image quality in overweight NEN patients? *Eur. J. Nucl. Med. Mol. Imaging* **2022**, *49*, 1607–1612. [CrossRef] [PubMed]
36. Krokos, G.; Pike, L.C.; Cook, G.J.R.; Marsden, P.K. Standardisation of conventional and advanced iterative reconstruction methods for Gallium-68 multi-centre PET-CT trials. *EJNMMI Phys.* **2021**, *8*, 52. [CrossRef] [PubMed]

Disclaimer/Publisher's Note: The statements, opinions and data contained in all publications are solely those of the individual author(s) and contributor(s) and not of MDPI and/or the editor(s). MDPI and/or the editor(s) disclaim responsibility for any injury to people or property resulting from any ideas, methods, instructions or products referred to in the content.

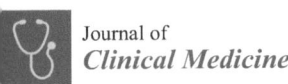

Article

Implications of Serum IgG4 Levels for Pancreatobiliary Disorders and Cancer

Ching-Tang Tseng [1,†], Yi-Jun Liao [1,2,†], Cheng-Li Lin [3] and Yen-Chun Peng [1,2,4,*]

1. Division of Gastroenterology and Hepatology, Department of Internal Medicine, Taichung Veterans General Hospital, Taichung 407, Taiwan; frank79503@hotmail.com (C.-T.T.); s19001029@gmail.com (Y.-J.L.)
2. Department of Post-Baccalaureate Medicine, School of Medicine, National Chung Hsing University, Taichung 402, Taiwan
3. Management Office for Health Data, Clinical Trial Center (CTC), China Medical University Hospital, Taichung 404, Taiwan; orangechengli@gmail.com
4. School of Medicine, National Yang Ming Chiao Tung University, Taipei 112, Taiwan
* Correspondence: pychunppp@gmail.com; Tel.: +886-4-23592525-3309
† These authors contributed equally to this work.

Abstract: Background/Objectives: Immunoglobulin G4-related disease (IgG4-RD) is an immune-mediated disorder presenting as mass-like lesions with obstructions. An elevated serum IgG4 level is identified in more than half of affected patients and is considered a diagnostic criterion. IgG4-RD is still easily misdiagnosed as neoplastic or infectious disease. We aimed to conduct a hospital-based study to illuminate the association between serum IgG4 levels and pancreatobiliary disorders and cancer. **Methods**: In this study, serum IgG4 levels were assessed at our hospital's immunology laboratory, utilizing data from the hospital's computer center, and the diagnostic codes used were based on ICD-9-CM. We analyzed IgG4 level data collected between April 2013 and April 2020, including patients' age, gender, and diseases, but excluding the rationale for IgG4 level assessment. Employing propensity score matching (PSM) at a 1:1 ratio to mitigate age and gender confounding, we analyzed 759 patients divided into groups by IgG4 levels ($\leq$140 and >140 mg/dL; and $\leq$140, 141–280, >280 mg/dL). We explored associations between IgG4 levels and conditions such as pancreatobiliary cancer (the group included cholangiocarcinoma, pancreatic cancer, and ampullary cancer), cholangitis, cholangiocarcinoma, pancreatitis, pancreatic cancer, and ampullary cancer. **Results**: Our study analyzed the demographics, characteristics, and serum IgG4 levels of participants and found no significant differences in serum IgG4 levels across various pancreatobiliary conditions. Nevertheless, the crude odds ratios (ORs) suggested a nuanced association between a higher IgG4 level > 280 mg/dL and increased risks of cancer and pancreatitis, with crude ORs of 1.52 (p = 0.03) and 1.49 (p = 0.008), respectively. After PSM matching, the further analysis of 759 matched patients showed no significant differences in IgG4 levels > 140 mg/dL between cancerous and non-cancerous groups, nor across other pancreatobiliary conditions. A higher serum IgG4 level > 280 mg/dL was significantly associated with pancreatobiliary cancer and cholangiocarcinoma, with crude ORs of 1.61 (p = 0.026) and 1.62 (p = 0.044), respectively. In addition, IgG4 > 280 mg/dL showed a greater association with pancreatic cancer compared with 141–280 mg/dL, with crude OR of 2.18 (p = 0.038). **Conclusions**: Our study did not find a clear association between serum IgG4 levels (>140 mg/dL) and pancreatobiliary cancer. We observed that higher IgG4 levels (>280 mg/dL) may be associated with cholangiocarcinoma and pancreatic cancer, as indicated by crude ORs. However, the adjusted analysis did not demonstrate the significant association between IgG4 level > 280 mg/dL and cancer. Considering IgG4-RD as a chronic and persistent inflammatory status, it is more closely associated with inflammatory diseases than with cancer. Therefore, further long-term cohort studies are necessary to evaluate the potential role of IgG4 levels in cancer risk among these patients.

Keywords: IgG4 levels; pancreatobiliary; inflammatory diseases; malignancy

Citation: Tseng, C.-T.; Liao, Y.-J.; Lin, C.-L.; Peng, Y.-C. Implications of Serum IgG4 Levels for Pancreatobiliary Disorders and Cancer. *J. Clin. Med.* **2024**, *13*, 3651. https://doi.org/10.3390/jcm13133651

Academic Editors: Hidekazu Suzuki and Stanley W. Ashley

Received: 29 March 2024
Revised: 26 May 2024
Accepted: 20 June 2024
Published: 22 June 2024

Copyright: © 2024 by the authors. Licensee MDPI, Basel, Switzerland. This article is an open access article distributed under the terms and conditions of the Creative Commons Attribution (CC BY) license (https://creativecommons.org/licenses/by/4.0/).

1. Introduction

IgG4 is the latest defined human IgG subclass in serum and an intriguing antibody with unique biological properties [1]. Clinically, IgG4-related disease (IgG4-RD) involves a chronic fibrous inflammatory process related to immunomodulation disorder, characterized as tumor-like lesions with dense lymphoplasmacytic infiltration with IgG4-positive plasma cells, and the most affected organs are the pancreas, bile duct, major salivary glands, lacrimal glands, retroperitoneum, kidneys, and lymphatic ducts. In addition to local inflammation-induced tissue fibrosis and injury, IgG4-RD has been recognized as a systemic disorder and was found to be linked to elevated serum IgG4 levels. As it is a newly defined disease, the global incidence and prevalence of IgG4-RD is underestimated. In addition, the natural history of IgG4-RD is also limited due its chronic nature and fluctuating clinical course [2–6]. The trigger of IgG4 production is thought to involve the activation of the innate immune response by microbe- and/or damage-associated molecular patterns that stimulate the production of the type I interferon and B cell-activating factor by innate immune cells, resulting in IgG4 production by B cells [7]. Thus, the serum IgG4 level is considered an important indicator for suspicion of the diagnosis of IgG4-RD.

Cancer is a multifactorial and complex disease process caused by cells that have lost their physiological control of cell overgrowth [8]. Chronic infection results in persistent stimulation and inflammation and, thus, is one of the main contributors to cancer development [9,10]. Most previous studies were related to the association of cancer concomitant with IgG4-RD [11,12]. Cancer could trigger autoantigen expression, leading to IgG4-RD, and an increased risk of IgG4-RD resulting from cancer treatment has also been proposed [13]. A recent multi-hospital study enrolled 121 patients and demonstrated that IgG4-sclerosing cholangitis carried potential risk for cancer [14]. There is also a lack of basic research on the molecular mechanism of IgG4 and carcinogenesis. A study of increased IgG4-containing lymphocytes in esophageal cancer implicated the role of IgG4 in the cancer micro-environment. The authors reported that IgG4 could play a role in cancer treatment [15].

The main histopathological features of IgG4-RD include a dense, polyclonal, lymphoplasmacytic infiltrate with an abundance of IgG4-positive plasma cells, storiform fibrosis, and obliterative phlebitis. These manifestations can range from mild to severe, and the natural history is wide-ranging and variable. The precise pathogenic mechanisms of IgG4-RD and its potential association with cancer risk remain unclear and require further investigation [6]. There are possible malignancies in patients with IgG4-RD at the time of diagnosis and follow-up in the natural course [16]. Thus, the differential diagnosis of IgG4-RD versus cancer with serum IgG4 level elevation may be difficult in some situations.

There is a lack of data showing the associations between IgG4-RD, serum IgG4 level, and cancer risk, particularly pancreatic, biliary, and ampullary cancers. Hence, we investigated the associations of serum IgG4 level with various cancers. We were interested in determining whether serum IgG4 level was associated with cancer and whether different serum levels were associated with a higher risk of cancer. Furthermore, we attempted to explore the association of a high serum IgG4 level, which indicates more definitive IgG4-RD, with carcinogenesis. While there is scanty clinical evidence, IgG4-RD could be associated with malignancy; IgG4-RD may present with a tumor-like focal tumefactive lesion, which could lead to misdiagnosis [17]. Thus, the evidence and risk of carcinogenesis related to IgG4-RD need to be clarified.

To address these questions, we conducted a hospital-based case–control study to analyze the association of IgG4 serum level among patients with cancer.

2. Materials and Methods

2.1. Data Source

Patients' serum IgG4 levels were checked at the laboratory of the immunology division in our hospital. The data were obtained from the database of our hospital computer center. The diagnostic codes used were based on the International Classification of Diseases, 9th

Revision, Clinical Modification (ICD-9-CM). This study was approved by the Institutional Review Board of our institution (Taichung Veterans General Hospital IRB: CE20314B).

2.2. Subjects

During April 2013 to April 2020, we collected data on serum IgG4 levels from our hospital database. Other data included the patients' age, gender, and diseases. The reason for checking the serum IgG4 level was according to the clinical physicians' judgment, and there was no prior record in the database. The diagnosis of cancer and pancreatobiliary disorders were determined using diagnostic codes based on ICD-9-CM (Figure 1). Cancer included cholangiocarcinoma (CCA), pancreatic cancer, and ampullary cancer. In pancreatobiliary disorders, we mainly focused on pancreatitis, including acute and chronic pancreatitis.

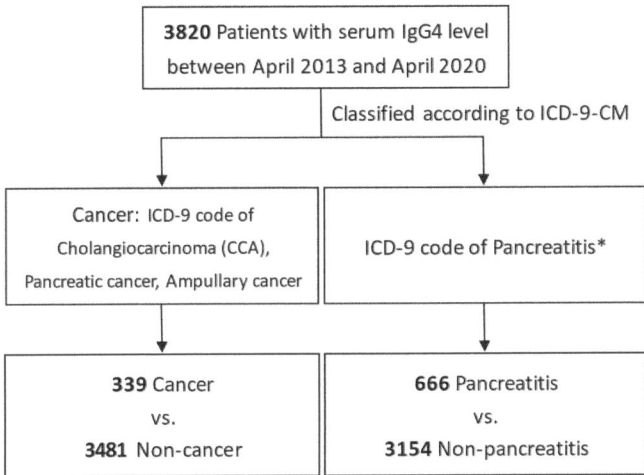

Figure 1. Flowchart for patients with cancer or pancreatitis. * Discusses pancreatobiliary disorders focusing on pancreatitis, including acute and chronic pancreatitis.

Definition of Pancreatobiliary Disorders

The diagnosis of cholangitis was made by Tokyo guidelines 2013/2018, including systemic inflammation, cholestasis, and imaging implying infection and biliary obstruction [18–20]. The diagnosis of acute pancreatitis required the presence of two of the following three criteria: the acute onset of persistent, severe, epigastric pain often radiating to the back; an elevation in serum lipase or amylase to three times or greater than the upper limit of normal; and characteristic findings of acute pancreatitis on imaging [21]. On the other hand, the diagnosis of chronic pancreatitis was based on exposure risk; underlying predisposition; clinical presentation, including chronic abdominal pain and/or a history of relapsing acute pancreatitis; symptoms of pancreatic exocrine insufficiency (diarrhea, steatorrhea, or weight loss); or pancreatogenic diabetes, and using other modalities, including cross-sectional imaging, and pancreatic function tests [22,23]. We linked the above diagnoses with ICD-9-CM.

2.3. The Associations between Serum IgG4 Levels and the Risk of Different Outcomes by Propensity Score Matching

To address the confounding effects of age and gender in our analysis, we employed propensity score matching (PSM) at a 1:1 ratio (Figure 2). This approach resulted in the selection of 759 patients, categorized into two groups based on their serum IgG4 levels: those with IgG4 $\leq$ 140 mg/dL and those with IgG4 > 140 mg/dL. These groups were then analyzed to investigate associations between serum IgG4 levels and various conditions, including cancer versus non-cancer, cholangitis versus non-cholangitis, cholangiocarcinoma versus non-cholangiocarcinoma, pancreatitis versus non-pancreatitis, pancreatic cancer versus non-pancreatic cancer, and ampullary cancer versus non-ampullary cancer, to facilitate a more detailed exploration of the relationships between serum IgG4 levels and these conditions. For further determination of the significant role in serum IgG4 levels in pancreatic and biliary diseases, we divided serum IgG4 levels into different groups, i.e., ≤140, 141–280, and >280 mg/dL, and determined the associations with pancreatic and biliary diseases, according to the International Consensus Diagnostic Criteria (ICDC), which indicated that the marked elevation of serum IgG4 (>2 times upper limit of normal; >280 mg/dL in our study) is strongly suggestive (Level 1 criteria) of autoimmune pancreatitis (AIP) in the setting of obstructive jaundice/pancreatic mass, and the serum IgG4 level between 141 and 280 mg/dL is Level 2 criteria [24].

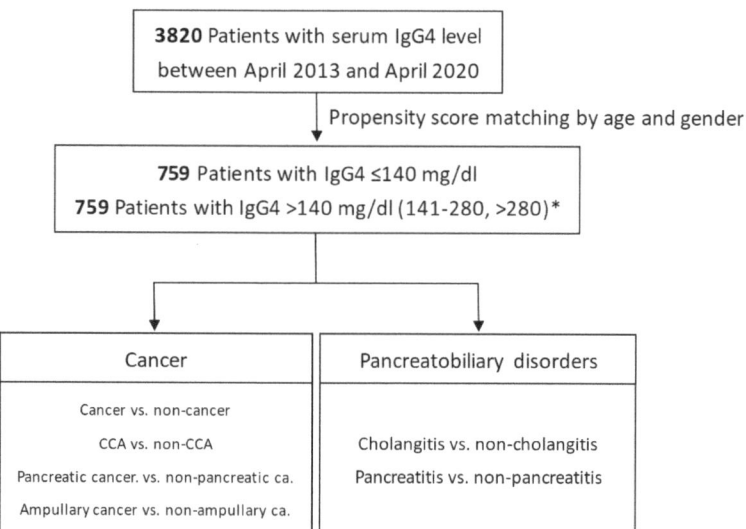

Figure 2. Flowchart for serum IgG4 levels and different outcomes after propensity score matching (PSM). * Serum IgG4 levels were divided into different groups, i.e., ≤140, 141–280, and >280 mg/dL.

2.4. Statistical Analysis

The statistical analyses were performed as follows: the Chi-square test was used to check the differences in categorical variables between the cancer and non-cancer groups, while the two-sample Student's t-test was used to examine continuous variables. Univariable and multivariable logistic regression were used to estimate the effect of serum IgG4 levels on the risk of cancer, as indicated by the odds ratio (OR) with a 95% confidence interval (CI). All analyses were performed using SAS statistical software (version 9.4; SAS Institute, Inc., Cary, NC, USA), and results were considered statistically significant when two-tailed p-values were less than 0.05.

3. Results

3.1. Demographics and Characteristics of Study Subjects

In Table 1, there was a higher proportion of females in the cancer group compared to the non-cancer group (57.82% vs. 38.50%, $p < 0.001$). Furthermore, the mean age of individuals in the cancer group was 63.81 (±14.19) years, which was considerably higher than the mean age of 53.3 (±16.69) years in the non-cancer control group and showed a statistically significant difference ($p < 0.001$). In terms of serum IgG4 levels (categorized as ≤140, 141–280, and >280 mg/dL), a notable disparity was found between cancer and non-cancer patients, accounting for 80.24%, 12.90%, and 6.87% of patients in the non-cancer group and 74.93%, 15.34%, and 9.73% in the cancer group, which was statistically significant

($p < 0.05$). These findings provide valuable insights into the differences between cancer and non-cancer patients across various demographic and IgG4 measures. A higher proportion of cancer patients had higher serum IgG4 levels compared with non-cancer patients.

Table 1. Baseline characteristics of serum IgG4 levels in cancer and non-cancer patients.

Variable	Non-Cancer (N = 3481)		Cancer [2] (N = 339)		p-Value
	N	%	N	%	
Sex					<0.0001
Female	1340	38.50	196	57.82	
Male	2141	61.51	143	42.18	
Age (years)					<0.0001
0–39	776	22.29	16	4.72	
40–59	1390	39.93	110	32.45	
60–79	1146	32.92	173	51.03	
>79	169	4.86	40	11.80	
Mean, (SD) [1]	53.3	(16.69)	63.81	(14.19)	<0.0001
IgG4 value (mg/dL)					0.048
≤140	2793	80.24	254	74.93	
141–280	449	12.90	52	15.34	
>280	239	6.87	33	9.73	
Mean, (SD) [1]	118.5	(223)	173.95	(483.31)	0.038

[1] Student's t-test; [2] cancer: cholangiocarcinoma, pancreatic cancer, ampullary cancer. Abbreviations: N, numbers of patients; SD, standard deviation.

3.2. Risk of Cancer Associated with Serum Level of IgG4

Table 2 displays the odds ratios (ORs) representing the estimated cancer risk associated with different IgG4 levels (≤140, 141–280, and >280 mg/dL). In the crude analysis, the ORs for IgG4 levels 141–280 mg/dL and >280 mg/dL were 1.27 (95% CI: 0.93–1.74, $p = 0.13$) and 1.52 (95% CI: 1.03–2.23, $p = 0.03$), respectively. Following adjustment for age and gender, the adjusted ORs for cancer risk in the IgG4 141–280 mg/dL and IgG4 > 280 mg/dL categories were 1.20 and 1.17, with 95% confidence intervals of 0.87–1.66 and 0.78–1.73, respectively. Interestingly, it was observed that cancer patients exhibited significantly higher IgG4 levels compared to non-cancer patients based on the crude OR analysis. These findings point to a potential association between higher IgG4 levels and increased cancer risk, particularly in the higher IgG4 category.

Table 2. Odds ratios of cancer.

Variable	Non-Cancer		Cancer [1]		Crude			Adjusted		
	N	%	N	%	cOR	(95% CI)	p-Value	aOR [†]	(95% CI)	p-Value
IgG4 value (mg/dL)										
≤140	2793	80.24	254	74.93	1.00	(reference)	-	1.00	(reference)	-
141–280	449	12.90	52	15.34	1.27	(0.93, 1.74)	0.13	1.20	(0.87, 1.66)	0.26
>280	239	6.87	33	9.73	1.52	(1.03, 2.23) *	0.03	1.17	(0.78, 1.73)	0.45

[†] Adjusted by age and gender; * $p < 0.05$. [1] Cancer: cholangiocarcinoma, pancreatic cancer, ampullary cancer. Abbreviations: N, numbers of patients; cOR, crude odds ratio; aOR, adjusted odds ratio; CI, confidence interval.

3.3. Odds of Pancreatitis Associated with Serum Level of IgG4

In our investigation, we aimed to elucidate the relationship between serum IgG4 levels and the incidence of pancreatitis. Our objective was to quantify the association between different concentrations of IgG4 (≤140, 141–280, and >280 mg/dL) and the likelihood of developing pancreatitis. According to Table 3, the preliminary analysis yielded odds ratios (ORs) of 0.92 (95% CI: 0.71–1.19, $p = 0.52$) for IgG4 levels between 141 and 280 mg/dL and 1.49 (95% CI: 1.11–2.00, $p = 0.008$) for levels above 280 mg/dL. Adjusting for age and gender, the adjusted ORs for IgG4 levels in the 141–280 mg/dL and >280 mg/dL categories were 0.85 and 1.21, with 95% confidence intervals of 0.66–1.11 and 0.89–1.64, respectively. These findings suggest a nuanced link between increased IgG4 levels and a heightened risk of pancreatitis, especially at higher IgG4 concentrations.

Table 3. Odds ratios of pancreatitis.

Variable	Non-Pancreatitis		Pancreatitis		Crude			Adjusted		
	N	%	N	%	cOR	(95% CI)	p-Value	aOR [†]	(95% CI)	p-Value
IgG4 value (mg/dL)										
≤140	2525	80.06	522	78.38	1.00	(reference)	-	1.00	(reference)	-
141–280	421	13.35	80	12.01	0.92	(0.71, 1.19)	0.52	0.85	(0.66, 1.11)	0.24
>280	208	6.59	64	9.61	1.49	(1.11, 2.00) **	0.008	1.21	(0.89, 1.64)	0.23

[†] Adjusted by age and gender; ** $p < 0.01$. Abbreviations: N, numbers of patients; cOR, crude odds ratio; aOR, adjusted odds ratio; CI, confidence interval.

3.4. Serum IgG4 Level >140 mg/dL in Different Pancreatobiliary Patient Groups after Propensity Score Matching

Following propensity score matching (PSM) with a 1:1 ratio, we identified 759 patients with IgG4 ≤ 140 mg/dL and another 759 with serum IgG4 levels > 140 mg/dL for in-depth analysis (Figure 2; Supplementary Table S1 shows the baseline characteristics after PSM). In Table 4, our findings indicate that IgG4 levels did not significantly differ between cancer patients and their non-cancer counterparts, with a crude OR of 1.20 (95% CI: 0.86–1.67, p = 0.276) and an adjusted OR of 1.21 (95% CI: 0.86–1.69, p = 0.266).

Similarly, for patients with cholangitis, the IgG4 levels were not significantly different from those without the condition, with both crude and adjusted ORs of 1.07 (95% CI: 0.80–1.44, p = 0.652; and 0.79–1.45, p = 0.644, respectively). The analysis of cholangiocarcinoma (CCA) patients also revealed no significant difference in IgG4 levels compared to non-CCA patients, with both crude and adjusted ORs of 1.18 (95% CI: 0.81–1.72, p = 0.391; and 0.81–1.73, p = 0.383, respectively).

The investigation of pancreatitis patients demonstrated no significant elevation in IgG4 levels compared to non-pancreatitis individuals, with ORs of 0.85 (95% CI: 0.66–1.09, p = 0.202) in the crude analysis and 0.84 (95% CI: 0.65–1.09, p = 0.193) upon adjustment. The assessment of pancreatic cancer patients also showed no significant difference in IgG4 levels, with both crude and adjusted ORs of 1.12 (95% CI: 0.66–1.90, p = 0.686; and 0.66–1.91, p = 0.683, respectively). Lastly, the analysis of ampullary cancer patients found no significant variation in IgG4 levels, with both crude and adjusted ORs of 1.00 (95% CI: 0.39–2.53, p = 1; and 0.39–2.54, p = 1, respectively).

3.5. The Association of Higher Serum IgG4 Level >280 mg/dL with Pancreatic and Biliary Diseases

Following propensity score matching (PSM) with a 1:1 ratio, we further determined the association of different IgG4 levels (≤140, 141–280, and >280 mg/dL) with pancreatic and biliary diseases (Figure 2). In Table 5, our findings indicate that IgG4 level > 280 mg/dL was significantly associated with cancer and cholangiocarcinoma, with crude ORs of 1.61 (95% CI: 1.06–2.44, p = 0.026) and 1.62 (95% CI: 1.01–2.59, p = 0.044), respectively. For pancreatic cancer, IgG4 > 280 mg/dL showed a greater association with pancreatic cancer compared with 141–280 mg/dL, with crude OR of 2.18 (95% CI: 1.05–4.53, p = 0.038). There was no significant correlation with IgG4 > 280 mg/dL in ampullary cancer compared with ≤140 mg/dL and 141–280 mg/dL, with crude ORs of 0.63 (95% CI: 0.14–2.93, p = 0.555) and 0.52 (95% CI: 0.11–2.54, p = 0.421), respectively.

Table 4. The associations between IgG4 values (≤140 and >140 mg/dL) and risks of different outcomes, after propensity score matching (a matching ratio of 1:1).

Variable	Non-Outcome N	%	Outcome N	%	Crude OR (95% CI)		p-Value	Adjusted OR † (95% CI)		p-Value
					Cancer					
IgG4 value (mg/dL)										
≤140	686	50.48	73	45.91	1.00	(reference)	-	1.00	(reference)	-
>140	673	49.52	86	54.09	1.20	(0.86, 1.67)	0.276	1.21	(0.86, 1.69)	0.266
Sex										
Female	632	46.50	42	26.42	1.00	(reference)	-	1.00	(reference)	-
Male	727	53.50	117	73.58	2.42	(1.68, 3.50) ***	<0.001	2.09	(1.44, 3.05) ***	<0.001
Age (years)										
18–50	492	36.20	16	10.06	1.00	(reference)	-	1.00	(reference)	-
51–64	400	29.43	62	38.99	4.77	(2.71, 8.39) ***	<0.001	4.50	(2.55, 7.95) ***	<0.001
65–92	467	34.36	81	50.94	5.33	(3.07, 9.25) ***	<0.001	4.65	(2.67, 8.11) ***	<0.001
					Cholangitis					
IgG4 value (mg/dL)										
≤140	660	50.23	99	48.53	1.00	(reference)	-	1.00	(reference)	-
>140	654	49.77	105	51.47	1.07	(0.80, 1.44)	0.652	1.07	(0.79, 1.45)	0.644
Sex										
Female	618	47.03	56	27.45	1.00	(reference)	-	1.00	(reference)	-
Male	696	52.97	148	72.55	2.35	(1.69, 3.25) ***	<0.001	2.01	(1.44, 2.80) ***	<0.001
Age (years)										
18–50	480	36.53	28	13.73	1.00	(reference)	-	1.00	(reference)	-
51–64	395	30.06	67	32.84	2.91	(1.83, 4.61) ***	<0.001	2.73	(1.72, 4.34) ***	<0.001
65–92	439	33.41	109	53.43	4.26	(2.76, 6.58) ***	<0.001	3.71	(2.39, 5.77) ***	<0.001
					Cholangiocarcinoma					
IgG4 value (mg/dL)										
≤140	704	50.32	55	46.22	1.00	(reference)	-	1.00	(reference)	-
>140	695	49.68	64	53.78	1.18	(0.81, 1.72)	0.391	1.18	(0.81, 1.73)	0.383
Sex										
Female	640	45.75	34	28.57	1.00	(reference)	-	1.00	(reference)	-
Male	759	54.25	85	71.43	2.11	(1.40, 3.18) ***	<0.001	1.78	(1.17, 2.72) **	0.007
Age (years)										
18–50	498	35.6	10	8.4	1.00	(reference)	-	1.00	(reference)	-
51–64	415	29.66	47	39.5	5.64	(2.82, 11.30) ***	<0.001	5.33	(2.66, 10.71) ***	<0.001
65–92	486	34.74	62	52.1	6.35	(3.22, 12.53) ***	<0.001	5.62	(2.84, 11.15) ***	<0.001

Table 4. Cont.

Variable	Non-Outcome		Outcome		Crude			Adjusted		
	N	%	N	%		OR (95% CI)	p-Value		OR [†] (95% CI)	p-Value
					Pancreatitis					
IgG4 value (mg/dL)										
≤140	595	49.17	164	53.25	1.00	(reference)	-	1.00	(reference)	-
>140	615	50.83	144	46.75	0.85	(0.66, 1.09)	0.202	0.84	(0.65, 1.09)	0.193
Sex										
Female	593	49.01	81	26.30	1.00	(reference)	-	1.00	(reference)	-
Male	617	50.99	227	73.70	2.69	(2.04, 3.56) ***	<0.001	2.50	(1.89, 3.32) ***	<0.001
Age (years)										
18–50	430	35.54	78	25.32	1.00	(reference)	-	1.00	(reference)	-
51–64	366	30.25	96	31.17	1.45	(1.04, 2.01) *	0.028	1.33	(0.95, 1.86)	0.096
65–92	414	34.21	134	43.51	1.78	(1.31, 2.43) ***	<0.001	1.49	(1.08, 2.05) *	0.014
					Pancreatic cancer					
IgG4 value (mg/dL)										
≤140	732	50.10	27	47.37	1.00	(reference)	-	1.00	(reference)	-
>140	729	49.90	30	52.63	1.12	(0.66, 1.90)	0.686	1.12	(0.66, 1.91)	0.683
Sex										
Female	662	45.31	12	21.05	1.00	(reference)	-	1.00	(reference)	-
Male	799	54.69	45	78.95	3.11	(1.63, 5.92) ***	<0.001	2.72	(1.41, 5.23) **	0.003
Age (years)										
18–50	501	34.29	7	12.28	1.00	(reference)	-	1.00	(reference)	-
51–64	438	29.98	24	42.11	3.92	(1.67, 9.19) **	0.002	3.54	(1.50, 8.34) **	0.004
65–92	522	35.73	26	45.61	3.56	(1.53, 8.29) **	0.003	2.90	(1.24, 6.79) *	0.014
					Ampullary cancer					
IgG4 value (mg/dL)										
≤140	750	50.00	9	50.00	1.00	(reference)	-	1.00	(reference)	-
>140	750	50.00	9	50.00	1.00	(0.39, 2.53)	1	1.00	(0.39, 2.54)	1
Sex										
Female	668	44.53	6	33.33	1.00	(reference)	-	1.00	(reference)	-
Male	832	55.47	12	66.67	1.61	(0.60, 4.30)	0.346	1.30	(0.48, 3.53)	0.612
Age (years)										
18–50	506	33.73	2	11.11	1.00	(reference)	-	1.00	(reference)	-
51–64	460	30.67	2	11.11	1.10	(0.15, 7.84)	0.924	1.12	(0.16, 8.03)	0.907
65–92	534	35.6	14	77.78	6.63	(1.50, 29.33) *	0.013	6.70	(1.50, 30.02) *	0.013

Abbreviations: N, numbers of patients; OR, odds ratio; CI, confidence interval. [†] Adjusted OR: multivariable analysis including age and gender; * p-value < 0.05, ** p < 0.01, *** p < 0.001.

Table 5. The associations between IgG4 values ($\leq$140, 141–280, and >280 mg/dL) and risks of different outcomes after propensity score matching (a matching ratio of 1:1).

IgG4 Value (mg/dL)	Non-Outcome N	Non-Outcome %	Outcome N	Outcome %	Crude OR (95% CI)	Crude p-Value	Adjusted OR [†] (95% CI)	Adjusted p-Value	Crude OR (95% CI)	Crude p-Value	Adjusted OR [†] (95% CI)	Adjusted p-Value
Cancer												
$\leq$140	686	50.48	73	45.91	1.00 (reference)	-	1.00 (reference)	-	1.00 (reference)	-	1.00 (reference)	-
141–280	445	32.74	47	29.56	0.99 (0.68, 1.46)	0.970	1.09 (0.74, 1.62)	0.656				
>280	228	16.78	39	24.53	1.61 (1.06, 2.44) *	0.026	1.39 (0.91, 2.13)	0.128	1.62 (1.03, 2.55) *	0.037	1.20 (0.75, 1.93)	0.444
Cholangitis												
$\leq$140	660	50.23	99	48.53	1.00 (reference)	-	1.00 (reference)	-	1.00 (reference)	-	1.00 (reference)	-
141–280	436	33.18	56	27.45	0.86 (0.60, 1.21)	0.384	0.93 (0.65, 1.33)	0.691				
>280	218	16.59	49	24.02	1.50 (1.03, 2.18) *	0.035	1.31 (0.89, 1.93)	0.168	1.75 (1.15, 2.65) **	0.008	1.40 (0.91, 2.16)	0.122
Cholangiocarcinoma												
$\leq$140	704	50.32	55	46.22	1.00 (reference)	-	1.00 (reference)	-	1.00 (reference)	-	1.00 (reference)	-
141–280	458	32.74	34	28.57	0.95 (0.61, 1.48)	0.821	1.04 (0.66, 1.63)	0.868				
>280	237	16.94	30	25.21	1.62 (1.01, 2.59) *	0.044	1.41 (0.88, 2.28)	0.157	1.71 (1.02, 2.85) *	0.042	1.31 (0.77, 2.24)	0.314
Pancreatitis												
$\leq$140	595	49.17	164	53.25	1.00 (reference)	-	1.00 (reference)	-	1.00 (reference)	-	1.00 (reference)	-
141–280	415	34.3	77	25	0.67 (0.50, 0.91) **	0.009	0.71 (0.52, 0.96) *	0.027				
>280	200	16.53	67	21.75	1.22 (0.88, 1.68)	0.241	1.09 (0.78, 1.52)	0.614	1.81 (1.25, 2.61) **	0.002	1.54 (1.05, 2.25) *	0.027
Pancreatic cancer												
$\leq$140	732	50.10	27	47.37	1.00 (reference)	-	1.00 (reference)	-	1.00 (reference)	-	1.00 (reference)	-
141–280	478	32.72	14	24.56	0.79 (0.41, 1.53)	0.491	0.87 (0.45, 1.69)	0.682				
>280	251	17.18	16	28.07	1.73 (0.92, 3.26)	0.091	1.49 (0.78, 2.83)	0.224	2.18 (1.05, 4.53) *	0.038	1.66 (0.78, 3.52)	0.187
Ampullary cancer												
$\leq$140	750	50.00	9	50.00	1.00 (reference)	-	1.00 (reference)	-	1.00 (reference)	-	1.00 (reference)	-
141–280	485	32.33	7	38.89	1.20 (0.44, 3.25)	0.716	1.31 (0.48, 3.56)	0.598				
>280	265	17.67	2	11.11	0.63 (0.14, 2.93)	0.555	0.55 (0.12, 2.57)	0.444	0.52 (0.11, 2.54)	0.421	0.37 (0.08, 1.82)	0.221

Abbreviations: N, numbers of patients; OR, odds ratio; CI, confidence interval. * p-value < 0.05, ** p < 0.01. [†] Adjusted OR: multivariable analysis including age and gender.

For cholangitis, IgG4 > 280 mg/dL was also significantly correlated, with a crude OR of 1.50 (95% CI: 1.03–2.18, $p = 0.035$). For pancreatitis, IgG4 > 280 mg/dL showed a greater association with pancreatitis compared with 141–280 mg/dL, with a crude OR of 1.81 (95% CI: 1.25–2.61, $p = 0.002$) and an adjusted OR of 1.54 (95% CI: 1.05–2.25, $p = 0.027$).

4. Discussion

Our analysis revealed that IgG4 levels showed distinct features among patients diagnosed with cholangitis, pancreatitis, and biliary–pancreatic–ampullary cancer. Markedly elevated serum IgG4 levels (>280 mg/dL) were found in patients undergoing IgG4 testing for other reasons for cholangiocarcinoma and pancreatic cancer, but not ampullary cancer. The analysis of biliary–pancreatic–ampullary cancer risk in relation to IgG4 levels showed a notably significant crude odds ratio (OR) for patients with higher IgG4 levels (>280 mg/dL). However, this significance lessened after accounting for age and gender, suggesting that the initial observed relationship was influenced by these demographic factors. These findings underscore potential connections between specific demographic and clinical characteristics in patients with biliary, pancreatic, or ampullary cancer and the levels of IgG4.

In clinical practice, it may be unclear whether patients with biliary or pancreatic obstructive diseases have cancer or not. Patients with IgG4-RD could just have a concomitantly elevated serum IgG4 level or they may indeed have an occult cancer component. The challenge for the physician is to assess the risk or odds of cancer, particularly biliary or pancreatic cancer, in patients with elevated serum IgG4 levels. Our results demonstrated that the association of serum IgG4 levels with biliary–pancreatic–ampullary cancer was not significant. These results may help physicians to make decisions for patients with obstructive disease and elevated serum IgG4 levels. A study has demonstrated the increasing clinical importance of both autoimmune pancreatitis and cholangitis, which can mimic pancreatic cancer and biliary cancer. IgG4 levels in tissue or blood cannot be used alone to diagnose IgG4-RD, and they should be adjunct to clinical, radiological, and histological features. There is importance in the differential diagnosis of inflammation and cancer, resulting in a significant impact on the clinical management of affected patients [25].

For diagnosing AIP, the International Association of Pancreatology proposed the ICDC, which combined pancreatic parenchyma and ductal changes at abdominal imaging, the serum IgG4 level, other organ involvement, histology, and the response to steroid treatment to reach a diagnosis [24]. Endoscopic ultrasound (EUS) and EUS-guided fine-needle aspiration/biopsy (EUS-FNA/B) were the tissue-acquisition techniques most used for AIP. In the clinical practice of one cohort study, endoscopic cytohistology was available in 46.2% of cases, and diagnostics for AIP was available in 35.2%. EUS-FNA/B of the pancreas was conducted mostly in the focal form of AIP (85% of cases) to exclude pancreatic cancer [26].

IgG4 may contribute to tumor-associated escape from immune surveillance and have implications for cancer immunotherapy [16,27]. In a case report, lung tumor with lung IgG4 interstitial infiltration was observed [11]. However, there are no large series of cases or surveys of IgG4 tumors in patients with lung disease in the literature. It has been reported that there is a potential for lymphoma to develop in patients with IgG4-RD. The co-occurrence of IgG4-RD and lymphoma has also been reported [28]. In another study, a negative association between IgG4 expression and cutaneous marginal zone lymphoma was found [29]. Regarding immunity, IgG4 antibodies and IgG4+ B cells in different cancers could involve IgG4 in tumor escape from immune surveillance through a number of potential mechanisms, including the IgG4 blockade of IgG1-mediated effector functions [15,27]. A proposed mechanism by which IgG4 may contribute to tumor-associated escape from human immune surveillance involves the possibility that inflammatory conditions may exist in tumors that support IgG4 [27]. IgG4 in inflammatory and cancer conditions is thus complex and sometimes confusing. As such, elevated IgG4 levels could result in malignancies being overlooked or misdiagnosed.

In an earlier survey of a general population for malignancies in IgG4-RD, malignancies were observed in 10.4% of the IgG4-RD patients. The malignancies were all different and included lung cancer, colon cancer, and lymphoma [16]. Except for age at the time the IgG4-RD diagnosis was made, there were no common features in patients with cancer. The frequency of history of malignancy was >3-fold higher in IgG4-RD patients, according to an analysis of an epidemiological database [13]. By timeframe, the results revealed that a history of malignancy was linked with a risk of IgG4-RD. There is a lack of evidence showing any causal relationships between IgG4-RD and malignancy.

In pancreatobiliary type IgG4-RD, there was a greater risk of developing cancer [14,16]. In the aforementioned multiple-hospital-based retrospective study, the authors concluded that IgG4-sclerosing cholangitis patients had a high risk of pancreatic and bile duct cancer. The risk of cancer was high <1 year and >5 years after the diagnosis of IgG4-sclerosing cholangitis. The higher risk at less than 1 year may have been due to the diagnosis of IgG4-RD and cancer at the same time. The present study found that a mildly elevated IgG4 level (>140 mg/dL) was not associated with pancreatobiliary disorders and cancer. A marked elevation of IgG4 levels (>280 mg/dL) was nuanced and associated with cholangiocarcinoma and pancreatic cancer, but not ampullary cancer.

The main strengths of this hospital-based study were the use of a validated database and disease diagnoses. There were some limitations in this study. First, the associations of patients' serum IgG4 levels with diagnoses of cancer were based solely on claims data. There was no definitive diagnosis of IgG4-RD by pathological proof in the analysis of associations with cancer. Second, as this was a case–control study, we did not determine the causal relationship between serum IgG4 level and cancer. Third, the treatments of both IgG4-RD and cancer were not included in this study.

5. Conclusions

Our study did not find a clear association between serum IgG4 levels (>140 mg/dL) and pancreatobiliary cancer. We observed that higher serum IgG4 levels (>280 mg/dL) may be associated with cholangiocarcinoma and pancreatic cancer, as indicated by crude odds ratios (ORs). However, the adjusted analysis did not demonstrate the significant association between IgG4 level > 280 mg/dL and cancer. Considering IgG4-RD as a chronic and persistent inflammatory status, it is more closely associated with inflammatory diseases than with cancer. Therefore, further long-term cohort studies are necessary to evaluate the potential role of IgG4 levels in cancer risk among these patients.

Supplementary Materials: The following supporting information can be downloaded at https://www.mdpi.com/article/10.3390/jcm13133651/s1: Table S1: Baseline characteristics after propensity score matching by age and gender.

Author Contributions: Conceptualization, C.-T.T., Y.-J.L. and Y.-C.P.; methodology, C.-T.T., Y.-J.L. and Y.-C.P.; formal analysis, C.-T.T., Y.-J.L. and C.-L.L.; investigation, C.-T.T. and C.-L.L.; resources, Y.-J.L. and C.-L.L.; writing—original draft preparation, C.-T.T. and Y.-J.L.; writing—review and editing, Y.-C.P.; supervision, Y.-C.P. All authors have read and agreed to the published version of the manuscript.

Funding: This research received no external funding.

Institutional Review Board Statement: The study was conducted in accordance with the Declaration of Helsinki and approved by the Institutional Review Board (or Ethics Committee) of Taichung Veterans General Hospital (Number: CE20314B, Date of approval: 21 October 2020).

Informed Consent Statement: The requirement for informed consent from the participants was waived due to all data being de-identified prior to analysis.

Data Availability Statement: The data presented in this study are available on request from the corresponding author.

Conflicts of Interest: The authors declare no conflicts of interest.

References

1. Davies, A.M.; Sutton, B.J. Human IgG4: A structural perspective. *Immunol. Rev.* **2015**, *268*, 139–159. [CrossRef]
2. Sánchez-Oro, R.; Alonso-Muñoz, E.M.; Martí Romero, L. Review of IgG4-related disease. *Gastroenterol. Hepatol.* **2019**, *42*, 638–647. [CrossRef] [PubMed]
3. Lanzillotta, M.; Mancuso, G.; Della-Torre, E. Advances in the diagnosis and management of IgG4 related disease. *BMJ (Clin. Res. Ed.)* **2020**, *369*, m1067. [CrossRef] [PubMed]
4. Maritati, F.; Peyronel, F.; Vaglio, A. IgG4-related disease: A clinical perspective. *Rheumatology* **2020**, *59*, iii123–iii131. [CrossRef]
5. Perugino, C.A.; Stone, J.H. IgG4-related disease: An update on pathophysiology and implications for clinical care. *Nat. Rev. Rheumatol.* **2020**, *16*, 702–714. [CrossRef] [PubMed]
6. Stone, J.H.; Zen, Y.; Deshpande, V. IgG4-related disease. *N. Engl. J. Med.* **2012**, *366*, 539–551. [CrossRef]
7. Watanabe, T.; Yamashita, K.; Kudo, M. IgG4-Related Disease and Innate Immunity. *Curr. Top. Microbiol. Immunol.* **2017**, *401*, 115–128. [CrossRef]
8. Yang, Y.M.; Kim, S.Y.; Seki, E. Inflammation and Liver Cancer: Molecular Mechanisms and Therapeutic Targets. *Semin. Liver Dis.* **2019**, *39*, 26–42. [CrossRef]
9. Balkwill, F.; Mantovani, A. Inflammation and cancer: Back to Virchow? *Lancet* **2001**, *357*, 539–545. [CrossRef]
10. Greten, F.R.; Grivennikov, S.I. Inflammation and Cancer: Triggers, Mechanisms, and Consequences. *Immunity* **2019**, *51*, 27–41. [CrossRef]
11. Inoue, T.; Hayama, M.; Kobayashi, S.; Oyaizu, T.; Nakazato, Y.; Honma, K.; Chida, M. Lung cancer complicated with IgG4-related disease of the lung. *Ann. Thorac. Cardiovasc. Surg.* **2014**, *20*, 474–477. [CrossRef] [PubMed]
12. Kazantseva, I.A.; Lishchuk, S.V.; Gribunov, Y.P.; Shestakova, I.N.; Pavlov, K.A. Gastric cancer concurrent with IgG4-related disease: A clinical case and a review of literature. *Arkh. Patol.* **2016**, *78*, 43–47. [CrossRef] [PubMed]
13. Wallace, Z.S.; Wallace, C.J.; Lu, N.; Choi, H.K.; Stone, J.H. Association of IgG4-Related Disease With History of Malignancy. *Arthritis Rheumatol.* **2016**, *68*, 2283–2289. [CrossRef] [PubMed]
14. Kurita, Y. IgG4-related sclerosing cholangitis may be a risk factor for cancer. *J. Immunother. Cancer* **2021**, *28*, 524–532. [CrossRef] [PubMed]
15. Wang, H.; Xu, Q.; Zhao, C.; Zhu, Z.; Zhu, X.; Zhou, J.; Zhang, S.; Yang, T.; Zhang, B.; Li, J.; et al. An immune evasion mechanism with IgG4 playing an essential role in cancer and implication for immunotherapy. *J. Immunother. Cancer* **2020**, *8*, e000661. [CrossRef] [PubMed]
16. Yamamoto, M.; Takahashi, H.; Tabeya, T.; Suzuki, C.; Naishiro, Y.; Ishigami, K.; Yajima, H.; Shimizu, Y.; Obara, M.; Yamamoto, H.; et al. Risk of malignancies in IgG4-related disease. *Mod. Rheumatol.* **2012**, *22*, 414–418. [CrossRef] [PubMed]
17. Dzhus, M.; Ivashkivsky, O.; Mikukst, V.; Parkishen, S.; Diadyk, O. IgG4-Related Disease Misdiagnosed as Neoplasm. *J. Clin. Rheumatol.* **2021**, *27*, e71–e72. [CrossRef] [PubMed]
18. Kimura, Y.; Takada, T.; Kawarada, Y.; Nimura, Y.; Hirata, K.; Sekimoto, M.; Yoshida, M.; Mayumi, T.; Wada, K.; Miura, F.; et al. Definitions, pathophysiology, and epidemiology of acute cholangitis and cholecystitis: Tokyo Guidelines. *J. Hepatobiliary Pancreat. Surg.* **2007**, *14*, 15–26. [CrossRef]
19. Kiriyama, S.; Takada, T.; Strasberg, S.M.; Solomkin, J.S.; Mayumi, T.; Pitt, H.A.; Gouma, D.J.; Garden, O.J.; Büchler, M.W.; Yokoe, M.; et al. TG13 guidelines for diagnosis and severity grading of acute cholangitis (with videos). *J. Hepatobiliary Pancreat. Sci.* **2013**, *20*, 24–34. [CrossRef]
20. Yokoe, M.; Hata, J.; Takada, T.; Strasberg, S.M.; Asbun, H.J.; Wakabayashi, G.; Kozaka, K.; Endo, I.; Deziel, D.J.; Miura, F.; et al. Tokyo Guidelines 2018: Diagnostic criteria and severity grading of acute cholecystitis (with videos). *J. Hepatobiliary Pancreat. Sci.* **2018**, *25*, 41–54. [CrossRef]
21. Banks, P.A.; Bollen, T.L.; Dervenis, C.; Gooszen, H.G.; Johnson, C.D.; Sarr, M.G.; Tsiotos, G.G.; Vege, S.S. Classification of acute pancreatitis--2012: Revision of the Atlanta classification and definitions by international consensus. *Gut* **2013**, *62*, 102–111. [CrossRef] [PubMed]
22. Garg, P.K. Chronic pancreatitis. *Gut* **2012**, *61*, 932. [CrossRef] [PubMed]
23. Rickels, M.R.; Bellin, M.; Toledo, F.G.; Robertson, R.P.; Andersen, D.K.; Chari, S.T.; Brand, R.; Frulloni, L.; Anderson, M.A.; Whitcomb, D.C. Detection, evaluation and treatment of diabetes mellitus in chronic pancreatitis: Recommendations from PancreasFest 2012. *Pancreatology* **2013**, *13*, 336–342. [CrossRef] [PubMed]
24. Shimosegawa, T.; Chari, S.T.; Frulloni, L.; Kamisawa, T.; Kawa, S.; Mino-Kenudson, M.; Kim, M.H.; Klöppel, G.; Lerch, M.M.; Löhr, M.; et al. International consensus diagnostic criteria for autoimmune pancreatitis: Guidelines of the International Association of Pancreatology. *Pancreas* **2011**, *40*, 352–358. [CrossRef]
25. Al-Dhahab, H.; McNabb-Baltar, J.; Al-Busafi, S.; Barkun, A.N. Immunoglobulin G4-related pancreatic and biliary diseases. *Can. J. Gastroenterol. Hepatol.* **2013**, *27*, 523–530. [CrossRef] [PubMed]
26. Barresi, L.; Tacelli, M.; Crinò, S.F.; Attili, F.; Petrone, M.C.; De Nucci, G.; Carrara, S.; Manfredi, G.; Capurso, G.; De Angelis, C.G.; et al. Multicentric Italian survey on daily practice for autoimmune pancreatitis: Clinical data, diagnosis, treatment, and evolution toward pancreatic insufficiency. *United Eur. Gastroenterol. J.* **2020**, *8*, 705–715. [CrossRef]
27. Crescioli, S.; Correa, I.; Karagiannis, P.; Davies, A.M.; Sutton, B.J.; Nestle, F.O.; Karagiannis, S.N. IgG4 Characteristics and Functions in Cancer Immunity. *Curr. Allergy Asthma Rep.* **2016**, *16*, 7. [CrossRef] [PubMed]

28. Bledsoe, J.R.; Wallace, Z.S.; Stone, J.H.; Deshpande, V.; Ferry, J.A. Lymphomas in IgG4-related disease: Clinicopathologic features in a Western population. *Virchows Arch.* **2018**, *472*, 839–852. [CrossRef]
29. De Souza, A.; Ferry, J.A.; Burghart, D.R.; Tinguely, M.; Goyal, A.; Duncan, L.M.; Kutzner, H.; Kempf, W. IgG4 Expression in Primary Cutaneous Marginal Zone Lymphoma: A Multicenter Study. *Appl. Immunohistochem. Mol. Morphol.* **2018**, *26*, 462–467. [CrossRef]

Disclaimer/Publisher's Note: The statements, opinions and data contained in all publications are solely those of the individual author(s) and contributor(s) and not of MDPI and/or the editor(s). MDPI and/or the editor(s) disclaim responsibility for any injury to people or property resulting from any ideas, methods, instructions or products referred to in the content.

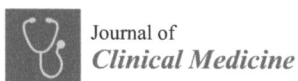 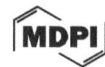

Article

Sequencing Treatments in Patients with Advanced Well-Differentiated Pancreatic Neuroendocrine Tumor (pNET): Results from a Large Multicenter Italian Cohort

Francesco Panzuto [1,2,†], Elisa Andrini [3,†], Giuseppe Lamberti [3,4,*], Sara Pusceddu [5], Maria Rinzivillo [1,2], Fabio Gelsomino [6], Alessandra Raimondi [5], Alberto Bongiovanni [7], Maria Vittoria Davì [8], Mauro Cives [9,10], Maria Pia Brizzi [11], Irene Persano [11], Maria Chiara Zatelli [12], Ivana Puliafito [13], Salvatore Tafuto [14] and Davide Campana [3,4]

[1] Digestive Disease Unit, Sant'Andrea University Hospital, ENETS Center of Excellence, 00189 Rome, Italy; francesco.panzuto@uniroma1.it (F.P.); mrinzivillo@ospedalesantandrea.it (M.R.)
[2] Department of Medical-Surgical Sciences and Translational Medicine, Sapienza University of Roma, 00189 Roma, Italy
[3] Department of Medical or Surgical Sciences, University of Bologna, 40126 Bologna, Italy; elisa.andrini3@unibo.it (E.A.); davide.campana@unibo.it (D.C.)
[4] Division of Medical Oncology, IRCCS Azienda Ospedaliera–Universitaria Bologna, Neuroendocrine Tumor Team Bologna, ENETS Center of Excellence Bologna, 40138 Bologna, Italy
[5] Department of Medical Oncology, Fondazione IRCCS Istituto Nazionale dei Tumori di Milano, European Neuroendocrine Tumor Society (ENETS) Center of Excellence, 20133 Milan, Italy; sara.pusceddu@istitutotumori.mi.it (S.P.); alessandra.raimondi@istitutotumori.mi.it (A.R.)
[6] Department of Oncology and Hematology, Division of Oncology, University Hospital of Modena, 41121 Modena, Italy; fabiogelsomino83@yahoo.it
[7] Osteoncology and Rare Tumors Center, IRCCS Istituto Romagnolo per lo Studio dei Tumori "Dino Amadori", 47014 Meldola, Italy; alberto.bongiovanni@irst.emr.it
[8] Department of Medicine, Section of Endocrinology, University and Hospital Trust of Verona, ENETS Center of Excellence, 37129 Verona, Italy; mariavittoria.davi@aovr.veneto.it
[9] Department of Interdisciplinary Medicine, University of Bari, 70121 Bari, Italy; mauro.cives@uniba.it
[10] Division of Medical Oncology, A.O.U. Consorziale Policlinico di Bari, 70124 Bari, Italy
[11] Division of Medical Oncology, Azienda Ospedaliera Universitaria San Luigi Gonzaga, 10143 Orbassano, Italy; brizzimariapia@gmail.com (M.P.B.); irene.persano@unito.it (I.P.)
[12] Department of Medical Sciences, Section of Endocrinology, Geriatrics and Internal Medicine, University of Ferrara, 44121 Ferrara, Italy; ztlmch@unife.it
[13] Oncologia Medica, Istituto Oncologico del Mediterraneo, 95029 Viagrande, Italy; ivana.puliafito@grupposamed.com
[14] Oncologia Clinica e Sperimentale Sarcomi e Tumori Rari, Istituto Nazionale Tumori IRCCS, Fondazione G. Pascale, 80131 Naples, Italy; s.tafuto@istitutotumori.na.it
* Correspondence: giuseppe.lamberti8@unibo.it
† These authors contributed equally to this work.

Citation: Panzuto, F.; Andrini, E.; Lamberti, G.; Pusceddu, S.; Rinzivillo, M.; Gelsomino, F.; Raimondi, A.; Bongiovanni, A.; Davì, M.V.; Cives, M.; et al. Sequencing Treatments in Patients with Advanced Well-Differentiated Pancreatic Neuroendocrine Tumor (pNET): Results from a Large Multicenter Italian Cohort. J. Clin. Med. 2024, 13, 2074. https://doi.org/10.3390/jcm13072074

Academic Editor: Antonio M. Caballero-Mateos

Received: 11 February 2024
Revised: 16 March 2024
Accepted: 28 March 2024
Published: 3 April 2024

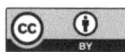

Copyright: © 2024 by the authors. Licensee MDPI, Basel, Switzerland. This article is an open access article distributed under the terms and conditions of the Creative Commons Attribution (CC BY) license (https://creativecommons.org/licenses/by/4.0/).

Abstract: Background: The optimal treatment sequencing for advanced, well-differentiated pancreatic neuroendocrine tumors (pNETs) is unknown. We performed a multicenter, retrospective study to evaluate the best treatment sequence in terms of progression-free survival to first-line (PFS1) and to second-line (PFS2), and overall survival among patients with advanced, well-differentiated pNETs. **Methods:** This multicenter study retrospectively analyzed the prospectively collected data of patients with sporadic well-differentiated pNETs who received at least two consecutive therapeutic lines, with evidence of radiological disease progression before change of treatment lines. **Results:** Among 201 patients, 40 (19.9%) had a grade 1 and 149 (74.1%) a grade 2 pNET. Primary tumor resection was performed in 98 patients (48.8%). First-line therapy was performed in 128 patients with somatostatin analogs (SSA), 35 received SSA + radioligand therapy (RLT), 21 temozolomide-based chemotherapy, and 17 SSA + targeted therapy. PFS was significantly longer in patients with grade 1 pNETs compared to those with grade 2, in patients who received primary tumor surgery, and in patients treated with RLT compared to other treatments. At multivariate analysis, the use of upfront RLT was independently associated with improved PFS compared to SSA. Second-line therapy was performed in 94 patients with SSA + targeted therapy, 35 received chemotherapy, 45

SSA + RLT, and 27 nonconventional-dose SSA or SSA switch. PFS was significantly longer in patients treated with RLT compared to other treatments. At multivariate analysis, the type of second-line therapy was independently associated with the risk for progression. OS was significantly longer in patients who received primary tumor surgery, with Ki67 < 10%, without extrahepatic disease, and in patients who received SSA–RLT sequence compared to other sequences. **Conclusions**: In this large, multicenter study, RLT was associated with better PFS compared to other treatments, and the SSA–RLT sequence was associated with the best survival outcomes in patients with pNETs with Ki67 < 10%. Primary tumor surgery was also associated with improved survival.

Keywords: pancreatic NET; SSA; RLT; targeted therapy; GEP-NENs; treatment sequence

1. Introduction

Neuroendocrine neoplasms (NENs) are a heterogeneous group of tumors, characterized by a variable range of differentiation, grading, primary sites, and functional status. According to the 2019 World Health Organization (WHO), NENs are classified into well-differentiated tumors, with grading G1, G2, or G3 based on Ki67 value (<3%, ≥3–20%, and >20%, respectively), and poorly-differentiated neuroendocrine carcinomas (NECs) [1]. Over the past few decades, NEN incidence has increased, with an age-adjusted incidence rate of 6.4-fold increase from 1973 to 2012, and prevalence increase from 0.006% in 1993 to 0.048% in 2012, including all tumor sites, stages, and grades [2]. The increased incidence is primarily due to improved detection of early-stage disease, whereas increased prevalence is linked to improvement of treatment strategies and survival outcomes, but also to improvement of diagnostic techniques detecting more incidental tumors and to a greater awareness among pathologists [3]. Historically, NENs are considered tumors with an indolent behavior and favorable long-term outcomes [4]. However, the prognosis is widely variable based on several factors, including tumor histology, grading, primary site of tumor, and stage at diagnosis. Currently available treatment strategies in well-differentiated advanced NETs include somatostatin analogs (SSA), targeted therapies (i.e., everolimus and sunitinib), chemotherapy, such as temozolomide-based treatment, and radioligand therapy (RLT) with lutetium 177 (^{177}Lu)-DOTATATE. Because of the lack of head-to-head comparison studies, the optimal treatment sequencing has not yet been defined. According to clinical practice, the sequencing of systemic treatments is still individualized and based on tumor type, grading, somatostatin receptor (SSTR) expression, extent of disease, and patient-related characteristics (e.g., age, performance status, comorbidities, presence of symptoms, and patient preferences). Therefore, the clinical decision-making and management of NENs is complex and requires discussion within a multidisciplinary team, which should include medical and radiation oncologists, surgeons, radiologists, and nuclear medicine specialists, at high-volume referral centers. This is particularly important for patients with advanced, well-differentiated pancreatic neuroendocrine tumors (pNETs), considering that the NETTER-1 trial proved the safety and efficacy of RLT as a second-line therapy after progression on standard SSA only in patients with well-differentiated midgut NENs [5]. Recently, preliminary results from the phase II randomized OCLURANDOM trial of RLT vs. sunitinib in patients with pNETs have been presented, showing an almost double progression-free survival rate at 12 months, the primary endpoint, but the final report is still awaited [6]. Thus, prospective data on the efficacy of RLT compared to chemotherapy or targeted therapy in patients with pNETs are still lacking. The identification of the best treatment timing and sequence in patients with advanced well-differentiated pNETs represents a critical unmet clinical need. Here, we performed a multicenter, retrospective study involving 11 Italian NET referral centers to evaluate the optimal treatment sequencing in a large population of patients with advanced well-differentiated pNETs.

2. Materials and Methods

2.1. Study Design

The study included all consecutive patients at 11 Italian NEN referral centers who had a histological diagnosis of well-differentiated pancreatic NETs (pNETs), no evidence or history of familiar NEN syndromes, treated with at least two consecutive therapeutic lines with approved agents, and evidence of progressive disease according to Response Evaluation Criteria in Solid Tumors (RECIST) criteria, version 1.1 [7] before change of treatment. The following baseline characteristics have been collected: sex, age at the time of the start of first-line treatment, pathology and grading, presence of symptoms secondary to hormone hypersecretion, surgical resection of primary tumor, disease stage at the time of first-line treatment start, presence of metastases outside of liver (extrahepatic disease extension), type of treatment received and outcomes (start and end date, best response, date of evidence of radiological progression of disease or last radiological evaluation), and date of death or last follow-up. The histological specimens were examined by a NEN-dedicated pathologist at each center. Tumors were classified according to the WHO 2019 classification and the ENETS grading system [1,8]. The Ki67 proliferation index was expressed as a percentage based on the count of Ki67-positive cells on 2000 tumor cells in the areas of the highest immunostaining. Clinical and radiological work-up has been performed according to the most recently available ENETS guidelines [9–13]. Objective response rate (ORR) was defined as the proportion of patients who achieved complete response (CR) or partial response (PR) as the best radiological response during each treatment line. Progression-free survival (PFS) was defined as the interval between the start of the therapy and the time of progression of disease (PD) or death by any cause, whichever occurred first. Overall survival (OS) was defined as the time between first-line treatment start and death by any cause. All patients or their legal representatives provided written informed consent for anonymous review of their data for research purposes. The study protocol was approved by the local Institution Review Board (Comitato Etico Indipendente, S.Orsola-Malpighi University Hospital, Bologna) and was conducted in accordance with the principles of the Declaration of Helsinki (6th revision, 2008).

2.2. Statistical Analysis

Categorical variables were expressed as numbers (percentage). Continuous variables were reported as median and range. Survival estimates were made using the Kaplan–Meier method, and the results were compared using the log-rank test. Predictive risk factors for PD and death were evaluated by univariate and multivariate analysis using the Cox proportional hazards method. Risk factors were expressed as hazard ratios (HRs) and 95% confidence interval (95% CI). The multivariate model was fitted using the forward stepwise method after including all variables. All analyses carried out for predictive and risk factors are listed in the tables. The p value was considered significant when inferior to 0.05. Statistical analysis was performed using dedicated software (IBM—SPSS Statistics v. 22).

3. Results

3.1. Study Population

Between January 1997 and December 2020, 237 consecutive patients with pNETs matched the inclusion criteria, but 36 were excluded because they had received investigational treatments. Thus, 201 patients were included in the study, whose baseline characteristics are summarized in Table 1. One hundred eighteen patients (58.7%) were males. Median age at diagnosis was 55 years (range 20–86), while median age at start of the first line of therapy was 58 (range 21–86). As for WHO classification, 40 patients (19.9%) had a G1 NET, while 149 (74.1%) had a G2 NET; data were missing in 12 cases (6.0%). Median Ki67 was 5% (range 0.6–20%); 144 patients (71.6%) had Ki67 $\leq$ 10%, whereas 45 (22.4%) had Ki67 > 10%. Twenty-seven patients (13.4%) had symptoms related to hormone hypersecretion: 9 hyperinsulinemic hypoglycaemia, 6 carcinoid syndrome, 4 Cushing syndrome, 4 Zollinger–Ellison syndrome, 2 glucagone hypersecretion, and 2 VIP hypersecretion. Primary tumor was resected in 98 patients (48.8%), and 48 patients (23.9%) had extrahepatic disease extension at diagnosis. Among patients undergoing surgery of primary tumors, 58 received radical surgery (R0), while 40 underwent surgery in the context of metastatic disease. At the beginning of first-line treatment, 192 patients had stage IV disease, whereas 9 had stage IIIB disease.

Table 1. Patient characteristics.

Characteristic	Patients (no. 201)
Demographic:	
Gender (male), no. (%)	118 (58.7%)
Median age (range) at therapy start, years	58 (21–86)
WHO classification:	
G1, no. (%)	40 (19.9%)
G2, no. (%)	149 (74.1%)
Missing data, no. (%)	12 (6.0%)
Median Ki67%	5 (0.6–20)
Ki67 > 10%	45 (22.4%)
Functioning tumors, no. (%):	27 (13.4%)
Primary tumor surgery, no. (%)	98 (48.8%)
Extrahepatic disease, no. (%)	48 (23.9%)
ttggd	

3.2. First-Line Therapy

In the first-line setting, 128 patients (63.7%) received standard-dose SSA alone, 35 (17.4%) SSA + RLT, 21 (10.4%) temozolomide (TMZ)-based chemotherapy, and 17 (10.4%) SSA + targeted therapy (TT) (n = 16 everolimus, n = 1 sunitinib). Overall, median PFS to first-line treatment (PFS1) was 13.9 months (95% CI: 10.2–17.6), while ORR was 14.9%: 4 patients achieved CR and 26 PR. In particular, ORR was 9.1% in patients who received SSA, 37.1% in those who received RLT, 0% in those who received TT, and 31.6% in those treated with chemotherapy. A difference in PFS was observed according to grading (G1: 22.0 months [95% CI: 15.3–28.7] vs. G2: 11.0 months [95% CI: 7.6–14.4]; p = 0.002; Figure 1A), surgery of primary tumor (yes: 17.6 months [95% CI: 12.1–23.1] vs. no: 11.7 months [95% CI: 8.1–15.3]; p = 0.044; Figure 1B), Ki67 $\leq$ 10% (yes: 15.9 months [95% CI: 10.0–21.8] vs. no: 5.9 months [95% CI: 1.6–10.2]; Figure 1C), and type of treatment (SSA: 9.7 months [95% CI: 6.9–12.5; RLT 34.3 [95% CI: 27.3–41.2]; TT: 10.1 [95% CI: 7.3–12.9]; CHT 9.1 [95% CI: 10.2–17.6]; p < 0.001; Figure 1D). No significant PFS difference according to sex (p = 0.189), presence of syndrome (p = 0.651), or presence of extrahepatic metastatic disease (p = 0.175) was observed. A higher risk for progression was associated with Ki67 > 10% (HR 2.04; p < 0.001) and first-line therapy with chemotherapy compared to SSA (HR 1.70; p = 0.029, Table 2). A lower risk of progression was associated with resection of primary tumor (HR 0.75; p = 0.046) and first-line therapy with RLT compared to SSA (HR 0.54; p = 0.001). Sex, presence of symptoms related to hormone hypersecretion, presence of extrahepatic metastatic disease, and first-line therapy with TKI were not significantly associated with the risk of progression. After adjusting for potential confounding factors, Ki67 > 10% (HR: 1.98; p < 0.001), resection of primary tumor (HR: 0.69; p = 0.019), and first-line therapy with RLT (HR: 0.49; p < 0.001) retained significant associations with the risk of progression.

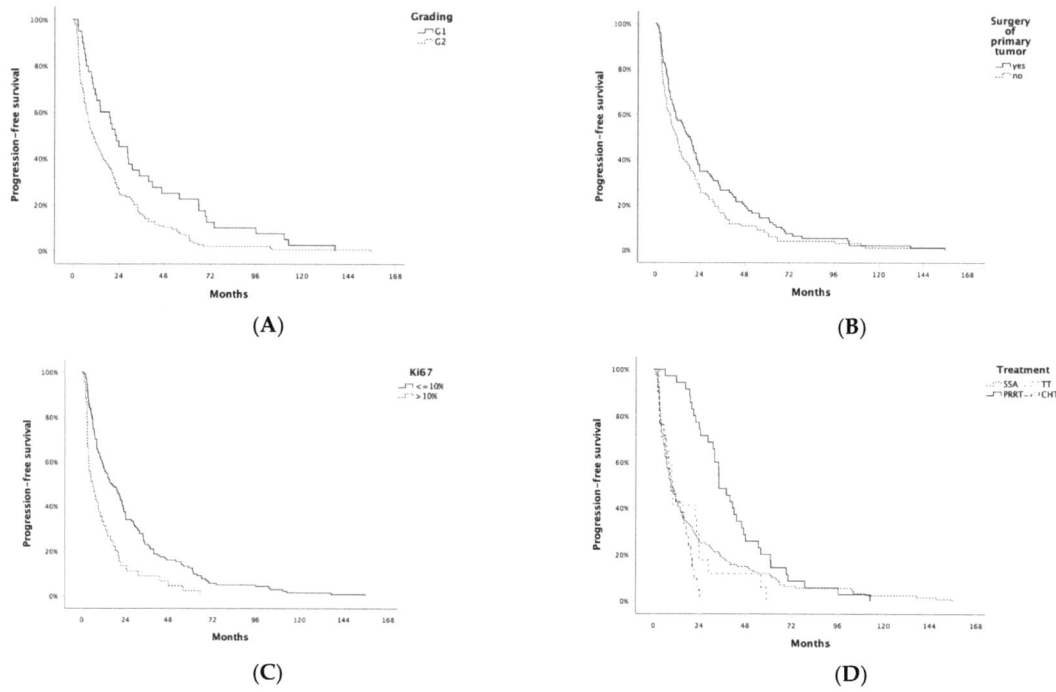

Figure 1. Progression-free survival to first-line treatment (PFS1) by (**A**) grading, (**B**) resection of primary tumor, (**C**) Ki67, and (**D**) type of first-line treatment. SSA: somatostatin analog; PRRT: peptide radionuclide receptor therapy; TT: targeted therapy; CHT: chemotherapy.

Table 2. Predictive risk factors for disease progression during first-line therapy.

Characteristic	Univariate Analysis			Multivariate Analysis		
	HR	95% CI	p Value	HR	95% CI	p Value
Gender (male)	1.21	0.91–1.60	0.191	-	-	-
Non-functioning tumor	1.10	0.73–1.65	0.653	-	-	-
Ki67 > 10%	2.04	1.45–2.88	<0.001	1.98	1.36–2.87	<0.001
Primary tumor resection	0.75	0.57–0.99	0.046	0.69	0.51–0.94	0.019
Extrahepatic disease	1.25	0.90–1.74	0.178	-	-	-
Type of therapy						
SSA	1			1		
RLT	0.54	0.37–0.79	0.001	0.49	0.33–0.72	<0.001
TT	1.20	0.72–2.01	0.479	1.12	0.67–1.88	0.662
CHT	1.70	1.06–2.74	0.029	1.15	0.67–1.99	0.608

Abbreviations: HR: hazard ratio; 95% CI: 95% confidence interval; SSA: somatostatin analogs; RLT: radioligand therapy; TT: targeted therapy; CHT: chemotherapy.

3.3. Second-Line Therapy

Ninety-four patients (46.8%) received SSA + targeted therapy, 35 chemotherapy (either TMZ- or oxaliplatin-based) (17.4%), 45 SSA + RLT (22.4%), and 27 SSA alone-based strategy (either non-conventional-dose SSA or switched SSA; 13.4%) as second-line treatment. Overall, median PFS to second-line treatment (PFS2) was 15.0 months (95% CI: 10.7–19.3 months), while ORR was 5.5%: 1 patient achieved CR and 10 PR. Significantly longer PFS2 was associated with grading (G1: 24.1 months [95% CI: 14.4–33.8] vs. G2: 12.0 months [95% CI: 9.2–14.8]; p = 0.006; Figure 2A), Ki67 ≤ 10% (18.4 months [95% CI: 12.5–24.3] vs. 9.9 months [95% CI: 6.2–13.6]; p = 0.025; Figure 2B) and type of therapy (SSA

HD/switch 10.0 months; RLT 26.0 months; TT: 16.0 months; chemotherapy 7.7 months; $p = 0.001$; Figure 2C). No significant PFS2 difference according to sex ($p = 0.232$), presence of syndrome ($p = 0.961$), surgery of primary tumor ($p = 0.141$), or presence of extrahepatic metastatic disease ($p = 0.204$) was observed. A higher risk of progression to second-line treatment was associated with Ki67 > 10% (HR 1.54; $p = 0.027$), while a lower risk of progression was associated with second-line treatment with RLT as compared to other therapeutic strategies (Table 3). Sex, presence of symptoms related to hormone hypersecretion, surgery of primary tumor, and presence of extrahepatic metastatic disease were not associated with the risk of progression to second-line treatment. At multivariate analysis, type of second-line therapy was independently associated with the risk of progression (HD-SSA vs. RLT HR: 2.06; $p = 0.019$ and chemotherapy vs. RLT HR: 2.23; $p = 0.003$; Table 3).

Table 3. Predictive risk factors for disease progression during second-line therapy.

Characteristic	Univariate Analysis			Multivariate Analysis		
	HR	95% CI	p Value	HR	95% CI	p Value
Gender (male)	1.21	0.88–1.68	0.234	-	-	-
Non-functioning tumor	1.01	0.64–1.59	0.961	-	-	-
Ki67 > 10%	1.54	1.05–2.26	0.027	1.42	0.96–2.12	0.081
Primary tumor resection	0.79	0.57–1.08	0.143	-	-	-
Extrahepatic disease	1.26	0.88–1.82	0.207	-	-	-
Type of therapy						
RLT	1			1		
SSA HD/Switch	1.80	1.02–3.15	0.041	2.06	1.13–3.75	0.019
TT	1.62	1.07–2.47	0.023	1.48	0.96–2.23	0.074
CHT	2.67	1.62–4.42	<0.001	2.23	1.31–3.80	0.003

Abbreviations: HR: hazard ratio; 95% CI: 95% confidence interval; SSA: somatostatin analogs; HD: high dose; RLT: radioligand therapy; TT: targeted therapy; CHT: chemotherapy.

3.4. Overall Survival

Median OS was 94.7 months (95% CI: 78.8–110.6 months). To investigate the impact of treatment sequencing on OS, we grouped patients by the three most-used treatment strategies, which encompassed 82.1% of patients (n = 165/201), as follows: SSA–RLT in 35 patients (21.2%), RLT–other in 35 (21.2%) and SSA–other in 95 (57.6%). Overall, median OS in those 165 patients was 107.9 months (95% CI: 88.2–127.5 months). Significantly longer OS was associated with sex (female: 109.1 months [95% CI: 67.9–150.3] vs. male: 86.2 months [95% CI: 67.3–105.1]; $p = 0.031$), Ki67 $\leq$ 10% (99.9 months [95% CI: 80.6–119.1] vs. 67.9 months [95% CI: 53.2–82.4]; $p = 0.001$), surgery of primary tumor (yes: 146.1 months [95% CI: 108.3–183.8] vs. no: 69.4 months [95% CI: 58.7–80.0]; $p < 0.001$), presence of extrahepatic metastatic disease (no: 105.2 months [95% CI: 81.7–128.6] vs. yes: 69.0 months [95% CI: 41.0–97.0]; $p = 0.012$), and type of treatment (SSA–RLT: 151.1 months; RLT–other: 86.2 months; SSA–other: 96.1 months; $p = 0.025$; Figure 3). No significant OS difference according to the presence of syndrome ($p = 0.576$) was observed. A higher risk of death was associated with male sex (HR: 1.58; $p = 0.032$), Ki67 > 10% (HR 2.18; $p = 0.001$), presence of extrahepatic metastatic disease (HR: 1.77; $p = 0.013$), and therapeutic sequence (Table 4). In particular, the RLT–other (HR: 1.80; $p = 0.041$) and SSA–other (HR: 1.62; $p = 0.023$) sequences were associated with an increased risk for death when compared to SSA–RLT (Table 5). A lower risk of death was associated with surgery of the primary tumor (HR: 0.38; $p < 0.001$). At multivariate analysis, Ki67 > 10% (HR: 2.24; $p = 0.005$) and primary tumor resection (HR: 0.40; $p = $ <0.001) were independently associated with the risk of death (Table 4).

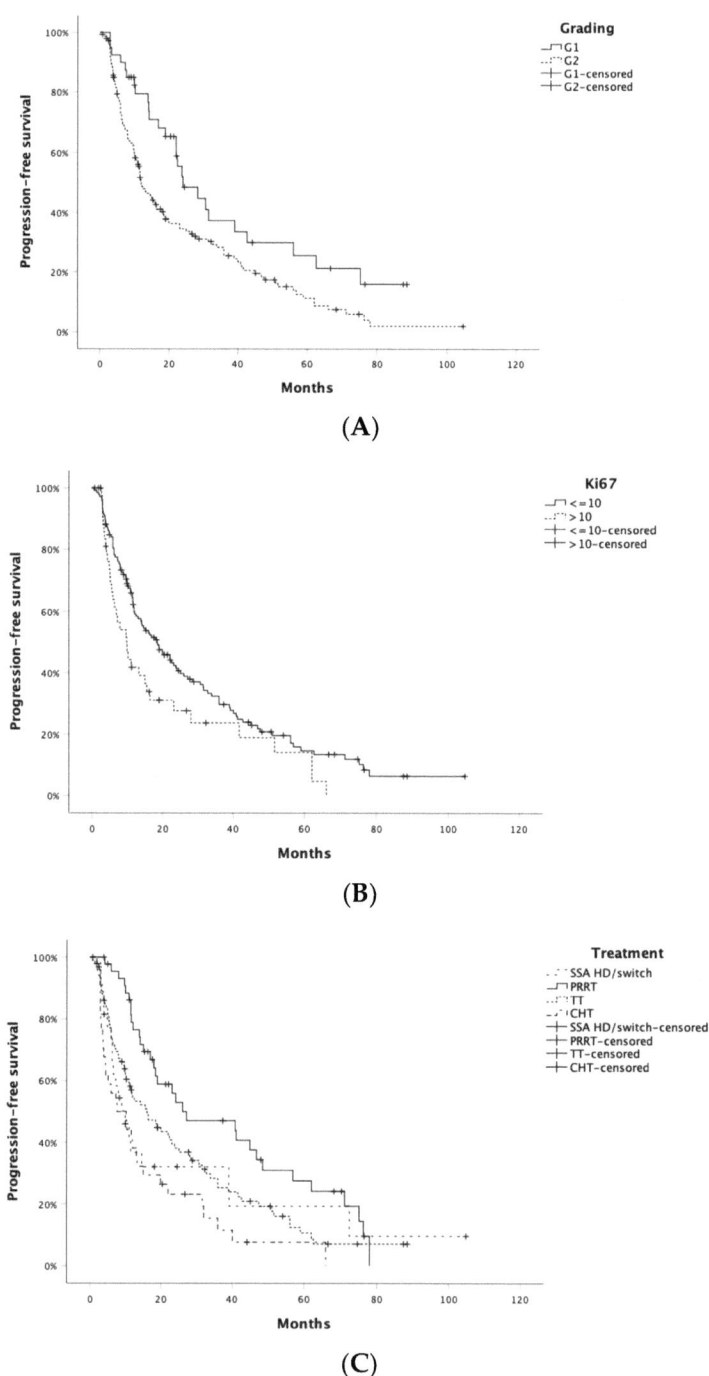

Figure 2. PFS to second-line treatment (PFS2) according to grade (**A**), Ki67 ≤ 10% (**B**) and type of therapy (**C**).

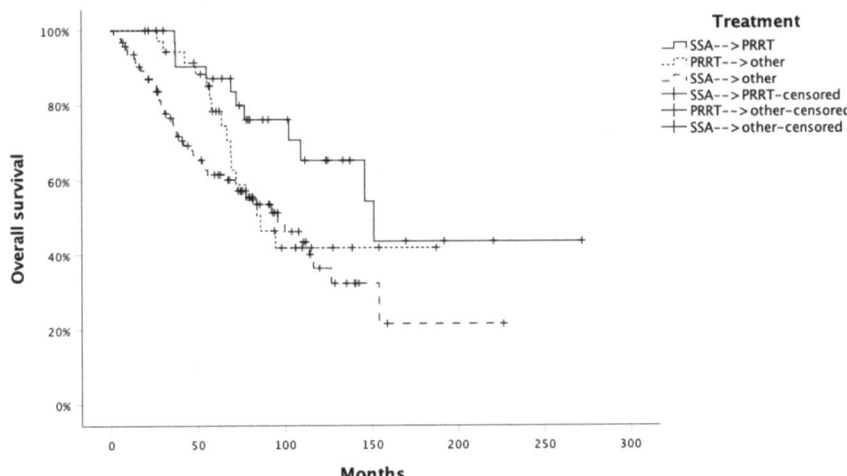

Figure 3. Overall survival (OS) by treatment sequence. SSA: somatostatin analog; PRRT: peptide radionuclide receptor therapy; Other includes targeted therapy, temozolomide-based or oxaliplatin-based chemotherapy, non-conventional doses SSA, or SSA switch.

Table 4. Predictive risk factors for death.

Characteristic	Univariate Analysis			Multivariate Analysis		
	HR	95% CI	p Value	HR	95% CI	p Value
Gender (male)	1.58	1.04–2.04	0.032	-	-	ns
Non-functioning tumor	1.18	0.66–2.12	0.576	-	-	-
Ki67 > 10%	2.18	1.35–3.52	0.001	2.24	1.28–3.94	0.005
Primary tumor resection	0.38	0.25–0.57	<0.001	0.40	0.24–0.66	<0.001
Extrahepatic disease	1.77	1.13–2.78	0.013	-	-	-
Type of therapy						
SSA–RLT	1			1		
RLT–Other	1.80	1.02–3.15	0.041	-	-	ns
SSA–Other	1.62	1.07–2.47	0.023	-	-	ns

Abbreviations: HR: hazard ratio; 95% CI: 95% confidence interval; SSA: somatostatin analogs; RLT: radioligand therapy; ns: not significant.

Table 5. Outcomes according to treatment sequences.

	N. (%)	PFS Months (95% CI)	OS Months (95% CI)
SSA–RLT	35 (21.2)	62.5 (42.2–82.7)	151.1 (97.4–204.8)
RLT–Other	35 (21.2)	38.1 (28.4–47.8)	86.2 (60.8–111.7)
SSA–Other	95 (57.6)	31.2 (17.0–45.3)	96.1 (66.4–125.8)

Abbreviations: PFS: progression-free survival; OS: overall survival; 95% CI: 95% confidence interval; SSA: somatostatin analogs; RLT: radioligand therapy.

3.5. Overall Survival in Patients with Ki67 ≤ 10%

Because the most relevant sequences in our cohort involved the use of SSA and RLT, which are mainly adopted in the treatment of pNETs with Ki67 ≤ 10%, we investigated the impact of treatment sequencing in this subgroup, which comprised 80.6% of patients (n = 133/165) whose median OS was 116.4 months (95% CI: 81.4–151.3). In this subgroup, a higher risk of death was associated with the presence of extrahepatic metastatic disease (HR: 1.77; p = 0.045) and therapeutic sequences with SSA–other compared to SSA–RLT (Table 6), while a lower risk of death was associated with primary tumor surgery

(HR: 0.34; $p < 0.001$). At multivariate analysis, primary tumor resection (HR 0.38; $p = 0.001$) and therapeutic sequence (HR 2.26; $p = 0.039$) were independently associated with the risk of death (Table 6).

Table 6. Predictive risk factors for death in patients with Ki67 ≤ 10%.

Characteristic	Univariate Analysis			Multivariate Analysis		
	HR	95% CI	p Value	HR	95% CI	p Value
Gender (male)	1.32	0.80–2.20	0.280	-	-	ns
Non-functioning tumor	1.08	0.56–2.07	0.817	-	-	-
Ki67	1.04	0.96–1.13	0.371	-	-	ns
Primary tumor resection	0.34	0.20–0.57	<0.001	0.38	0.21–0.69	0.001
Extrahepatic disease	1.77	1.01–3.10	0.045	-	-	ns
Type of therapy						
SSA–RLT	1			1		
RLT–Other	2.02	0.85–4.77	0.110	1.65	0.69–3.97	0.264
SSA–Other	2.39	1.18–5.12	0.025	2.26	1.04–4.88	0.039

Abbreviations: HR: hazard ratio; 95% CI: 95% confidence interval; SSA: somatostatin analogs; RLT: radioligand therapy; ns: not significant.

3.6. Overall Survival in Patients with Ki67 > 10%

Finally, we investigated the impact of treatment sequencing in the subgroup of patients with Ki67 > 10%, which comprised 19.4% of patients (n = 32/165) whose median OS was 69.0 months (95% CI: 51.2–86.8). In this subgroup, no factor was found to be correlated with an increase in the risk of death in both univariate and in multivariate analysis.

4. Discussion

The definition of the optimal therapeutic sequence in patients with advanced, unresectable GEP-NENs remains challenging, considering the extreme heterogeneity of NETs and the lack of solid evidence supporting the choice of the most effective treatment option as first-line or beyond. We report on prospectively-collected data from a large multicenter cohort of patients with well-differentiated pNETs who received at least two treatment lines switched upon evidence of radiological progression. RLT was associated with both prolonged PFS1 and PFS2 as compared to other therapeutic strategies, namely SSA and chemotherapy, which is consistent with the findings of a recent, multicenter, large retrospective study of 508 patients with entero-pancreatic NENs and a network meta-analysis of phase III trials of different treatment strategies in GEP-NET [14,15]. The RLT–other and the SSA–other sequences were associated with an increased risk of death when compared to SSA–RLT. This is because treatment with upfront RLT in patients who had experienced disease progression with SSA is associated with significantly improved survival outcomes compared to upfront chemotherapy or targeted therapy, as demonstrated in a recent multicenter retrospective study [14]. SSAs (i.e., octreotide and lanreotide) are widely recommended by the current guidelines as first-line therapy in patients with well-differentiated, slowly progressive, G1, and G2 GEP-NENs [16–19]. Nevertheless, sequencing treatment after disease progression on SSA has not been established. The available therapeutic options beyond first-line SSA are limited, including everolimus, sunitinib, temozolomide-based chemotherapy, and nonconventional-doses SSA and RLT with lutetium 177 (^{177}Lu)-DOTATATE [5,20–22]. Everolimus was approved based on the RADIANT 3 study, which showed a significant improvement of PFS among progressive metastatic pNET patients treated with everolimus compared to placebo (mPFS of 11.0 months vs. 4.6 months, $p < 0.001$) [23]. Similarly, sunitinib was approved based on a phase III trial showing a statistically significant improvement in PFS in progressive metastatic pNET patients treated with sunitinib compared to placebo (mPFS of 11.4 months vs. 5.5 months, $p < 0.001$) [21]. The combination of capecitabine plus temozolomide was recently compared with single-agent temozolomide in a randomized phase II trial including patients with progressive pNETs [22]. The study showed a significant improvement of PFS for the combination compared to single-agent (mPFS of 22.7 months vs. 14.4 months, $p < 0.02$), with a confirmed radiographic response rate of 40%. Furthermore, the efficacy of RLT as second-line treatment has been investigated in the NETTER-1 trial, an open-label, randomized, phase III trial, comparing RLT to high-doses octreotide among 229 patients with advanced, well-differentiated, progressive midgut NETs [5]. The primary endpoint of PFS was reached, with an estimated PFS at 20 months of 65.2% for RLT compared to 10.8% in the control arm. The final long-term analysis of NETTER-1 has shown an 11.7-month prolongation in survival among patients receiving RLT (mOS of 48 months in the experimental arm compared to 36.3 months in the control arm), although a statistically significant benefit was not achieved, likely attenuated by crossover to RLT in over a third of patients from the control arm. Although RLT is worldwide approved for both small-intestine and pNETs, prospective randomized evidence supporting its efficacy specifically in pNET is lacking. RLT use in patients with pNET has been mostly supported by retrospective data [24], or non-randomized trials, which reported that the efficacy of RLT in pNETs was similar to that reported in NETTER-1 [25]. Preliminary results from the OCLURANDOM study, a phase II randomized trial of RLT vs. sunitinib in patients with pNETs, have recently been presented [26]. Despite being a phase II trial, in contrast to the phase III NETTER-1 study, the OCLURANDOM study represents the first prospective randomized evidence of RLT in patients with pNET. The trial enrolled 84 patients (n = 41 receiving RLT and n = 43 receiving sunitinib) and demonstrated an almost double progression-free survival rate at 12 months, the primary endpoint, in the RLT arm when compared to the sunitinib arm (80.5% vs. 42%, respectively). Although definitive data are eagerly awaited, the preliminary report further supports the use of RLT in patients with pNETs.

To date, there is no evidence supporting the superiority of RLT over chemotherapy with capecitabine plus temozolomide. However, chemotherapy should be the preferred option in patients with high tumor burden requiring rapid cytoreduction. In addition, clinical trial to investigate the best sequence are challenging, as demonstrated by the SEQTOR study, which aimed to establish the better treatment sequence between everolimus followed by chemotherapy with streptozotocin-5fluoro-uracil (STZ/5-FU) and the opposite sequence in patients with pNET [27]. Slow accrual rate made the comparison of the two treatment sequences not possible, and the trial was amended to change the progression-free survival rate to first-line treatment at 12 months (12-m PFS1) as the primary endpoint. Both arms showed similar 12-m PFS1 ($p = 0.425$). STZ-5FU assigned as the first-line treatment achieved a statistically significant higher ORR compared to everolimus (30% vs. 11%, $p = 0.014$). Based on these data, STZ/5-FU should be considered as first-line treatment, especially in patients with good performance status and grade 2, when tumor shrinkage is needed.

Notably, primary tumor resection was significantly associated with longer survival. Currently, the role of surgical treatment of metastatic NENs is still controversial, considering the heterogeneous behavior of these tumors and the lack of definitive clinical evidence. However, a retrospective analysis of data from the Surveillance, Epidemiology, and End Results (SEER) database, including 897 patients with GEP-NENs and liver metastases who underwent primary tumor resection, has shown that the surgery of the primary tumor is an independent prognostic factor for survival [28]. Another retrospective analysis of data from the National Cancer Database (NCDB) has shown that the resection of the primary tumor is associated with prolonged survival among patients with G1–G2 advanced GEP-NENs [29]. Because retrospective surgical studies are subjected to bias, prospective studies are needed to clearly define the role of the surgery of the primary tumor in this setting, which might be considered in selected patients with pNET. Despite being classified as G2 pNET, tumors with Ki67 $\leq$ 10% have a more indolent behavior than those with higher Ki67. Since pNETs with Ki67 $\leq$ 10% represented the majority of our sample, we conducted a separated analysis in this group. Interestingly, the OS of pNET patients with Ki67 $\leq$ 10% treated with SSA–RLT was significantly longer compared to that of patients treated with other therapeutic sequences (i.e., RLT–other, SSA–other), thus suggesting that in this more indolent pNET population upfront SSA followed by RLT upon disease progression might be the best treatment choice, as recommended by ENETS Guidelines [16]. On the other hand, earlier use of RLT in the first-line setting might be more beneficial in pNETs with Ki67 > 10%. To elucidate this topic, the randomized phase III NETTER-2 trial is currently ongoing and evaluating the role of RLT as first-line treatment of patients with newly diagnosed GEP-NET and high proliferation rate (i.e., G2 >10% and G3) compared to treatment with high-dose long-acting octreotide (NCT03972488). The preliminary results of the NETTER-2 trial were recently presented at the 2024 American Society of Clinical Oncology (ASCO) Gastrointestinal Cancers Symposium [30]. The majority of tumors originated from the pancreas (54.4%) or small intestine (29.2%), whereas G3 tumors were reported in 35% of cases. Median PFS was significantly prolonged by 14.3 months, from 8.5 months in the control arm to 22.8 months in the RLT arm ($p < 0.0001$), thus reducing the risk of disease progression or death by 72%. Moreover, the ORR was significantly improved in the RLT arm (43.0%) compared to the control arm (9.3%). However, no data regarding OS are still available. Regarding the role of nonconventional-dose SSA (either by increased administered dose (dose intensity) or shortened interval between administrations (dose density), conflicting results have been reported in NEN patients after failure of the standard SSA dose. Indeed, earlier retrospective studies [31,32] reported better outcomes associated with the use of nonconventional-dose SSA as second-line treatment compared to third- or later-line treatment, which were not clearly confirmed by the recently published phase II CLARINET FORTE study. This trial investigated the efficacy of doubled-dose lanreotide (120 mg/2 weeks) among 99 patients with advanced G1 or G2 midgut NENs or pancreatic NENs, after progressing on the standard dose (120 mg/4 weeks) [33]. The median PFS was 8.3 months in midgut NENs and 5.6 months in pancreatic NENs. Overall, the estimated probability to achieve disease control rate (mostly obtained as disease stabilization) is 45%, as reported by a recent systematic review and meta-analysis evaluating the pooled data on the efficacy of increasing SSA dose in patients with progressive GEP-NENs after standard dose SSA [32]. In general, the efficacy of targeted agents (i.e., everolimus and sunitinib) in progressive GEP-NENs is well known, based on the findings reported more than ten years ago by the regulatory phase III trials, which showed an 11–16 month advantage in terms of PFS as compared to placebo [20,21,23]. However, solid data on a direct comparison between RLT and targeted agents as second-line therapy in patients with progressive disease after SSA are currently not available. A phase III, randomized trial (COMPETE trial) addressing this question is currently ongoing by comparing the efficacy of RLT and everolimus in progressive somatostatin receptor (SSTR)-positive GEP-NETs (NCT03049189). The study has recently completed accrual and results are awaited.

5. Conclusions

To date, the optimal management of advanced pNETs is controversial, given the heterogeneity of these tumors and the near absence of randomized trials comparing available treatment options. In patients with pNETs who received at least two treatment lines because of radiological disease progression, RLT is associated with better PFS in both first- and second-line setting. Similarly, surgical resection of the primary tumor is associated with improved survival. In the subgroup of patients with pNETs with Ki67 <10%, the best treatment sequence is represented by first-line SSA followed by RLT upon disease progression. Thus, the best treatment sequence should include upfront RLT in patients who experienced disease progression after SSA and target therapies or chemotherapy in later lines. Defining the management and treatment sequencing of advanced pancreatic NENs could be challenging and requires discussion within a multidisciplinary team, including medical and radiation oncologists, surgeons, radiologists, and nuclear medicine specialists, at referring and high-volume centers. However, larger, prospective, phase III clinical trials are needed to define the correct timing and the optimal treatment sequence of available systemic treatments in these patients.

Author Contributions: Conceptualization, F.P., E.A. and D.C.; methodology, D.C. and G.L.; software, G.L. and S.P.; validation, F.P., A.R. and D.C.; formal analysis, D.C., M.R., M.C.Z. and F.G.; investigation, A.B. and M.V.D.; resources, E.A. and M.C.; data curation, M.C. and M.P.B.; writing—original draft preparation, F.P., G.L., S.T. and E.A.; writing—review and editing, E.A. and G.L.; visualization, M.C.Z., A.B. and I.P. (Irene Persano); supervision, F.P., I.P. (Ivana Puliafito) and D.C.; project administration, G.L. All authors have read and agreed to the published version of the manuscript.

Funding: This research received no external funding.

Institutional Review Board Statement: The study was conducted in accordance with the Declaration of Helsinki and approved by the Institutional Review Board (or Ethics Committee) of Comitato Etico Indipendente, S.Orsola-Malpighi University Hospital, Bologna (protocol code 626/2020/Oss/AOUBo, 18 June 2020).

Informed Consent Statement: Informed consent was obtained from all subjects involved in the study.

Data Availability Statement: The data presented in this study are available on request from the corresponding author due to ethical reasons.

Conflicts of Interest: The authors declare no conflicts of interest.

References

1. Klimstra, D.S.; Kloppell, G.; La Rosa, S.; Rindi, G. Classification of neuroendocrine neoplasms of the digestive system. In *WHO Classification of Tumours: Digestive System Tumours*, 5th ed.; International Agency for Research on Cancer: Lyon, France, 2019; Volume 1.
2. Dasari, A.; Shen, C.; Halperin, D.; Zhao, B.; Zhou, S.; Xu, Y.; Shih, T.; Yao, J.C. Trends in the Incidence, Prevalence, and Survival Outcomes in Patients with Neuroendocrine Tumors in the United States. *JAMA Oncol.* **2017**, *3*, 1335. [CrossRef] [PubMed]
3. Stensbøl, A.B.; Krogh, J.; Holmager, P.; Klose, M.; Oturai, P.; Kjaer, A.; Hansen, C.P.; Federspiel, B.; Langer, S.W.; Knigge, U.; et al. Incidence, Clinical Presentation and Trends in Indication for Diagnostic Work-Up of Small Intestinal and Pancreatic Neuroendocrine Tumors. *Diagnostics* **2021**, *11*, 2030. [CrossRef] [PubMed]
4. Öberg, K.E. Gastrointestinal neuroendocrine tumors. *Ann. Oncol.* **2010**, *21*, vii72–vii80. [CrossRef] [PubMed]
5. Strosberg, J.R.; Caplin, M.E.; Kunz, P.L.; Ruszniewski, P.B.; Bodei, L.; Hendifar, A.; Mittra, E.; Wolin, E.M.; Yao, J.C.; Pavel, M.E.; et al. 177Lu-Dotatate plus long-acting octreotide versus high-dose long-acting octreotide in patients with midgut neuroendocrine tumours (NETTER-1): Final overall survival and long-term safety results from an open-label, randomised, controlled, phase 3 trial. *Lancet Oncol.* **2021**, *22*, 1752–1763. [CrossRef] [PubMed]
6. Baudin, E.; Walter, T.A.; Beron, A.; Smith, D.; Hadoux, J.; Lachachi, C.; Taieb, D.; Ansquer, C.; Dierickx, L.O.; du Bourg, L.D.M.; et al. 887O First multicentric randomized phase II trial investigating the antitumor efficacy of peptide receptor radionucleide therapy with 177Lutetium-Octreotate (OCLU) in unresectable progressive neuroendocrine pancreatic tumor: Results of the OCLURANDOM trial. *Ann. Oncol.* **2022**, *33* (Suppl. S7), S954. [CrossRef]
7. Eisenhauer, E.A.; Therasse, P.; Bogaerts, J.; Schwartz, L.H.; Sargent, D.; Ford, R.; Dancey, J.; Arbuck, S.; Gwyther, S.; Mooney, M.; et al. New response evaluation criteria in solid tumours: Revised RECIST guideline (version 1.1). *Eur. J. Cancer* **2009**, *45*, 228–247. [CrossRef] [PubMed]
8. Rindi, G.; Klöppel, G.; Couvelard, A.; Komminoth, P.; Körner, M.; Lopes, J.M.; McNicol, A.-M.; Nilsson, O.; Perren, A.; Scarpa, A.; et al. TNM staging of midgut and hindgut (neuro) endocrine tumors: A consensus proposal including a grading system. *Virchows Arch.* **2007**, *451*, 757–762. [CrossRef] [PubMed]
9. Panzuto, F.; Ramage, J.; Pritchard, D.M.; van Velthuysen, M.F.; Schrader, J.; Begum, N.; Sundin, A.; Falconi, M.; O'Toole, D. European Neuroendocrine Tumor Society (ENETS) 2023 guidance paper for gastroduodenal neuroendocrine tumours (NETs) G1–G3. *J. Neuroendocrinol.* **2023**, *35*, e13306. [CrossRef] [PubMed]
10. Kos-Kudła, B.; Castaño, J.P.; Denecke, T.; Grande, E.; Kjaer, A.; Koumarianou, A.; de Mestier, L.; Partelli, S.; Perren, A.; Stättner, S.; et al. European Neuroendocrine Tumour Society (ENETS) 2023 guidance paper for nonfunctioning pancreatic neuroendocrine tumours. *J. Neuroendocrinol.* **2023**, *35*, e13343. [CrossRef]
11. Rinke, A.; Ambrosini, V.; Dromain, C.; Garcia-Carbonero, R.; Haji, A.; Koumarianou, A.; van Dijkum, E.N.; O'Toole, D.; Rindi, G.; Scoazec, J.; et al. European Neuroendocrine Tumor Society (ENETS) 2023 guidance paper for colorectal neuroendocrine tumours. *J. Neuroendocrinol.* **2023**, *35*, e13309. [CrossRef]
12. Hofland, J.; Falconi, M.; Christ, E.; Castaño, J.P.; Faggiano, A.; Lamarca, A.; Perren, A.; Petrucci, S.; Prasad, V.; Ruszniewski, P.; et al. European Neuroendocrine Tumor Society 2023 guidance paper for functioning pancreatic neuroendocrine tumour syndromes. *J. Neuroendocrinol.* **2023**, *35*, e13318. [CrossRef] [PubMed]

13. Kaltsas, G.; Walter, T.; Knigge, U.; Toumpanakis, C.; Santos, A.P.; Begum, N.; Pape, U.F.; Volante, M.; Frilling, A.; Couvelard, A. European Neuroendocrine Tumor Society (ENETS) 2023 guidance paper for appendiceal neuroendocrine tumours (aNET). *J. Neuroendocrinol.* **2023**, *35*, e13332. [CrossRef] [PubMed]
14. Pusceddu, S.; Prinzi, N.; Tafuto, S.; Ibrahim, T.; Filice, A.; Brizzi, M.P.; Panzuto, F.; Baldari, S.; Grana, C.M.; Campana, D.; et al. Association of Upfront Peptide Receptor Radionuclide Therapy with Progression-Free Survival Among Patients with Enteropancreatic Neuroendocrine Tumors. *JAMA Netw. Open* **2022**, *5*, e220290. [CrossRef] [PubMed]
15. Ricci, C.; Lamberti, G.; Ingaldi, C.; Mosconi, C.; Pagano, N.; Alberici, L.; Ambrosini, V.; Manuzzi, L.; Monari, F.; Malvi, D.; et al. Treatment of Advanced Gastro-Entero-Pancreatic Neuro-Endocrine Tumors: A Systematic Review and Network Meta-Analysis of Phase III Randomized Controlled Trials. *Cancers* **2021**, *13*, 358. [CrossRef] [PubMed]
16. Pavel, M.; O"Toole, D.; Costa, F.; Capdevila, J.; Gross, D.; Kianmanesh, R.; Krenning, E.; Knigge, U.; Salazar, R.; Pape, U.-F.; et al. ENETS Consensus Guidelines Update for the Management of Distant Metastatic Disease of Intestinal, Pancreatic, Bronchial Neuroendocrine Neoplasms (NEN) and NEN of Unknown Primary Site. *Neuroendocrinology* **2016**, *103*, 172–185. [CrossRef] [PubMed]
17. Kulke, M.H.; Anthony, L.B.; Bushnell, D.L.; de Herder, W.W.; Goldsmith, S.J.; Klimstra, D.S.; Marx, S.J.; Pasieka, J.L.; Pommier, R.F.; Yao, J.C.; et al. NANETS Treatment Guidelines. *Pancreas* **2010**, *39*, 735–752. [CrossRef] [PubMed]
18. Boudreaux, J.P.; Klimstra, D.S.; Hassan, M.M.; Woltering, E.A.; Jensen, R.T.; Goldsmith, S.J.; Nutting, C.; Bushnell, D.L.; Caplin, M.E.; Yao, J.C. The NANETS Consensus Guideline for the Diagnosis and Management of Neuroendocrine Tumors. *Pancreas* **2010**, *39*, 753–766. [CrossRef] [PubMed]
19. Strosberg, J.R.; Halfdanarson, T.R.; Bellizzi, A.M.; Chan, J.A.; Dillon, J.S.; Heaney, A.P.; Kunz, P.L.; O'Dorisio, T.M.; Salem, R.; Segelov, E.; et al. The north American neuroendocrine tumor society consensus guidelines for surveillance and medical management of midgut neuroendocrine tumors. *Pancreas* **2017**, *46*, 707–714. [CrossRef] [PubMed]
20. Yao, J.C.; Fazio, N.; Singh, S.; Buzzoni, R.; Carnaghi, C.; Wolin, E.; Tomasek, J.; Raderer, M.; Lahner, H.; Voi, M.; et al. Everolimus for the treatment of advanced, non-functional neuroendocrine tumours of the lung or gastrointestinal tract (RADIANT-4): A randomised, placebo-controlled, phase 3 study. *Lancet* **2016**, *387*, 968–977. [CrossRef]
21. Raymond, E.; Dahan, L.; Raoul, J.-L.; Bang, Y.-J.; Borbath, I.; Lombard-Bohas, C.; Valle, J.; Metrakos, P.; Smith, D.; Vinik, A.; et al. Sunitinib Malate for the Treatment of Pancreatic Neuroendocrine Tumors. *N. Engl. J. Med.* **2011**, *364*, 501–513. [CrossRef]
22. Kunz, P.L.; Graham, N.; Catalano, P.J.; Nimeiri, H.; Fisher, G.A.; Longacre, T.A.; Suarez, C.J.; Rubin, D.; Yao, J.C.; Kulke, M.H.; et al. A randomized study of temozolomide or temozolomide and capecitabine in patients with advanced pancreatic neuroendocrine tumors: Final analysis of efficacy and evaluation of MGMT (ECOG-ACRIN E2211). *J. Clin. Oncol.* **2022**, *40*, 4004. [CrossRef]
23. Yao, J.C.; Shah, M.H.; Ito, T.; Bohas, C.L.; Wolin, E.M.; Van Cutsem, E.; Hobday, T.J.; Okusaka, T.; Capdevila, J.; de Vries, E.G.E.; et al. Everolimus for Advanced Pancreatic Neuroendocrine Tumors. *N. Engl. J. Med.* **2011**, *364*, 514–523. [CrossRef]
24. Brabander, T.; van der Zwan, W.A.; Teunissen, J.J.M.; Kam, B.L.R.; Feelders, R.A.; de Herder, W.W.; van Eijck, C.H.J.; Franssen, G.J.H.; Krenning, E.P.; Kwekkeboom, D.J. Long-Term Efficacy, Survival, and Safety of [177Lu-DOTA0,Tyr3]octreotate in Patients with Gastroenteropancreatic and Bronchial Neuroendocrine Tumors. *Clin. Cancer Res.* **2017**, *23*, 4617–4624. [CrossRef]
25. Ramage, J.; Naraev, B.G.; Halfdanarson, T.R. Peptide receptor radionuclide therapy for patients with advanced pancreatic neuroendocrine tumors. *Semin. Oncol.* **2018**, *45*, 236–248. [CrossRef]
26. Baudin, E.; Walter, T.; Docao, C.; Haissaguerre, M.; Hadoux, J.; Taieb, D.; Ansquer, C.; Dierickx, L.; De Mestier, L.; Deshayes, E.; et al. First multicentric randomized phase II trial investigating the antitumor efficacy of peptide receptor radionuclide therapy with 177Lutetium—Octreotate (OCLU) in unresectable progressive neuroendocrine pancreatic tumor: Results of the OCLURANDOM trial. In *Annales d"Endocrinologie*; Elsevier: Amsterdam, The Netherlands, 2022; Volume 83, pp. 289–290. [CrossRef]
27. Salazar, R.; Tafuto, S.; Krogh, M.; Teule, A.; Garcia-Carbonero, R.; Klumpen, H.J.; Cremer, B.; Sevilla, I.; Eriksson, B.; Tabaksblat, E.; et al. LBA45 Randomized open label phase III study comparing the efficacy and safety of everolimus followed by chemotherapy (CT) with streptozotocin (STZ)-5FU upon progression or the reverse sequence, in advanced progressive panNETs: The SEQTOR study (GETNE 1206. *Ann. Oncol.* **2022**, *33*, S1412. [CrossRef]
28. Zheng, M.; Li, Y.; Li, T.; Zhang, L.; Zhou, L. Resection of the primary tumor improves survival in patients with gastro-enteropancreatic neuroendocrine neoplasms with liver metastases: A SEER-based analysis. *Cancer Med.* **2019**, *8*, 5128–5136. [CrossRef]
29. Tierney, J.F.; Chivukula, S.V.; Wang, X.; Pappas, S.G.; Schadde, E.; Hertl, M.; Poirier, J.; Keutgen, X.M. Resection of primary tumor may prolong survival in metastatic gastroenteropancreatic neuroendocrine tumors. *Surgery* **2019**, *165*, 644–651. [CrossRef]
30. Singh, S.; Halperin, D.M.; Myrehaug, S.; Herrmann, K.; Pavel, M.; Kunz, P.L.; Chasen, B.; Capdevila, J.; Tafuto, S.; Oh, D.-Y.; et al. [177Lu]Lu-DOTA-TATE in newly diagnosed patients with advanced grade 2 and grade 3, well-differentiated gastroenteropancreatic neuroendocrine tumors: Primary analysis of the phase 3 randomized NETTER-2 study. *J. Clin. Oncol.* **2024**, *42*, LBA588. [CrossRef]
31. Diamantopoulos, L.N.; Laskaratos, F.M.; Kalligeros, M.; Shah, R.; Navalkissoor, S.; Gnanasegaran, G.; Banks, J.; Smith, J.; Jacobs, B.; Galanopoulos, M.; et al. Antiproliferative Effect of Above-Label Doses of Somatostatin Analogs for the Management of Gastroenteropancreatic Neuroendocrine Tumors. *Neuroendocrinology* **2021**, *111*, 650–659. [CrossRef]

32. Panzuto, F.; Ricci, C.; Rinzivillo, M.; Magi, L.; Marasco, M.; Lamberti, G.; Casadei, R.; Campana, D. The Antiproliferative Activity of High-Dose Somatostatin Analogs in Gastro-Entero-Pancreatic Neuroendocrine Tumors: A Systematic Review and Meta-Analysis. *J. Clin. Med.* **2022**, *11*, 6127. [CrossRef]
33. Pavel, M.; Ćwikła, J.B.; Lombard-Bohas, C.; Borbath, I.; Shah, T.; Pape, U.F.; Capdevila, J.; Panzuto, F.; Truong Thanh, X.M.; Houchard, A.; et al. Efficacy and safety of high-dose lanreotide autogel in patients with progressive pancreatic or midgut neuroendocrine tumours: CLARINET FORTE phase 2 study results. *Eur. J. Cancer* **2021**, *157*, 403–414. [CrossRef]

Disclaimer/Publisher's Note: The statements, opinions and data contained in all publications are solely those of the individual author(s) and contributor(s) and not of MDPI and/or the editor(s). MDPI and/or the editor(s) disclaim responsibility for any injury to people or property resulting from any ideas, methods, instructions or products referred to in the content.

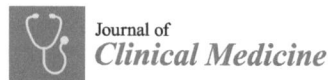 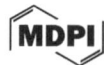

Review

Urgent Endoscopic Biliary Procedures: "Run Like the Wind"?

Francesca Lodato *, Stefano Landi, Marco Bassi, Stefania Ghersi and Vincenzo Cennamo

Department of Gastroenterology and Interventional Endoscopy, AUSL Bologna Bellaria, Maggiore Hospital, 40133 Bologna, Italy; stefano.landi@ausl.bo.it (S.L.); marco.bassi@ausl.bo.it (M.B.); stefania.ghersi@ausl.bo.it (S.G.); vincenzo.cennamo@ausl.bo.it (V.C.)
* Correspondence: francesca.lodato@ausl.bo.it

Abstract: Emergency endoscopy is an activity that must be guaranteed 7 days a week and 24 h a day. The pathologies of endoscopic interest that require emergency intervention are mainly hemorrhages of the upper digestive tract, the removal of foreign bodies, and the ingestion of caustics. The emergency endoscopist must therefore be experienced in the management of these pathologies. Nowadays, however, we know that even some biliary tract pathologies must be managed within a variable period between 12 and 72 h, in particular acute cholangitis (Ach), acute biliary pancreatitis (ABP), biliary duct leaks (BDLs), and acute cholecystitis (AC). If, on one hand, there is little awareness among doctors about which pathologies of the biliary tract really deserve urgent treatment, on the other, the international guidelines, although not uniformly, have acquired the results of the studies and have clarified that only severe Ach should be treated within 12 h; in other cases, endoscopic treatment can be delayed up to 72 h according to the specific condition. This obviously has a significant organizational implication, as not all endoscopists have training in biliary tract endoscopy, and guaranteeing the availability of a biliary endoscopist 24/7 may be incompatible with respecting the working hours of individual professionals. This review aims to evaluate which pathologies of the biliary tract really require an endoscopic approach in emergency or urgency and the organizational consequences that this can determine. Based on the guidelines, we can conclude that a daytime availability for urgent biliary tract procedures 7 days a week should be provided for the management of severe ACh. Patients with ABP, AC unfit for surgery, and not responsive to medical therapy or BDLs can be treated over a longer period, allowing its scheduling on the first available day of the week.

Keywords: biliary endoscopy; emergency; organization

1. Introduction

The organization of digestive endoscopy units provides for an on-call endoscopist 24 h a day. This figure is needed to manage urgent and emergent conditions such as digestive hemorrhages, caustic ingestion, or the ingestion of foreign bodies. In these cases, the promptness of the procedure plays a role in the patient's prognosis depending on the clinical situation [1–4]. Therefore, the emergency endoscopist must be trained in the management of endoluminal urgencies.

Urgent endoscopic procedures are also often required for some biliopancreatic diseases. Training in biliopancreatic endoscopy is specific, and not all endoscopists can perform such procedures. In addition, indications for performing emergency or urgent procedures in biliopancreatic diseases are uncertain, and it is unclear if promptness of the procedure has a prognostic impact.

This review focuses on biliopancreatic diseases that may benefit from performing endoscopic procedures in emergency/urgent setting, namely acute cholangitis (ACh), acute biliary pancreatitis (ABP), biliary duct leaks (BDLs), and acute cholecystitis (AC); moreover, we discuss the practical–organizational impact that the proper management of biliary emergencies can have.

2. Acute Cholangitis (Ach)

ACh is a common clinical complication of biliary obstruction associated with significant morbidity and mortality. The mortality rate ranges from 10% to 40%, depending on disease severity [5]. Thus, severity assessment is a cornerstone for ACh management.

The 2013 revision of the Tokyo Guidelines [6], confirmed in 2018 [7], divides ACh into severe, moderate, and mild, considering severe ACh associated with other organ systemic dysfunctions (Table 1).

Table 1. Severity classification of Ach according to TG18/TG13 Guidelines [6,8].

Grade III (Severe)	Ach associated with dysfunction at least in one of the following: 1. Cardiovascular: hypotension requiring dopamine $\geq$ 5 Lg/kg per min, or any dose of norepinephrine; 2. Neurological: disturbance of consciousness; 3. Respiratory: PaO_2/FiO_2 ratio < 300; 4. Renal: oliguria, serum creatinine > 2.0 mg/dL; 5. Hepatic: PT-INR > 1.5; 6. Hematological: platelet count < 100,000/mm.
Grade II (Moderate)	Ach associated with any two of the following: 1. Abnormal WBC count (>12,000/mm^3, <4000/mm^3); 2. High fever ($\geq$39 °C); 3. Age ($\geq$75 years old); 4. Hyperbilirubinemia (total bilirubin $\geq$ 5 mg/dL); 5. Hypoalbuminemia (<STD $\times$ 0.7 [a]).
Grade I (Mild)	Grade I Ach does not meet the criteria of "Grade III" or "Grade II" ACh at initial diagnosis

[a] STD: lower limit of normal value.

Most patients with ACh have mild-to-moderate disease responding to antibiotics therapy, which is a cornerstone in these cases [9,10]; but in 15–30% of cases, ACh is severe, requiring prompt biliary decompression; therefore, a correct classification of cholangitis severity is fundamental to selecting the appropriate treatment.

Endoscopic retrograde cholangiopancreatography (ERCP) remains the procedure of choice for biliary drainage, and its superiority over surgical procedures in terms of mortality and morbidity has already been established in many studies [10].

A further advantage of ERCP is the possibility of performing a biliary culture; this may be of particular importance given the increasing occurrence of resistance to third-generation cephalosporins, the most used antibiotics in patients with acute cholangitis [11,12].

In case of ERCP failure or unfavourable anatomy, percutaneous transhepatic biliary drainage (PTBD) or, more recently, endoscopic ultrasound-guided biliary drainage (EUS-BD) is an alternative approach to ERCP recommended by international guidelines [5,13].

The questions are as follows: When should ERCP be performed? How urgent is the procedure? In this topic, the literature is not in complete consensus.

The current Tokyo guidelines recommend biliary drainage in severe ACh "as soon as possible after patients' conditions allows"; in cases of mild and moderate ACh not responding to medical treatment, early biliary drainage is recommended but no specific timing for procedure is given [7].

Most studies chose to compare procedures when performed before or after 48 h mostly because they address the workforce and financial concerns of weekend procedures [14].

No randomized trials have compared ERCP before 48 h versus >48 h but a recent systematic review and meta-analysis by Iqbal et al. [14] defined "emergent ERCP" as a procedure performed within 48 h and found that in severe ACh, this procedural timeframe was associated with significantly lower in-hospital mortality and a shorter duration of hospital stay. Emergent ERCP was not only beneficial in patients with severe ACh but it was associated with better outcomes in patients with mild to moderate ACh in terms of 30-day mortality and organ failure. The meta-analysis included studies with patients who underwent ERCP within 24 or 48 h, but it was impossible to evaluate any mortality difference in patients with ACh who underwent ERCP within 24 h and patients who underwent ERCP between 24 and 48 h, because the mortality data for patients who underwent ERCP between 24 and 48 h was inconsistently reported in the studies [15–25]. Accordingly, the American Society of Gastrointestinal Endoscopy (ASGE) guidelines on the management of acute cholangitis recommend the performance of ERCP within 48 h for biliary decompression [5].

Nevertheless, the opportunity of performing ERCP "as soon as possible" as suggested by Tokyo Guidelines is also supported by a 2016 international study [26] including 260 patients with septic shock; the authors found that biliary drainage performed more than 12 h after the onset of shock was associated with higher in-hospital mortality (OR 3.4, 95% CI 1.12–10.31).

As a result, the European Society of Gastrointestinal Endoscopy (ESGE) Guidelines [13] are more detailed in the definition of timing for biliary drainage and recommends performing ERCP as soon as possible in severe ACh and within 12 h for patients with septic shock. When ACh is moderate, it is suggested to be performed within 48–72 h. For mild cases, the procedure could be elective.

Another important point is whether the timing of biliary drainage is equally important in malignant diseases. Malignant biliary obstruction (MBO), such as pancreatic cancer, cholangiocarcinoma, or metastatic cancer, is observed in 10–30% of cholangitis [22,23,27].

Neoplastic patients are certainly more complex than those suffering from lithiasis; their performance status is compromised by malnutrition related to concomitant chemotherapies and neoplastic cachexia [28–30]. Overall, they have a worse prognosis with a higher risk of readmission within 30 days [31] and, when ACh is present, it is associated with higher mortality and morbidity [32].

Moreover, when a biliary stricture is present, an additional endoscopic treatment is required to achieve an effective biliary decompression, such as stent placement, which could be more challenging in these patients due to anatomical alterations related to underlying disease [33,34].

A retrospective study [35] including 421 patients with ACh and distal MBO evaluated three time frames for ERCP: the authors chose to define "urgent" as the procedures performed within 24 h from admission; "early" as the procedures performed between 24 and 48 h; and "late" as the procedures performed after 48 h. ERCP performed by 24 h was significantly related to lower 30-day mortality (urgent 2.2%, early 4.3%, late 13.5%; $p < 0.001$) and 180-day mortality (39.4%, 44.8%, 60.8%; $p = 0.006$); these results were confirmed in subgroup analysis both for 30- and 180-day mortality, for patients with primary MBO and with moderate-to-severe cholangitis.

These data should support increased attention and urgency in patients with MBO, who may have a clinical presentation less conspicuous of ACh than patients with lithiasis. Nevertheless, a retrospective study comparing the waiting time for ERCP in patients with ACh and MBO compared to those with ACh and lithiasis showed that it is significantly longer in patients with MBO [36]. In this study, MBO-related ACh had a significantly higher 30-day mortality than lithiasis-related Ach, with time to ERCP, but not MBO itself, being an independent factor associated with 30 d mortality in the multivariate analysis. Other relevant findings were the significantly higher ICU admission and the 30-day readmission rates in patients with MBO. Therefore, we can conclude that more attention should be paid to neoplastic patients with MBO, offering these patients urgent procedures that guarantee better outcomes.

3. Acute Biliary Pancreatitis (ABP)

Acute pancreatitis (AP) is a frequent condition that can have different presentations with a benign outcome in most cases. In 20% of patients, however, the presentation is severe and is associated with high mortality and morbidity because patients may develop cholangitis, organ failure, and other severe complications [37].

The main etiology of AP is biliary, due to obstruction of the biliary tract by stones. This may result in obstruction and bile reflux into the pancreatic duct, which can trigger the processes of self-digestion by pancreatic enzymes. Clinical and experimental studies have shown that the severity of pancreatitis depends on the duration of biliary obstruction [38,39], with 80% of severe pancreatitis reported when an obstruction persists more than 48 h. Therefore, the need to drain the biliary tract by endoscopic decompression, mainly using ERCP with or without sphincterotomy, is mandatory.

The timing of the procedure, however, is debated; while it may be intuitive that the sooner the cause is removed, the sooner the pancreatitis is resolved, this is not universally true nor is it substantiated by clear evidence.

The first trial on the use of urgent ERCP in ABP was in 1988 [40]; the study evaluated the outcome of patients hospitalized for ABP and showed a significant reduction in complications (fluid collection rate and organ failure rate) and mortality in patients with severe ABP treated by ERCP within 72 h from ABP onset, compared with those treated conservatively. In 1993, Fan et al. [41] confirmed these results in a group of patients admitted with AP with various etiologies, mainly biliary. In this study, patients were randomly assigned to the early ERCP or conservative group even though gallstone diagnosis was not confirmed. Early ERCP was established in 24 h.

Later, other studies confirmed these results, albeit with some differences especially on the definition of the time of urgency (24 vs. 72 h) [42–47], as summarized in Table 2.

Regarding possible complications of the procedure, the advantage of biliary clearance remains significant: the main post-procedural complication was represented by bleeding, which, however, does not appear to increase mortality in a large cohort study comparing mortality in patients that underwent early or late ERCP with ABP (1.1 vs. 0.57, OR 2.08) [48].

Table 2. Main studies comparing early ERCP (at different timepoints) with conservative treatment for AP with cholangitis.

Author	Year	Patients (ERCP/Control)	Timing (h)	Mortality (%)	Morbidity (%)	Pancreatic Fluid Collection (%)	Organ Failure/Sepsis (%)
Neoptolemos [40]	1988	59/62	<72	1.7/8.1	22/62.9	11.9/21.0	10.2/37.1
Fan [41]	1993	97/98	<24	5.2/9.4	20.6/38.8	10.3/12.2	10.3/26.5
Nowak [47]	1998	178/102	<24	2.2/12.8	16.9/38.2	-	-
Zhou [46]	2002	20/25	<24	0/0	5/16	5.0/16.0	-
Acosta [45]	2006	30/31	<48	0/0	3.3/25.8	3.3/22.6	0/3.2
Chen [44]	2010	21/32	<72	0/6.3	4.8/18.8	4.8/18.8	-
Zhou [43]	2011	50/55	<72	0/1.8	12/30.6	2.0/0	6.0/18.2
Yang [42]	2012	60/60	<72	1.7/10	10/26.7	1.7713.3	1.7/13.3

Modified from Mukai et al. [49].

Considering the above, it might seem clear, therefore, that ABP always needs a rapid ERCP with biliary drainage, even considering the greater technical and procedural difficulty observed in these patients [50].

On the other hand, if we think about the pathogenesis of pancreatitis, it is necessary to remember that, after stones migrate into the main bile duct and trigger pancreatitis, the same stone may pass spontaneously due to increased bile pressure in the duct, without causing cholangitis.

All studies described above have in common that they mostly included patients with cholangitis, jaundice, or cholestasis. ABP without cholangitis should be considered a different condition compared to ABP with cholangitis, and the efficacy of ERCP in this context has been evaluated in recent studies [51–53] and, as a result, no benefit has been shown from performing urgent biliary clearance, neither in terms of mortality nor major complications (Table 3).

Table 3. Main studies comparing early ERCP (at different timepoints) with conservative treatment for AP without cholangitis.

Author	Year	Patients (ERCP/Control)	Timing (h)	Mortality (%)	Morbidity (%)	Pancreatic Fluid Collection (%)	Organ Failure/Sepsis (%)
Folsch [53]	1997	126/112	<72	7.9/3.6	46/50.9	23/22.3	34.1/25.9
Oria [52]	2007	51/51	<72	5.9/2	37.3/29.4	11.8/9.8	25.5/19.6
Schepers [51]	2020	117/113	<24	6.8/8.8	28.5/44.2	14.5/15.9	18.8/15

Modified from Mukai et al. [49].

A recent multicentre randomized trial on this issue published by Shepers et al. [51], which included only patients with predicted severe ABP without cholangitis, concluded that urgent ERCP with sphincterotomy did not reduce the composite endpoint of major complications or mortality, compared with conservative treatment. Their findings support a conservative strategy in patients with predicted severe ABP with an ERCP indicated only in patients with cholangitis or persistent cholestasis.

The same conclusions were proposed by an earlier Cochrane review in 2012 [54] that, pooling together seven RCTs including patients with and without severe pancreatitis, failed to show a significant benefit of early ERCP in terms of mortality (RR 0.74, 95% CI 0.18 to 3.03) and local and systemic complications as defined by the Atlanta Classification (RR 0.86, 95% CI 0.52 to 1.43; and RR 0.59, 95% CI 0.31 to 1.11, respectively), except for patients with cholangitis and cholestasis in whom early routine ERCP significantly reduced mortality (RR 0.20, 95% CI 0.06 to 0.68) and local and systemic complications as defined by the Atlanta Classification (RR 0.45, 95% CI 0.20 to 0.99; and RR 0.37, 95% CI 0.18 to 0.78, respectively).

Based on this evidence, ESGE recommends urgent ERCP in patients with ABP only in the presence of cholangitis or evidence of biliary obstruction [55].

As stated in ESGE guidelines, no study has been specifically designed to assess the timing of ERCP in biliary acute pancreatitis. The 2012 Cochrane systematic review did not show significant benefit when ERCP was performed as early as 24 h with respect to procedures delayed up to 72 h.

Considering this, the ESGE suggests performing ERCP within 24 h in cases of ABP with cholangitis, while delaying the procedure until 72 h in cases of biliary obstruction.

4. Biliary Duct Leak (BDL)

BDLs affects up to 1.5% of laparoscopic cholecystectomies [56–61]; it is moreover the most common surgical complication of liver transplantation [62–64], partial hepatectomy, and hepatic trauma [65].

ERCP with stenting, sphincterotomy, or a combination thereof is the first-line treatment for most BDLs, allowing the pressure gradient between the bile duct and the duodenum to be decreased; this creates a preferential transpapillary bile flow and allows the leak to heal [66,67]. The best approach to manage BDLs is not standardized, and current international guidelines recommend biliary decompression by either sphincterotomy alone or nasobiliary drain placement, with or without sphincterotomy (ASGE) [68] or biliary stent placement, only without sphincterotomy to avoid both short- and long-term adverse events (ESGEs) [69].

ERCP is effective in BDL treatment in up to 90% [70,71]; the remainder require additional treatment, with the location of the leak being reported as the main factor influencing the success of ERCP therapy [71]. In these cases, a second attempt could be performed with repeated stenting or the addition of a sphincterotomy if not previously performed. In refractory leaks, percutaneous transhepatic biliary drainage (PTBD) or surgical intervention should be proposed.

Some endoscopists and surgeons consider BDLs to be an emergency, whereas others treat patients on an elective basis [72].

No RCTs are available to evaluate the best timing for endoscopic treatment of biliary leaks. To the best of our knowledge, only three retrospective studies have studied the clinical impact of timing on ERCP outcome for the treatment of post-surgical BDL [73–75]. These studies divided patients into those exhibiting ERCP within 1 day, 2–3 days, and after 3 days from the onset of BDL. Studies are difficult to compare because of many differences: firstly, the BDL prevalence of post-cholecystectomy was 52%, 70.6%, and 100%, respectively; the rate of percutaneous abdominal drainage placement was as follows: not reported, 45%, and 9%, respectively. However, all three studies found that patients treated earlier have worst outcomes than those treated later, with lower overall adverse events after 3 days [75] and lower mortality when ERCP was performed between 48 and 72 h compared to those performed within 24 or after 72 h. These results could be explained with selection bias because it is likely that more severe patients underwent ERCP earlier while more stable cases were treated later with expectable better outcomes.

Nevertheless, in view of these data, there is no basis for considering BDLs as a matter of emergency and patients can mostly be managed within 3 days depending on the general clinical picture.

5. Acute Cholecystitis (AC)

AC is the most common complication of gallstone disease and the first presentation in up to 15% of cases [76,77].

According to the Tokyo guidelines, AC should be classified in three grades according to severity into mild, moderate, and severe [8], with grade 3 being associated with systemic dysfunction.

The definitive treatment of AC is cholecystectomy to be performed as soon as possible and within 7 days from admission, as stated by current guidelines [8,78], but in cases of patients unfit for surgery with severe AC not responding to antibiotics, non-surgical treatments (NSTs) should be proposed (Figure 1). The main factors predicting failure of NST in patients with absolute contraindication for surgery after 24 h of follow-up are age over 70 years, diabetes, tachycardia, and gallbladder empyema; after 48 h, predictors of failure are leucocytosis (>15,000 cell/mm^3), fever, and age over 70 years. Therefore, in patients unfit for surgery, gallbladder drainage should be proposed and performed within 24–48 h [79] in case of non-response to medical treatment.

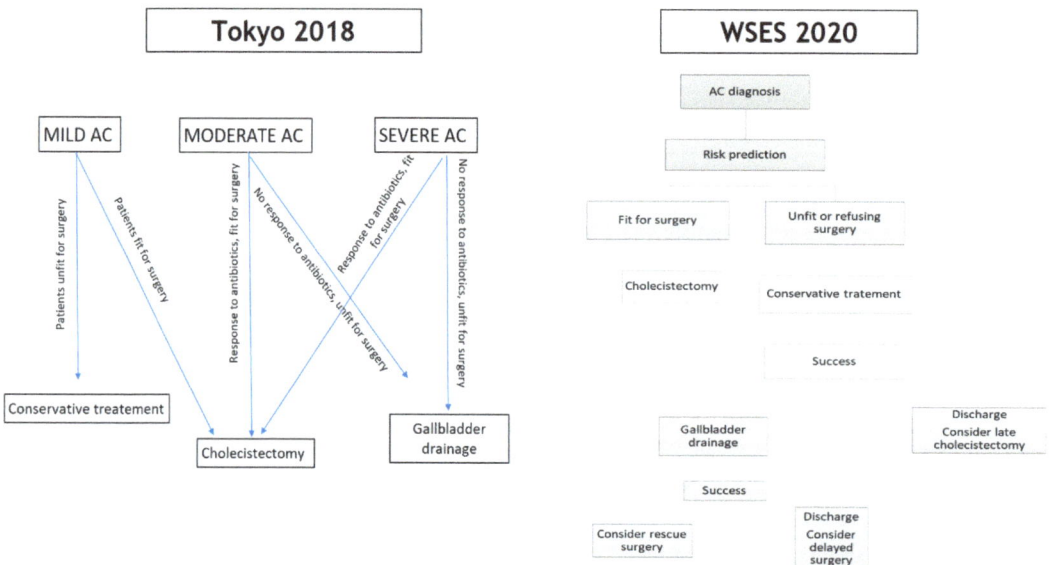

Figure 1. Flowchart of AC management according to Tokio and World Society of Emergency Surgery (WSES) Guidelines.

Among alternative approaches, AC could be treated by percutaneous transhepatic ultrasound/CT-guided biliary drainage (PT-GBD), transpapillary drainage by ERCP (TP-GBD), or EUS-guided transmural drainage (EUS-GBD).

PT-GBD is a feasible radiological procedure, with a rate of procedural success up to 86% [80,81]; however, mortality and morbidity is difficult to evaluate due to the significant heterogeneity of patients' inclusion in different studies, ranging, respectively, from 4 to 50% for mortality and from 8 to 62% for morbidity [82]. Moreover, it is not a definitive treatment, since the gallbladder is not removed and possible recurrent biliary complications may occur [83,84]. A recent RCT comparing laparoscopic cholecystectomy and PT-GBD reported a significantly higher rate of major complications, reinterventions, and recurrent biliary disease in the PT-GBD group compared to surgery, even in high-risk patients [85].

TP-GBD can be performed with two different methods: endoscopic naso-gallbladder drainage and endoscopic gallbladder stenting. These transpapillary procedures are used to place a drainage tube in the gallbladder via the cystic duct with ERCP [86,87]. This approach is clinically effective but technically challenging as it needs selective cystic duct cannulation and stent placement, in addition to the complexity of a standard ERCP; thus, it should be reserved to patients with contraindications to other drainage approaches, like patients with ascites, severe coagulopathy, thrombocytopenia, or an anatomically inaccessible location or in patients undergoing ERCP for common bile duct obstruction [88]. This approach could reasonably be performed in patients undergoing ERCP for biliary obstruction.

EUS-GBD is a relatively new technique; it is based on the creation of a fistula between the stomach or the duodenal bulb and the gallbladder using a stent, fixing the gallbladder wall directly to the intestinal lumen [89–91]. In the beginning, different devices were adapted from ERCP or transmural drainage, like self-expanding metal stents (SEMSs) or double pig-tail plastic stents (DPSs). Those devices have several problems when used for EUS-GBD, being designed for other purposes. SEMSs with radial expansion may be traumatic to visceral walls and might migrate due to the lack of anti-migratory systems; DPSs have a higher risk of leakage due to the lack of sealing of the fistula [91]. More recently, a novel technique for EUS-guided positioning of a lumen-apposing metal stent

(LAMS) was implemented. LAMSs are self-expanding metal stents with a dedicated design for transmural drainage; they have flanges to ensure lumen-to-lumen apposition, anti-migratory properties, and sealing of the fresh transmural tract, minimizing the risk of leakage [92].

The performance of EUS-GBD and PT-GBD has been evaluated in only one RCT [93]; both procedures had comparable technical and clinical success rates (97.4% vs. 100%, $p = 0.494$ and 92.3% vs. 92.5%, $p = 1$, respectively) with comparable 30-day mortality (7.7% vs. 10%, $p = 1$). Nevertheless, EUS-GBD was associated with significantly lower (25.6% vs. 77.5%, $p < 0.001$) 30-day adverse events (12.8% vs. 47.5%, $p = 0.010$), re-interventions after 30 days (2.6% vs. 30%, $p = 0.001$), readmissions (15.4% vs. 50%, $p = 0.002$), and recurrent cholecystitis (2.6% vs. 20%, $p = 0.029$). PT-GBD was also related to an increased risk of cholecystitis recurrence (OR 5.63).

NST techniques in high-risk surgical patients with acute cholecystitis have been compared by Mohan et al. in a large meta-analysis including 82 studies for a total of 15,131 patients (1223 treated with TP-GBD, 557 with EUS-GBD, and 13,351 with PGBD) [94]. The authors reported pooled technical and clinical successes for TP-GBD of 83% (95% confidence interval [CI]: 80.1–85.5) and 88.1% (95% CI: 83.6–91.4), respectively; for EUS-GBD, 95.3% (95% CI: 92.8–96.9) and 96.7% (95% CI: 94.0–98.2), respectively; and for PT-GBD, 98.7% (95% CI: 98.0–99.1) and 89.3% (95% CI: 86.6–91.5), respectively.

Current guidelines suggest, in centres experienced in the procedure, the use of EUS-GBD as the first choice in the drainage of AC unfit for surgery [8,78,95,96]. As said, the procedure should be performed within 24–48 h.

The endoscopic approach can indeed be considered a definitive treatment for patients unfit for surgery. Conversely, percutaneous drainage is the procedure of choice when expertise is not available for EUS-GBD in severely compromised patients with a surgical perspective, as a bridge before cholecystectomy. Delayed laparoscopic cholecystectomy in patients with PT-GBD is suggested in all those patients recovering from the conditions that previously discouraged surgical intervention after at least 6 weeks from the gallbladder drainage [97].

6. Conclusions

The endoscopic on-call system provides a trained endoscopist for urgent procedures, available 24/7.

Endoscopic procedures of the biliopancreatic tract, however, require specialized training that not all endoscopists, even those with much experience, may have.

An analysis of the literature shows that some diseases of the biliary tract require endoscopic treatment in an emergency, raising a challenging organization of trained personnel in the Gastroenterology Units.

Severe ACh is a disease of greater emergency, which, according to the ESGE guidelines, should be treated with ERCP within 12 h; in the case of ABP associated with cholangitis, the available studies show an extended operative window of up to 24 h. All other conditions evaluated could be delayed between 24 and 72 h (Figure 2).

Thus, it can be assumed that a full weekend can be waited for most procedures, whereas for severe cholangitis, with or without associated acute pancreatitis, a biliary endoscopist, available at least during daytime hours 7 days a week, should be provided.

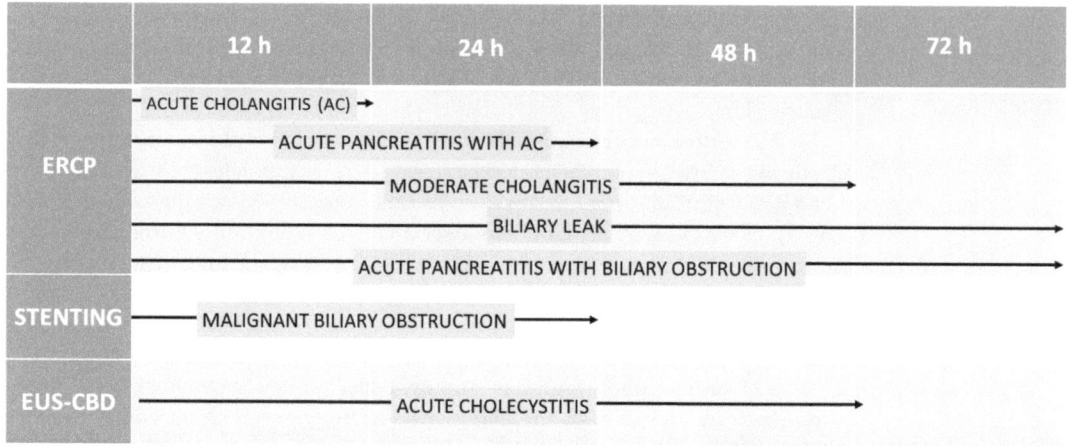

Figure 2. Performance time of procedures according to type and clinical condition.

The organization is more complex; in fact, it is not only necessary to consider the need for a specifically trained gastroenterologist—ERCP requires a dedicated team made by nursing staff and, in some hospitals, radiology technologists to manage the fluoroscopy equipment. Furthermore, most ECRPs are nowadays performed with anesthesia, thus requiring an additional nurse and an anesthesiologist. In summary, it is a procedure that requires the coordination of numerous professional figures and the use of advanced equipment.

Multiple studies have shown that ERCP performed after-hours or over the weekend is as safe as those performed during standard weekday hours [98–100]; thus, considering the guidelines and the clinical benefit of patients, the organization of the Gastroenterology Units should be reviewed.

In conclusion, every Gastroenterology Unit should provide at least a daytime availability for urgent biliary tract procedures 7 days a week for the management of severe ACh. Patients with ABP, AC unfit for surgery, and not responsive to medical therapy or BDLs can be treated over a longer period, allowing its scheduling on the first available day of the week.

Author Contributions: Conceptualization: F.L.; methodology: F.L., S.L and M.B.; writing—original draft preparation: F.L.; writing—review and editing: F.L., S.L., M.B. and S.G.; supervision: V.C. All authors have read and agreed to the published version of the manuscript.

Funding: This research received no external funding.

Data Availability Statement: No new data were created or analyzed in this study.

Conflicts of Interest: The authors declare no conflicts of interest.

Abbreviations

The following abbreviations are used in this manuscript:

ABP	Acute biliary pancreatitis
AP	Acute pancreatitis
AC	Acute cholecystitis
ACh	Acute cholangitis
ASGE	American Society of Gastrointestinal Endoscopy
BDL	Biliary duct leak
DPS	Double pig-tail stent
ESGE	European Society of Gastrointestinal Endoscopy

ERCP	Endoscopic retrograde cholangiopancreatography
EUS	Endoscopic ultrasound
EUS-BD	Endoscopic ultrasound-guided biliary drainage
EUS-GBD	EUS-guided gallbladder drainage
LAMS	Lumen-apposing metal stent
MBO	Malignant biliary obstruction
PTBD	Percutaneous transhepatic biliary drainage
PT-GBD	Percutaneous transhepatic gallbladder drainage
TP-GBD	Trans-papillary gallbladder drainage
SEMS	Self-expanding metal stent
WSES	World Society of Emergency Surgery

References

1. Gralnek, I.; Dumonceau, J.-M.; Kuipers, E.; Lanas, A.; Sanders, D.; Kurien, M.; Rotondano, G.; Hucl, T.; Dinis-Ribeiro, M.; Marmo, R.; et al. Diagnosis and Management of Nonvariceal Upper Gastrointestinal Hemorrhage: European Society of Gastrointestinal Endoscopy (ESGE) Guideline. *Endoscopy* **2015**, *47*, a1–a46. [CrossRef] [PubMed]
2. Birk, M.; Bauerfeind, P.; Deprez, P.; Häfner, M.; Hartmann, D.; Hassan, C.; Hucl, T.; Lesur, G.; Aabakken, L.; Meining, A. Removal of Foreign Bodies in the Upper Gastrointestinal Tract in Adults: European Society of Gastrointestinal Endoscopy (ESGE) Clinical Guideline. *Endoscopy* **2016**, *48*, 489–496. [CrossRef]
3. ASGE Standards of Practice Committee; Ikenberry, S.O.; Jue, T.L.; Anderson, M.A.; Appalaneni, V.; Banerjee, S.; Ben-Menachem, T.; Decker, G.A.; Fanelli, R.D.; Fisher, L.R.; et al. Management of Ingested Foreign Bodies and Food Impactions. *Gastrointest. Endosc.* **2011**, *73*, 1085–1091.
4. Lau, J.Y.W.; Yu, Y.; Tang, R.S.Y.; Chan, H.C.H.; Yip, H.-C.; Chan, S.M.; Luk, S.W.Y.; Wong, S.H.; Lau, L.H.S.; Lui, R.N.; et al. Timing of Endoscopy for Acute Upper Gastrointestinal Bleeding. *N. Engl. J. Med.* **2020**, *382*, 1299–1308. [CrossRef]
5. Buxbaum, J.L.; Buitrago, C.; Lee, A.; Elmunzer, B.J.; Riaz, A.; Ceppa, E.P.; Al-Haddad, M.; Amateau, S.K.; Calderwood, A.H.; Fishman, D.S.; et al. ASGE Guideline on the Management of Cholangitis. *Gastrointest. Endosc.* **2021**, *94*, 207–221.e14. [CrossRef]
6. Kiriyama, S.; Takada, T.; Strasberg, S.M.; Solomkin, J.S.; Mayumi, T.; Pitt, H.A.; Gouma, D.J.; Garden, O.J.; Büchler, M.W.; Yokoe, M.; et al. TG13 Guidelines for Diagnosis and Severity Grading of Acute Cholangitis (with Videos). *J. Hepato-Biliary-Pancreat. Sci.* **2013**, *20*, 24–34. [CrossRef] [PubMed]
7. Kiriyama, S.; Kozaka, K.; Takada, T.; Strasberg, S.M.; Pitt, H.A.; Gabata, T.; Hata, J.; Liau, K.-H.; Miura, F.; Horiguchi, A.; et al. Tokyo Guidelines 2018: Diagnostic Criteria and Severity Grading of Acute Cholangitis (with Videos). *J. Hepato-Biliary-Pancreat. Sci.* **2018**, *25*, 17–30. [CrossRef] [PubMed]
8. Okamoto, K.; Suzuki, K.; Takada, T.; Strasberg, S.M.; Asbun, H.J.; Endo, I.; Iwashita, Y.; Hibi, T.; Pitt, H.A.; Umezawa, A.; et al. Tokyo Guidelines 2018: Flowchart for the Management of Acute Cholecystitis. *J. Hepato-Biliary-Pancreat. Sci.* **2018**, *25*, 55–72. [CrossRef] [PubMed]
9. Srinu, D.; Shah, J.; Jena, A.; Jearth, V.; Singh, A.K.; Mandavdhare, H.S.; Sharma, V.; Irrinki, S.; Sakaray, Y.R.; Gupta, R.; et al. Conventional vs Short Duration of Antibiotics in Patients with Moderate or Severe Cholangitis: Noninferiority Randomized Trial. *Am. J. Gastroenterol.* **2024**, *119*, 176–182. [CrossRef]
10. Lai, E.C.S.; Mok, F.P.T.; Tan, E.S.Y.; Lo, C.; Fan, S.; You, K.; Wong, J. Endoscopic Biliary Drainage for Severe Acute Cholangitis. *N. Engl. J. Med.* **1992**, *326*, 1582–1586. [CrossRef]
11. Kruis, T.; Güse-Jaschuck, S.; Siegmund, B.; Adam, T.; Epple, H.-J. Use of Microbiological and Patient Data for Choice of Empirical Antibiotic Therapy in Acute Cholangitis. *BMC Gastroenterol.* **2020**, *20*, 65. [CrossRef]
12. Cozma, M.-A.; Găman, M.-A.; Srichawla, B.S.; Dhali, A.; Manan, M.R.; Nahian, A.; Marsool, M.D.M.; Suteja, R.C.; Kutikuppala, L.V.S.; Kipkorir, V.; et al. Acute Cholangitis: A State-of-the-Art Review. *Ann. Med. Surg.* **2024**, *86*, 4560–4574. [CrossRef] [PubMed]
13. Manes, G.; Paspatis, G.; Aabakken, L.; Anderloni, A.; Arvanitakis, M.; Ah-Soune, P.; Barthet, M.; Domagk, D.; Dumonceau, J.-M.; Gigot, J.-F.; et al. Endoscopic Management of Common Bile Duct Stones: European Society of Gastrointestinal Endoscopy (ESGE) Guideline. *Endoscopy* **2019**, *51*, 472–491. [CrossRef]
14. Iqbal, U.; Khara, H.S.; Hu, Y.; Khan, M.A.; Ovalle, A.; Siddique, O.; Sun, H.; Shellenberger, M.J. Emergent versus Urgent ERCP in Acute Cholangitis: A Systematic Review and Meta-Analysis. *Gastrointest. Endosc.* **2020**, *91*, 753–760.e4. [CrossRef] [PubMed]
15. Kiriyama, S.; Takada, T.; Hwang, T.; Akazawa, K.; Miura, F.; Gomi, H.; Mori, R.; Endo, I.; Itoi, T.; Yokoe, M.; et al. Clinical Application and Verification of the TG13 Diagnostic and Severity Grading Criteria for Acute Cholangitis: An International Multicenter Observational Study. *J. Hepato-Biliary-Pancreat. Sci.* **2017**, *24*, 329–337. [CrossRef] [PubMed]

16. Park, C.S.; Jeong, H.S.; Kim, K.B.; Han, J.-H.; Chae, H.B.; Youn, S.J.; Park, S.M. Urgent ERCP for Acute Cholangitis Reduces Mortality and Hospital Stay in Elderly and Very Elderly Patients. *Hepatobiliary Pancreat. Dis. Int.* **2016**, *15*, 619–625. [CrossRef] [PubMed]
17. Jang, S.E.; Park, S.W.; Lee, B.S.; Shin, C.M.; Lee, S.H.; Kim, J.-W.; Jeong, S.-H.; Kim, N.; Lee, D.H.; Park, J.K.; et al. Management for CBD Stone-Related Mild to Moderate Acute Cholangitis: Urgent Versus Elective ERCP. *Dig. Dis. Sci.* **2013**, *58*, 2082–2087. [CrossRef]
18. Mulki, R.; Shah, R.; Qayed, E. Early vs Late Endoscopic Retrograde Cholangiopancreatography in Patients with Acute Cholangitis: A Nationwide Analysis. *World J. Gastrointest. Endosc.* **2019**, *11*, 41–53. [CrossRef]
19. Tan, M.; Schaffalitzky de Muckadell, O.B.; Laursen, S.B. Association between Early ERCP and Mortality in Patients with Acute Cholangitis. *Gastrointest. Endosc.* **2018**, *87*, 185–192. [CrossRef]
20. Patel, H.K.; Gaduputi, V.; Chelimilla, H.; Makker, J.; Hashmi, H.R.T.; Irigela, M.; Dev, A.; Chilimuri, S. Acute Cholangitis: Does the Timing of ERCP Alter Outcomes? *J. Pancreas* **2016**, *17*, 504–509.
21. Alper, E.; Unsal, B.; Buyraç, Z.; Baydar, H.; Aslan, F.; Akça, S.; Ustundag, Y. Sa1520 Early ERCP Is Safe and Cost-Effective in the Treatment of Mild to Moderate Acute Cholangitis. *Gastrointest. Endosc.* **2011**, *73*, AB195. [CrossRef]
22. Lee, F.; Ohanian, E.; Rheem, J.; Laine, L.; Che, K.; Kim, J.J. Delayed Endoscopic Retrograde Cholangiopancreatography Is Associated with Persistent Organ Failure in Hospitalised Patients with Acute Cholangitis. *Aliment. Pharmacol. Ther.* **2015**, *42*, 212–220. [CrossRef]
23. Hou, L.A.; Laine, L.; Motamedi, N.; Sahakian, A.; Lane, C.; Buxbaum, J. Optimal Timing of Endoscopic Retrograde Cholangiopancreatography in Acute Cholangitis. *J. Clin. Gastroenterol.* **2017**, *51*, 534–538. [CrossRef] [PubMed]
24. Aboelsoud, M.; Siddique, O.; Morales, A.; Seol, Y.; Al-Qadi, M. Early Biliary Drainage Is Associated with Favourable Outcomes in Critically-Ill Patients with Acute Cholangitis. *Gastroenterol. Rev.* **2018**, *13*, 16–21. [CrossRef]
25. Parikh, M.P.; Wadhwa, V.; Thota, P.N.; Lopez, R.; Sanaka, M.R. Outcomes Associated With Timing of ERCP in Acute Cholangitis Secondary to Choledocholithiasis. *J. Clin. Gastroenterol.* **2018**, *52*, e97–e102. [CrossRef]
26. Karvellas, C.J.; Abraldes, J.G.; Zepeda-Gomez, S.; Moffat, D.C.; Mirzanejad, Y.; Vazquez-Grande, G.; Esfahani, E.K.; Kumar, A. The Impact of Delayed Biliary Decompression and Anti-microbial Therapy in 260 Patients with Cholangitis-associated Septic Shock. *Aliment. Pharmacol. Ther.* **2016**, *44*, 755–766. [CrossRef] [PubMed]
27. Navaneethan, U.; Gutierrez, N.G.; Jegadeesan, R.; Venkatesh, P.G.K.; Butt, M.; Sanaka, M.R.; Vargo, J.J.; Parsi, M.A. Delay in Performing ERCP and Adverse Events Increase the 30-Day Readmission Risk in Patients with Acute Cholangitis. *Gastrointest. Endosc.* **2013**, *78*, 81–90. [CrossRef]
28. Valle, J.; Wasan, H.; Palmer, D.H.; Cunningham, D.; Anthoney, A.; Maraveyas, A.; Madhusudan, S.; Iveson, T.; Hughes, S.; Pereira, S.P.; et al. Cisplatin plus Gemcitabine versus Gemcitabine for Biliary Tract Cancer. *N. Engl. J. Med.* **2010**, *362*, 1273–1281. [CrossRef] [PubMed]
29. Von Hoff, D.D.; Ervin, T.; Arena, F.P.; Chiorean, E.G.; Infante, J.; Moore, M.; Seay, T.; Tjulandin, S.A.; Ma, W.W.; Saleh, M.N.; et al. Increased Survival in Pancreatic Cancer with Nab-Paclitaxel plus Gemcitabine. *N. Engl. J. Med.* **2013**, *369*, 1691–1703. [CrossRef]
30. Conroy, T.; Hammel, P.; Hebbar, M.; Ben Abdelghani, M.; Wei, A.C.; Raoul, J.-L.; Choné, L.; Francois, E.; Artru, P.; Biagi, J.J.; et al. FOLFIRINOX or Gemcitabine as Adjuvant Therapy for Pancreatic Cancer. *N. Engl. J. Med.* **2018**, *379*, 2395–2406. [CrossRef]
31. Parikh, M.P.; Garg, R.; Chittajallu, V.; Gupta, N.; Sarvepalli, S.; Lopez, R.; Thota, P.N.; Siddiki, H.; Bhatt, A.; Chahal, P.; et al. Trends and Risk Factors for 30-Day Readmissions in Patients with Acute Cholangitis: Analysis from the National Readmission Database. *Surg. Endosc.* **2021**, *35*, 223–231. [CrossRef]
32. Singh, I.; Chou, J.F.; Capanu, M.; Park, J.; Yu, K.H.; Varghese, A.M.; Park, W.; Zervoudakis, A.; Keane, F.; Rolston, V.S.; et al. Morbidity and Mortality in Patients with Stage IV Pancreatic Adenocarcinoma and Acute Cholangitis: Outcomes and Risk Prognostication. *Pancreatology* **2024**, *24*, 608–615. [CrossRef] [PubMed]
33. Reddy Ginnaram, S. Comparative Efficacy of Endoscopic Ultrasound-Guided Biliary Drainage versus Endoscopic Retrograde Cholangiopancreatography as First-Line Palliation in Malignant Distal Biliary Obstruction: A Systematic Review and Meta-Analysis. *Ann. Gastroenterol.* **2024**, *37*, 1–8. [CrossRef]
34. Dhir, V.; Itoi, T.; Khashab, M.A.; Park, D.H.; Teoh, A.Y.B.; Attam, R.; Messallam, A.; Varadarajulu, S.; Maydeo, A. Multicenter Comparative Evaluation of Endoscopic Placement of Expandable Metal Stents for Malignant Distal Common Bile Duct Obstruction by ERCP or EUS-Guided Approach. *Gastrointest. Endosc.* **2015**, *81*, 913–923. [CrossRef] [PubMed]
35. Park, N.; Lee, S.H.; You, M.S.; Kim, J.S.; Huh, G.; Chun, J.W.; Cho, I.R.; Paik, W.H.; Ryu, J.K.; Kim, Y.-T. Optimal Timing of Endoscopic Retrograde Cholangiopancreatography for Acute Cholangitis Associated with Distal Malignant Biliary Obstruction. *BMC Gastroenterol.* **2021**, *21*, 175. [CrossRef]
36. Tsou, Y.-K.; Su, Y.-T.; Lin, C.-H.; Liu, N.-J. Acute Cholangitis: Does Malignant Biliary Obstruction vs Choledocholithiasis Etiology Change the Clinical Presentation and Outcomes? *World J. Clin. Cases* **2023**, *11*, 6984–6994. [CrossRef] [PubMed]

37. Banks, P.A.; Bollen, T.L.; Dervenis, C.; Gooszen, H.G.; Johnson, C.D.; Sarr, M.G.; Tsiotos, G.G.; Vege, S.S. Classification of Acute Pancreatitis—2012: Revision of the Atlanta Classification and Definitions by International Consensus. *Gut* **2013**, *62*, 102–111. [CrossRef]
38. Senninger, N.; Moody, F.G.; Coelho, J.C.; Van Buren, D.H. The Role of Biliary Obstruction in the Pathogenesis of Acute Pancreatitis in the Opossum. *Surgery* **1986**, *99*, 688–693. [PubMed]
39. Acosta, J.M.; Rubio Galli, O.M.; Rossi, R.; Chinellato, A.V.; Pellegrini, C.A. Effect of Duration of Ampullary Gallstone Obstruction on Severity of Lesions of Acute Pancreatitis. *J. Am. Coll. Surg.* **1997**, *184*, 499–505. [PubMed]
40. Neoptolemos, J.P.; Carr-Locke, D.L.; London, N.J.; Bailey, I.A.; James, D.; Fossard, D.P. Controlled Trial of Urgent Endoscopic Retrograde Cholangiopancreatography and Endoscopic Sphincterotomy versus Conservative Treatment for Acute Pancreatitis Due to Gallstones. *Lancet* **1988**, *2*, 979–983. [CrossRef]
41. Fan, S.-T.; Lai, E.; Mok, F.; Lo, C.-M.; Zheng, S.-S.; Wong, J. Early Treatment of Acute Biliary Pancreatitis by Endoscopic Papillotomy. *N. Engl. J. Med.* **1993**, *328*, 228–232. [CrossRef]
42. Yang, P.; Feng, K.-X.; Luo, H.; Wang, D.; Hu, Z.-H. Acute Biliary Pancreatitis Treated by Early Endoscopic Intervention. *Panminerva Med.* **2012**, *54*, 65–69.
43. Zhou, W.-C.; Li, Y.-M.; Zhang, H.; Li, X.; Zhang, L.; Meng, W.-B.; Zhu, K.-X.; Zhang, Q.-B.; He, M.-Y. Therapeutic Effects of Endoscopic Therapy Combined with Enteral Nutrition on Acute Severe Biliary Pancreatitis. *Chin. Med. J. (Engl.)* **2011**, *124*, 2993–2996. [PubMed]
44. Chen, P.; Hu, B.; Wang, C.; Kang, Y.; Jin, X.; Tang, C. Pilot Study of Urgent Endoscopic Intervention Without Fluoroscopy on Patients With Severe Acute Biliary Pancreatitis in the Intensive Care Unit. *Pancreas* **2010**, *39*, 398–402. [CrossRef]
45. Acosta, J.M.; Katkhouda, N.; Debian, K.A.; Groshen, S.G.; Tsao-Wei, D.D.; Berne, T.V. Early Ductal Decompression Versus Conservative Management for Gallstone Pancreatitis with Ampullary Obstruction. *Ann. Surg.* **2006**, *243*, 33–40. [CrossRef] [PubMed]
46. Zhou, M.-Q.; Li, N.-P.; Lu, R.-D. Duodenoscopy in Treatment of Acute Gallstone Pancreatitis. *Hepatobiliary Pancreat. Dis. Int.* **2002**, *1*, 608–610. [PubMed]
47. Nowak, A.; Marek, T.A.; Nowakowska-Duława, E.; Rybicka, J.; Kaczor, R. Biliary Pancreatitis Needs Endoscopic Retrograde Cholangiopancreatography with Endoscopic Sphincterotomy for Cure. *Endoscopy* **1998**, *30*, A256–A259. [CrossRef] [PubMed]
48. Malli, A.; Durkin, C.; Groce, J.R.; Hinton, A.; Conwell, D.L.; Krishna, S.G. Unavailability of Endoscopic Retrograde Cholangiography Adversely Impacts Hospital Outcomes of Acute Biliary Pancreatitis. *Pancreas* **2020**, *49*, 39–45. [CrossRef]
49. Mukai, S.; Itoi, T.; Tsuchiya, T.; Ishii, K.; Tanaka, R.; Tonozuka, R.; Sofuni, A. Urgent and emergency endoscopic retrograde cholangiopancreatography for gallstone-induced acute cholangitis and pancreatitis. *Dig. Endosc.* **2023**, *35*, 47–57. [CrossRef] [PubMed]
50. Pécsi, D.; Gódi, S.; Hegyi, P.; Hanák, L.; Szentesi, A.; Altorjay, I.; Bakucz, T.; Czakó, L.; Kovács, G.; Orbán-Szilágyi, Á.; et al. ERCP Is More Challenging in Cases of Acute Biliary Pancreatitis than in Acute Cholangitis—Analysis of the Hungarian ERCP Registry Data. *Pancreatology* **2021**, *21*, 59–63. [CrossRef]
51. Schepers, N.J.; Hallensleben, N.D.L.; Besselink, M.G.; Anten, M.-P.G.F.; Bollen, T.L.; da Costa, D.W.; van Delft, F.; van Dijk, S.M.; van Dullemen, H.M.; Dijkgraaf, M.G.W.; et al. Urgent Endoscopic Retrograde Cholangiopancreatography with Sphincterotomy versus Conservative Treatment in Predicted Severe Acute Gallstone Pancreatitis (APEC): A Multicentre Randomised Controlled Trial. *Lancet* **2020**, *396*, 167–176. [CrossRef]
52. Oría, A.; Cimmino, D.; Ocampo, C.; Silva, W.; Kohan, G.; Zandalazini, H.; Szelagowski, C.; Chiappetta, L. Early Endoscopic Intervention versus Early Conservative Management in Patients with Acute Gallstone Pancreatitis and Biliopancreatic Obstruction: A Randomized Clinical Trial. *Ann. Surg.* **2007**, *245*, 10–17. [CrossRef] [PubMed]
53. Fölsch, U.R.; Nitsche, R.; Lüdtke, R.; Hilgers, R.A.; Creutzfeldt, W. Early ERCP and Papillotomy Compared with Conservative Treatment for Acute Biliary Pancreatitis. *N. Engl. J. Med.* **1997**, *336*, 237–242. [CrossRef]
54. Tse, F.; Yuan, Y. Early Routine Endoscopic Retrograde Cholangiopancreatography Strategy versus Early Conservative Management Strategy in Acute Gallstone Pancreatitis. In *Cochrane Database of Systematic Reviews*; Tse, F., Ed.; John Wiley & Sons, Ltd.: Chichester, UK, 2012.
55. Arvanitakis, M.; Dumonceau, J.-M.; Albert, J.; Badaoui, A.; Bali, M.; Barthet, M.; Besselink, M.; Deviere, J.; Oliveira Ferreira, A.; Gyökeres, T.; et al. Endoscopic Management of Acute Necrotizing Pancreatitis: European Society of Gastrointestinal Endoscopy (ESGE) Evidence-Based Multidisciplinary Guidelines. *Endoscopy* **2018**, *50*, 524–546. [CrossRef] [PubMed]
56. Viste, A.; Horn, A.; Øvrebø, K.; Christensen, B.; Angelsen, J.-H.; Hoem, D. Bile Duct Injuries Following Laparoscopic Cholecystectomy. *Scand. J. Surg.* **2015**, *104*, 233–237. [CrossRef] [PubMed]
57. Sanjay, P.; Weerakoon, R.; Shaikh, I.A.; Bird, T.; Paily, A.; Yalamarthi, S. A 5-Year Analysis of Readmissions Following Elective Laparoscopic Cholecystectomy—Cohort Study. *Int. J. Surg.* **2011**, *9*, 52–54. [CrossRef]
58. Manguso, N.; Zuckerman, R. Identification and Management of Bile Duct Injuries. *Surg. Clin. N. Am.* **2024**, *104*, 1229–1236. [CrossRef]

59. Khan, M.H.; Howard, T.J.; Fogel, E.L.; Sherman, S.; McHenry, L.; Watkins, J.L.; Canal, D.F.; Lehman, G.A. Frequency of Biliary Complications after Laparoscopic Cholecystectomy Detected by ERCP: Experience at a Large Tertiary Referral Center. *Gastrointest. Endosc.* 2007, 65, 247–252. [CrossRef]
60. Harboe, K.M.; Bardram, L. The Quality of Cholecystectomy in Denmark: Outcome and Risk Factors for 20,307 Patients from the National Database. *Surg. Endosc.* 2011, 25, 1630–1641. [CrossRef]
61. Wu, Y.V.; Linehan, D.C. Bile Duct Injuries in the Era of Laparoscopic Cholecystectomies. *Surg. Clin. N. Am.* 2010, 90, 787–802. [CrossRef] [PubMed]
62. Rerknimitr, R.; Sherman, S.; Fogel, E.L.; Kalayci, C.; Lumeng, L.; Chalasani, N.; Kwo, P.; Lehman, G.A. Biliary Tract Complications after Orthotopic Liver Transplantation with Choledochocholedochostomy Anastomosis: Endoscopic Findings and Results of Therapy. *Gastrointest. Endosc.* 2002, 55, 224–231. [CrossRef]
63. Morelli, J.; Mulcahy, H.E.; Willner, I.R.; Baliga, P.; Chavin, K.D.; Patel, R.; Payne, M.; Cotton, P.B.; Hawes, R.; Reuben, A.; et al. Endoscopic Treatment of Post-Liver Transplantation Biliary Leaks with Stent Placement across the Leak Site. *Gastrointest. Endosc.* 2001, 54, 471–475. [CrossRef]
64. Oh, D.; Lee, S.K.; Song, T.J.; Park, D.H.; Lee, S.S.; Seo, D.-W.; Kim, M.-H. Endoscopic Management of Bile Leakage after Liver Transplantation. *Gut Liver* 2015, 9, 417–423. [CrossRef] [PubMed]
65. Spinn, M.P.; Patel, M.K.; Cotton, B.A.; Lukens, F.J. Successful Endoscopic Therapy of Traumatic Bile Leaks. *Case Rep. Gastroenterol.* 2013, 7, 56–62. [CrossRef] [PubMed]
66. Canena, J.; Horta, D.; Coimbra, J.; Meireles, L.; Russo, P.; Marques, I.; Ricardo, L.; Rodrigues, C.; Capela, T.; Carvalho, D.; et al. Outcomes of Endoscopic Management of Primary and Refractory Postcholecystectomy Biliary Leaks in a Multicentre Review of 178 Patients. *BMC Gastroenterol.* 2015, 15, 105. [CrossRef]
67. Kim, K.H.; Kim, T.N. Endoscopic Management of Bile Leakage after Cholecystectomy: A Single-Center Experience for 12 Years. *Clin. Endosc.* 2014, 47, 248. [CrossRef]
68. Chathadi, K.V.; Chandrasekhara, V.; Acosta, R.D.; Decker, G.A.; Early, D.S.; Eloubeidi, M.A.; Evans, J.A.; Faulx, A.L.; Fanelli, R.D.; Fisher, D.A.; et al. The Role of ERCP in Benign Diseases of the Biliary Tract. *Gastrointest. Endosc.* 2015, 81, 795–803. [CrossRef] [PubMed]
69. Dumonceau, J.-M.; Tringali, A.; Blero, D.; Devière, J.; Laugiers, R.; Heresbach, D.; Costamagna, G. Biliary Stenting: Indications, Choice of Stents and Results: European Society of Gastrointestinal Endoscopy (ESGE) Clinical Guideline. *Endoscopy* 2012, 44, 277–298. [CrossRef] [PubMed]
70. Quintini, D.; Rizzo, G.E.M.; Tarantino, I.; Sarzo, G.; Fantin, A.; Miraglia, R.; Maruzzelli, L.; Ligresti, D.; Carrozza, L.; Rancatore, G.; et al. Endoscopic or Combined Management of Post-Surgical Biliary Leaks: A Two-Center Recent Experience. *Surg. Endosc.* 2024, 38, 7233–7242. [CrossRef]
71. Tewani, S.K.; Turner, B.G.; Chuttani, R.; Pleskow, D.K.; Sawhney, M.S. Location of Bile Leak Predicts the Success of ERCP Performed for Postoperative Bile Leaks. *Gastrointest. Endosc.* 2013, 77, 601–608. [CrossRef] [PubMed]
72. Bhattacharjya, S.; Puleston, J.; Davidson, B.R.; Dooley, J.S. Outcome of Early Endoscopic Biliary Drainage in the Management of Bile Leaks after Hepatic Resection. *Gastrointest. Endosc.* 2003, 57, 526–530. [CrossRef] [PubMed]
73. Abbas, A.; Sethi, S.; Brady, P.; Taunk, P. Endoscopic Management of Postcholecystectomy Biliary Leak: When and How? A Nationwide Study. *Gastrointest. Endosc.* 2019, 90, 233–241.e1. [CrossRef]
74. Adler, D.G.; Papachristou, G.I.; Taylor, L.J.; McVay, T.; Birch, M.; Francis, G.; Zabolotsky, A.; Laique, S.N.; Hayat, U.; Zhan, T.; et al. Clinical Outcomes in Patients with Bile Leaks Treated via ERCP with Regard to the Timing of ERCP: A Large Multicenter Study. *Gastrointest. Endosc.* 2017, 85, 766–772. [CrossRef] [PubMed]
75. Desai, A.; Twohig, P.; Trujillo, S.; Dalal, S.; Kochhar, G.S.; Sandhu, D.S. Clinical Efficacy, Timing, and Outcomes of ERCP for Management of Bile Duct Leaks: A Nationwide Cohort Study. *Endosc. Int. Open* 2021, 09, E247–E252. [CrossRef]
76. Shaffer, E.A. Epidemiology and Risk Factors for Gallstone Disease: Has the Paradigm Changed in the 21st Century? *Curr. Gastroenterol. Rep.* 2005, 7, 132–140. [CrossRef]
77. Kratzer, W.; Mason, R.A.; Kächele, V. Prevalence of Gallstones in Sonographic Surveys Worldwide. *J. Clin. Ultrasound* 1999, 27, 1–7. [CrossRef]
78. Pisano, M.; Allievi, N.; Gurusamy, K.; Borzellino, G.; Cimbanassi, S.; Boerna, D.; Coccolini, F.; Tufo, A.; Di Martino, M.; Leung, J.; et al. 2020 World Society of Emergency Surgery Updated Guidelines for the Diagnosis and Treatment of Acute Calculus Cholecystitis. *World J. Emerg. Surg.* 2020, 15, 61. [CrossRef]
79. Barak, O.; Elazary, R.; Appelbaum, L.; Rivkind, A.; Almogy, G. Conservative Treatment for Acute Cholecystitis: Clinical and Radiographic Predictors of Failure. *Isr. Med. Assoc. J.* 2009, 11, 739–743.
80. Winbladh, A.; Gullstrand, P.; Svanvik, J.; Sandström, P. Systematic Review of Cholecystostomy as a Treatment Option in Acute Cholecystitis. *HPB* 2009, 11, 183–193. [CrossRef]
81. Gurusamy, K.S.; Kumar, Y.; Farouk, M.; Davidson, B.R. Methods of Management of High-Risk Surgical Patients with Acute Cholecystitis. In *Cochrane Database of Systematic Reviews*; Gurusamy, K.S., Ed.; John Wiley & Sons, Ltd.: Chichester, UK, 2008.

82. Campanile, F.C.; Pisano, M.; Coccolini, F.; Catena, F.; Agresta, F.; Ansaloni, L. Acute Cholecystitis: WSES Position Statement. *World J. Emerg. Surg.* **2014**, *9*, 58. [CrossRef]
83. Jang, W.S.; Lim, J.U.; Joo, K.R.; Cha, J.M.; Shin, H.P.; Joo, S.H. Outcome of Conservative Percutaneous Cholecystostomy in High-Risk Patients with Acute Cholecystitis and Risk Factors Leading to Surgery. *Surg. Endosc.* **2015**, *29*, 2359–2364. [CrossRef] [PubMed]
84. Sanjay, P.; Mittapalli, D.; Marioud, A.; White, R.D.; Ram, R.; Alijani, A. Clinical Outcomes of a Percutaneous Cholecystostomy for Acute Cholecystitis: A Multicentre Analysis. *HPB* **2013**, *15*, 511–516. [CrossRef] [PubMed]
85. Loozen, C.S.; van Santvoort, H.C.; van Duijvendijk, P.; Besselink, M.G.; Gouma, D.J.; Nieuwenhuijzen, G.A.; Kelder, J.C.; Donkervoort, S.C.; van Geloven, A.A.; Kruyt, P.M.; et al. Laparoscopic Cholecystectomy versus Percutaneous Catheter Drainage for Acute Cholecystitis in High Risk Patients (CHOCOLATE): Multicentre Randomised Clinical Trial. *BMJ* **2018**, *363*, k3965. [CrossRef] [PubMed]
86. Kozarek, R.A. Selective Cannulation of the Cystic Duct at Time of ERCP. *J. Clin. Gastroenterol.* **1984**, *6*, 37–40. [PubMed]
87. Itoi, T.; Coelho-Prabhu, N.; Baron, T.H. Endoscopic Gallbladder Drainage for Management of Acute Cholecystitis. *Gastrointest. Endosc.* **2010**, *71*, 1038–1045. [CrossRef]
88. Itoi, T.; Sofuni, A.; Itokawa, F.; Tsuchiya, T.; Kurihara, T.; Ishii, K.; Tsuji, S.; Ikeuchi, N.; Tsukamoto, S.; Takeuchi, M.; et al. Endoscopic Transpapillary Gallbladder Drainage in Patients with Acute Cholecystitis in Whom Percutaneous Transhepatic Approach Is Contraindicated or Anatomically Impossible (with Video). *Gastrointest. Endosc.* **2008**, *68*, 455–460. [CrossRef] [PubMed]
89. James, T.; Baron, T. EUS-Guided Gallbladder Drainage: A Review of Current Practices and Procedures. *Endosc. Ultrasound* **2019**, *8*, 28. [CrossRef]
90. Choi, J.-H.; Lee, S.; Choi, J.; Park, D.; Seo, D.-W.; Lee, S.; Kim, M.-H. Long-Term Outcomes after Endoscopic Ultrasonography-Guided Gallbladder Drainage for Acute Cholecystitis. *Endoscopy* **2014**, *46*, 656–661. [CrossRef] [PubMed]
91. Anderloni, A.; Buda, A.; Vieceli, F.; Khashab, M.A.; Hassan, C.; Repici, A. Endoscopic Ultrasound-Guided Transmural Stenting for Gallbladder Drainage in High-Risk Patients with Acute Cholecystitis: A Systematic Review and Pooled Analysis. *Surg. Endosc.* **2016**, *30*, 5200–5208. [CrossRef]
92. Stefanovic, S.; Adler, D.G.; Arlt, A.; Baron, T.H.; Binmoeller, K.F.; Bronswijk, M.; Bruno, M.J.; Chevaux, J.-B.; Crinò, S.F.; Degroote, H.; et al. International Consensus Recommendations for Safe Use of LAMS for On- and Off-Label Indications Using a Modified Delphi Process. *Am. J. Gastroenterol.* **2023**, *119*, 671–681. [CrossRef] [PubMed]
93. Teoh, A.Y.B.; Kitano, M.; Itoi, T.; Pérez-Miranda, M.; Ogura, T.; Chan, S.M.; Serna-Higuera, C.; Omoto, S.; Torres-Yuste, R.; Tsuichiya, T.; et al. Endosonography-Guided Gallbladder Drainage versus Percutaneous Cholecystostomy in Very High-Risk Surgical Patients with Acute Cholecystitis: An International Randomised Multicentre Controlled Superiority Trial (DRAC 1). *Gut* **2020**, *69*, 1085–1091. [CrossRef] [PubMed]
94. Mohan, B.P.; Khan, S.R.; Trakroo, S.; Ponnada, S.; Jayaraj, M.; Asokkumar, R.; Adler, D.G. Endoscopic Ultrasound-Guided Gallbladder Drainage, Transpapillary Drainage, or Percutaneous Drainage in High Risk Acute Cholecystitis Patients: A Systematic Review and Comparative Meta-Analysis. *Endoscopy* **2020**, *52*, 96–106. [CrossRef] [PubMed]
95. Marya, N.B.; Pawa, S.; Thiruvengadam, N.R.; Ngamruengphong, S.; Baron, T.H.; Bun Teoh, A.Y.; Bent, C.K.; Abidi, W.; Alipour, O.; Amateau, S.K.; et al. American Society for Gastrointestinal Endoscopy Guideline on the Role of Therapeutic EUS in the Management of Biliary Tract Disorders: Methodology and Review of Evidence. *Gastrointest. Endosc.* **2024**, *100*, e79–e135. [CrossRef]
96. van der Merwe, S.W.; van Wanrooij, R.L.J.; Bronswijk, M.; Everett, S.; Lakhtakia, S.; Rimbas, M.; Hucl, T.; Kunda, R.; Badaoui, A.; Law, R.; et al. Therapeutic Endoscopic Ultrasound: European Society of Gastrointestinal Endoscopy (ESGE) Guideline. *Endoscopy* **2022**, *54*, 185–205. [CrossRef] [PubMed]
97. Coccolini, F.; Cucinotta, E.; Mingoli, A.; Zago, M.; Altieri, G.; Biloslavo, A.; Caronna, R.; Cengeli, I.; Cicuttin, E.; Cirocchi, R.; et al. Acute Cholecystitis Management in High-Risk, Critically Ill, and Unfit-for-Surgery Patients: The Italian Society of Emergency Surgery and Trauma (SICUT) Guidelines. *Updates Surg.* **2024**, *76*, 331–343. [CrossRef]
98. Hakuta, R.; Hamada, T.; Nakai, Y.; Kogure, H.; Uchino, R.; Takahara, N.; Mizuno, S.; Suzuki, T.; Sato, T.; Takeda, T.; et al. No Association of Timing of Endoscopic Biliary Drainage with Clinical Outcomes in Patients with Non-Severe Acute Cholangitis. *Dig. Dis. Sci.* **2018**, *63*, 1937–1945. [CrossRef]
99. Inamdar, S.; Sejpal, D.V.; Ullah, M.; Trindade, A.J. Weekend vs. Weekday Admissions for Cholangitis Requiring an ERCP: Comparison of Outcomes in a National Cohort. *Am. J. Gastroenterol.* **2016**, *111*, 405–410. [CrossRef]
100. Tabibian, J.H.; Yang, J.D.; Baron, T.H.; Kane, S.V.; Enders, F.B.; Gostout, C.J. Weekend Admission for Acute Cholangitis Does Not Adversely Impact Clinical or Endoscopic Outcomes. *Dig. Dis. Sci.* **2016**, *61*, 53–61. [CrossRef] [PubMed]

Disclaimer/Publisher's Note: The statements, opinions and data contained in all publications are solely those of the individual author(s) and contributor(s) and not of MDPI and/or the editor(s). MDPI and/or the editor(s) disclaim responsibility for any injury to people or property resulting from any ideas, methods, instructions or products referred to in the content.

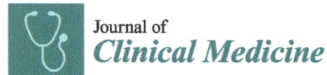 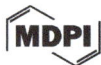

Review

Endoscopic-Ultrasound-Guided Radiofrequency Ablation for Pancreatic Tumors

Chiara Coluccio [1,*], Stefania Cappetta [2,3], Giovanna Romagnoli [1,3], Valentina Di Giorgio [2,3], Paolo Giuffrida [1], Stefano Fabbri [1], Carlo Fabbri [1] and Cecilia Binda [1]

1 Gastroenterology and Digestive Endoscopy Unit, Forlì-Cesena Hospitals, 47121 Romagna, Italy
2 IRCCS Azienda Ospedaliero-Universitaria di Bologna, Policlinico S. Orsola, 40138 Bologna, Italy
3 Department of Medical and Surgical Sciences, University of Bologna, 40138 Bologna, Italy
* Correspondence: chiara.coluccio@auslromagna.it

Abstract: Endoscopic ultrasound (EUS)-guided radiofrequency ablation (RFA) is a promising minimally invasive technique for the treatment of pancreatic lesions. This review first focuses on the technical aspects in EUS-RFA: the procedure typically employs EUS probes with integrated radiofrequency electrodes, enabling accurate targeting and ablation of pancreatic lesions. Different types of RFA devices, monopolar and bipolar energy delivery systems, are discussed, along with considerations for optimal ablation, including energy settings, procedure time, and pre- and post-procedural management. This paper presents a comprehensive literature review of EUS-RFA applied to both solid and cystic pancreatic lesions, including functioning and non-functioning pancreatic neuroendocrine tumors (pNETs), pancreatic cystic lesions (PCLs), pancreatic ductal adenocarcinoma (PDAC), and pancreatic metastases (PMs), discussing current evidence on safety, efficacy, clinical outcomes, and adverse events (AEs). EUS-RFA is an emerging technique with expanding potential for the treatment of both benign and malignant conditions; however, further studies are needed to better define patient selection criteria, assess long-term benefits, and establish definitive indications for its use.

Keywords: endoscopic ultrasound; radiofrequency; ablation; locoregional therapy; pancreas

1. Introduction

The increase in diagnoses of solid and cystic lesions of the pancreas is substantial worldwide, due to the improved diagnostic performance of cross-sectional imaging machines and the aging population.

At present, surgery is the treatment of choice for most pancreatic lesions, both for malignant forms such as pancreatic ductal adenocarcinoma (PDAC) as well as for benign forms with non-negligible evolutionary potential or for symptomatic benign lesions; this is the case for neuroendocrine tumors (pNETs) and pancreatic cystic lesions (PCLs). Although in high-volume centers, mortality associated with pancreatic surgery has been reduced over the years, surgery-related complications are still very common (up to 50% of patients), with the most frequent and feared being postoperative pancreatic fistula (POPF), which has an incidence ranging from 3% to 45% in specialized centers [1,2]. In addition, many pancreatic lesions with a low risk of malignancy often require long-term surveillance, leading to increased healthcare costs.

In the last twenty years, the endoscopic ultrasound (EUS) technique has increasingly evolved in an interventional and therapeutic sense, expanding its initial purely diagnostic purpose.

EUS-guided radiofrequency ablation (EUS-RFA) is a novel minimally invasive technique for the treatment of pancreatic focal lesions, which produces a high-resolution, real-time image of the target area and ablates lesions through the application of thermal energy via radiofrequency. This results in irreversible cell injury, and simultaneous control supports high accuracy, minimizing the effect on surrounding healthy tissue [3].

Among the thermoablative technologies, RFA is one of the most widely used in the field of oncology (i.e., hepatocellular carcinoma); however, its application for the treatment of focal lesions of the pancreas is relatively new and not yet fully understood. In summary, a high-frequency alternating current generates high thermal energy (60–100 °C), and thus cells undergo protein denaturation, leading to coagulative necrosis [4]. Through a mechanism of indirect tissue damage, RFA also promotes the activation of antitumor immunity by remodeling the cancer microenvironment, inflammatory cytokines' release, dendritic cells' activation, and CD4+ and CD8+ T cells' response [5].

The aim of this review was to collect literature data on the application of EUS-RFA, to both clarify technical aspects of the procedure itself, by grasping the common points and differences in the various published studies, and to gather information on all possible indications for EUS-RFA and the expected results from its employment in clinical practice.

2. Focus on the Technique

In 1999, Nahum Goldberg S. et al. first published the results of applying EUS-RFA with modified 19-gauge needle electrodes on healthy pancreatic tail tissue from 13 Yorkshire pigs using a transgastric approach, demonstrating that the method was technically feasible and safe [6].

Since then, the interest in this technique has gradually grown, leading to the production of dedicated devices and the publication of studies in animal models and later in humans. However, there is still no formal technical protocol accepted by scientific societies for EUS-RFA, and thus the technical details must be gathered from experts' opinions developed in recent years.

The procedure is performed under deep sedation or general anesthesia with the patient positioned in left lateral decubitus. A linear-array echoendoscope with a 3.8 mm operator channel is advanced along the upper digestive tract to visualize the target lesion and, after exclusion of vascular structures by color Doppler imaging, the device is inserted into the lesion under EUS guidance with a transgastric or transduodenal approach (bulb or second part of the duodenum). The generator is turned on and the wattage set, and immediately afterwards, the endosonographer proceeds with ablation. Then, the tool can be repositioned in another part of the lesion to perform further ablation and the procedure repeated until the entire lesion is covered.

2.1. EUSRA™ Endoscopic UltraSound Guided Radiofrequency Ablation Electrode (TaeWoong Medical, Goyang-si, Gyeonggi-do, Republic of Korea)

2.1.1. Description of Device

The EUSRA™ electrode is a modified 19 G needle for RFA consisting of a 140 cm flexible metal wire coated with an insulating cover, except for the exposed end portion of 5 mm, 7 mm, or 10 mm in length, and ending with a tapered, sharp tip capable of releasing energy in the form of heat (monopolar device).

The VIVA Combo™ RF Generator System (STARmed, TaeWoong Medical, Goyang-si, Gyeonggi-do, Republic of Korea), consisting of two components, is also required to carry out the procedure:

- VIVA Combo™ RF Generator, a current generator that operates at a frequency of 480 KHz, allowing the power setting to be varied from 0 to 200 watts, enables real-time monitoring of temperature (5–95 °C) and impendence (10–800 Ohms) of the tissue. It is connected via a cable to the upper end of the EUSRA™. Two grounding pads must be attached to the patient's skin before the procedure.

- VIVA Pump is an internal cooling system that, through two tubes connected to the handle of the needle, allows cold saline solution (0 °C) to be pumped into the needle (inflow tube), which circulates inside and then is expelled warm through the second tube (outflow tube) into an external container. Circulation of cold saline solution inside the needle allows continuous cooling of the active needle tip, preventing tissue charring [7,8]. Tissue carbonization is indeed associated with increasing tissue impedance and reaching an ablation plateau with disruption of coagulative necrosis; hence, the cooling system should improve performance by providing ablation of a larger volume of tissue.

The ablated volume depends both on device and preset characteristics (wattage setting, length of active tip, and application time) and on intrinsic characteristics of the tissue (temperature and humidity). Barret et al. compared two ad hoc devices for EUS-RFA on the pancreas in a porcine model; the data collected suggest using EUSRA™ at 30 W for 15 s of application to achieve an ablation volume of 302 mm^3, corresponding to an oval section of about 7 mm in diameter [9].

2.1.2. Technical Features

EUSRA™ is positioned directly inside the target lesion, likewise a fine needle aspiration (FNA) needle. After setting up the generator, the operator can control the start and end of the ablation with a foot switch.

2.2. Habib™ EUS RFA Endoscopic Ultrasound Radiofrequency Ablation Catheter (EMcision Ltd., London, UK)

2.2.1. Description of Device

The Habib™ EUS RFA is a "through-the-needle" device no longer commercially available since 2018; nonetheless, it deserves a mention as it has been used in several pioneering papers for EUS-RFA. The Habib™ EUS RFA is a flexible catheter with a diameter of 1 Fr (0.33 mm) and length of 220 cm; its distal end consists of an electrode with a length of 10 or 20 mm, and can be inserted through a 19 G or 22 G FNA needle. The probe is connected via an adapter cable to a regular electrosurgical generator with no cooling system. As a monopolar device, the attachment of a grounding pad on the patient is necessary.

2.2.2. Technical Features

After proper visualization of the pancreatic gland, a 19 G or 22 G FNA needle is advanced within the target lesion in a deep location. The stylet is removed, and the Habib probe is cautiously advanced inside the needle until resistance is sensed. At this point, the needle is slowly retracted a few centimeters to expose the active tip of the catheter, to avoid contact between the electrode and the metal part of the needle, representing a delicate phase for the endoscopist in seeking to maintain the position.

2.3. Hybrid-Therm® Probe HTP (ERBE, Tübingen, Germany)

Description of Device

Contrary to the description above, the HTP is a bipolar RF probe that combines cryotechnology with conventional thermoablation. The probe is fully covered with a protective tube 150 mm long; the stiff and pointed distal end is the electrically active part, with a diameter of 1.8 mm and a length of 20 mm. Connector cables for the current generator (VIO 300D, ERBE) and the internal carbon dioxide cooling system (ERBOKRYO

CA System, ERBE) branch off from the proximal side of the handle. The wattage setting and gas pressure can be controlled independently. Integration of cryotechnology is intended to increase the effectiveness of RF by decreasing the power of the generator and thus reducing the risk of damage to the tissue.

As already mentioned, there is currently no standardization of the procedure and the setup of equipment. Therefore, many questions remain open in this regard.

2.4. Electrode Insertion and End of Ablation

Differences are reported in the literature regarding the criterion used for inserting the electrode within the lesion; some echoendoscopists place it directly in the center of the mass [10], while others position the echogenic tip at the far end of the lesion [11–13]. In another technique, the echogenic tip is inserted first in the distal right portion of the lesion, and then the process is repeated in the left portion [14]. To perform multiple applications, the needle can be retracted slightly to repeat the procedure on the same trajectory, or a new puncture can be made to insert the needle at a different angle [15,16].

In most early studies, the RFA procedure was considered complete when echogenic bubbles began to appear around the needle tip and progressively covered the entire lesion after one or more applications. It is currently assumed that to increase the accuracy of thermoablation, another useful element to evaluate at this stage is the bioimpedance, continuously tracked by the generator, because a sudden rise in impedance may be an indicator of early tissue charring. Scopelliti et al. [8] considered a value of 500 Ohms adequate to end the ablation; concurrently, Barthet et al. [17] stopped the procedure when the impedance settled in the range of 100–500 Ohms and white bubbles appeared on the screen.

2.5. Power Setting and Application Time

A variety of wattage settings have been used on the pancreas in recent studies, both due to the technical specifications of the devices and the decisions of the operators.

The Habib™ EUS RFA has been described with a power range from 5 W to 25 W [11]; however, the most widely used is 10 W or ERBE SOFT COAG mode effect 4, with an application time between 90 and 120 s.

Using an early prototype 19 G EUSRA™, Lakhtakia et al. [12] published the results of three cases of patients with insulinoma (maximum diameter 22 mm) treated with EUS-RFA, using a power setting of 50 W for an application time of 10–15 s and a mean number of applications of 5. A similar technique was used in Song et al. on six patients with PDAC with an average diameter of 38 mm [14]. Differently, Crinò et al. [7] proposed a technical approach with EUSRA™, involving a wattage setting of 30 W for a mean application time of 50 s (not determined in advance) and a mean number of applications of 1.5 in seven cases of PDAC and one case of metastasis from clear-cell renal cell carcinoma. Reducing the power and extending the application time allowed the ablated volume to be increased as a result of slower thermal diffusion, thus reducing the number of applications and the need to reinsert the electrode into the tissue.

A recent ex vivo study on RFA conducted on 15 fresh surgical samples of patients with PDAC treated with neoadjuvant therapy failed to establish a correlation between power setting group (10 W, 30 W, and 50 W) and the mean short-axis diameter of coagulative necrosis, as determined by two blind expert pathologists [18].

In contrast, the Hybrid-Therm® Probe was set at 18 W power with a carbon dioxide gas pressure of 650 psi and an application time in the range of 240 to 480 s on PDAC lesions from 20 mm to more than 30 mm in diameter [19,20].

3. Pre- and Post-Procedural Issues

3.1. Antibiotic Use and Acute Post-Ablation Pancreatitis Prophylaxis

3.1.1. Antibiotic Prophylaxis and Rectal Non-Steroidal Anti-Inflammatory Drugs (NSAIDs)

Evidence on the usefulness of antibiotic prophylaxis in therapeutic EUS, particularly in EUS-RFA, is limited. At this juncture, the lack of a clear protocol has left the choice up to the operators; in most of the papers, the administration is reported of peri-procedural antibiotic prophylaxis with broad-spectrum antibiotics (ceftriaxone, amoxicillin/clavulanic acid). Barthet et al. [21] had not planned on using any prophylaxis; however, two moderate–severe post-procedural adverse events (AEs) occurred in the first two patients treated: an acute pancreatitis with early infected necrosis and a small bowel perforation with retroperitoneal fluid collection requiring surgery. These two cases led to the modification of the study protocol to include the administration of antibiotic prophylaxis and rectal diclofenac, producing a significant decrease in adverse events (from 13.79% to 7.4%).

Another issue concerns the use of NSAIDs as a preventive measure for acute post-ablation pancreatitis, following the recommendations for acute post-ERCP pancreatitis [22]. The largest multicenter retrospective analysis we have available [23], reporting data from 116 EUS-RFA sessions, showed that antibiotic prophylaxis was administered in 85.3% of cases and that rectal NSAIDs were administered in 88.8%. This study attempted to identify risk factors for EUS-RFA-related adverse events by univariate and multivariate analysis; with the limitations and potential bias of a retrospective study, the analyses failed to identify a potential protective action of antibiotic prophylaxis and rectal NSAIDs

3.1.2. Placement of Pancreatic Stent

The role of prophylactic placement of a pancreatic stent for lesions close to the main pancreatic duct (MPD) to prevent post-ablation pancreatitis remains controversial due to the procedure's inherent risk of pancreatitis. In fact, although in most cases, post-ERCP pancreatitis is mild, its overall incidence ranges from 3.5% to 9.7% and increases to about 15% in high-risk patients [24].

Therefore, there is debate about the minimum distance from the MPD for RFA to be considered safe, beyond which the benefits of pancreatic stent placement outweigh the risks. In this case, the French study showed a significant increase in the incidence of AEs (OR, 4.1) in lesions in close proximity to the MPD ($\leq$1 mm) [23]. Another large multicenter retrospective analysis by Crinò et al. [25] showed that in eight of nine cases of post-RFA acute pancreatitis, the distance between the lesion and the MPD was $\leq$2 mm, and although it did not reach statistical significance in a univariate analysis of risk factors for AEs, it remains an indispensable preprocedural parameter.

3.2. Fluid Component Suction Before EUS-RFA on PCLs and Cystic pNETs

In PCLs undergoing EUS-RFA, operators frequently reported making the choice to aspirate the liquid component using an FNA needle before the ablation, preserving only a thin layer of fluid. The purpose would be to reduce the overall volume of the lesion and avoid excessive application of current to the liquid component, thus reducing the risk of thermal damage and post-procedural infection [26]. However, it remains a debated practice due to the increased procedural time, number of passes and punctures, and also the potential reduced visibility of mural nodules and enhanced septa.

3.3. Role of Contrast Harmonic EUS (CH-EUS) and Follow-Up

CH-EUS has emerged as an evidence-based auxiliary diagnostic tool to optimize the characterization of solid lesions, improve the staging of malignancies, and target tissue acquisition. Recently, there has been a growing interest in the potential impact of CH-EUS in interventional procedures, including EUS-guided tumor ablation. Choi et al. [27] investigated its use to assist ablation, providing a delineated real-time visualization of the vascular lesion pattern, as well as its application in post-procedural monitoring. Technical success was achieved in all 19 patients (14 pNETs, 2 PCLs, 2 adrenal adenomas, and 1 adrenal metastasis from hepatocellular carcinoma); after approximately one week from the first RFA session, all patients underwent CH-EUS to check the treatment response, and 12 patients had residual tumor and therefore underwent further RFA sessions. At the one-year follow-up, 68.4% (13 patients) had a complete radiological response (CR). Borrelli de Andreis et al. [28] proposed CH-EUS-assisted RFA in 10 patients with insulinomas, injecting a new contrast bolus at the end of the ablation to verify vascularity, so that further RFA applications could be performed in the same session. At the 3-month follow-up, all patients had CR, and up to the end of follow-up (average 19.5 months), complete regression of symptoms was confirmed.

The timing of post-ablation surveillance with EUS or a CT scan or MRI is not supported by evidence; it could be useful to perform a first close work-up, within 1–3 months, to assess whether more RFA sessions are needed (see Figure 1).

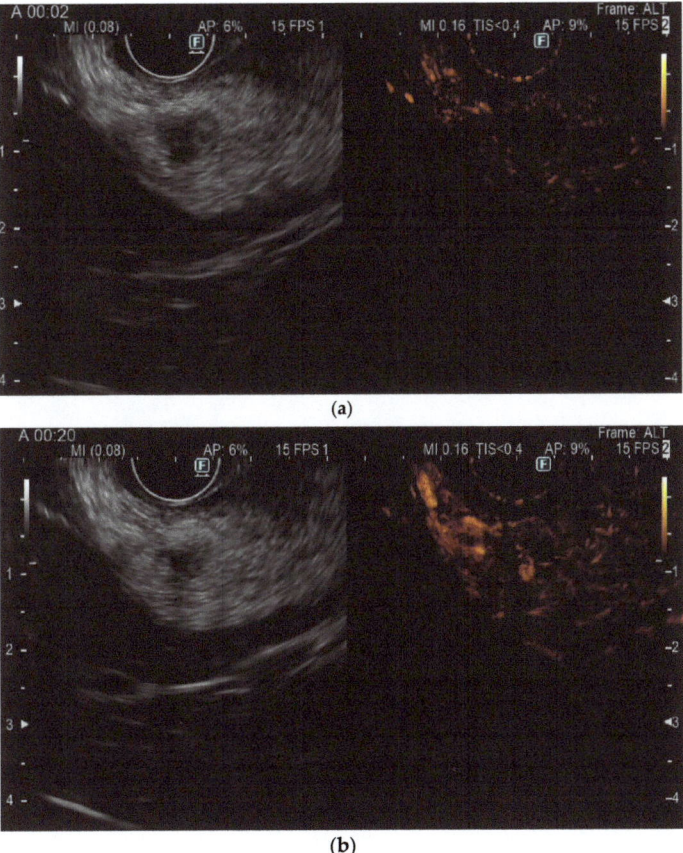

Figure 1. CH-EUS six-month follow-up in an asymptomatic patient after EUS-RFA on an insulinoma of the uncinate. (**a**) Time 0 corresponding to the injection of SonoVue®, (**b**) arterial phase with suspicion of millimetric residual disease, hypervascular in the image.

4. EUS-RFA in Pancreatic Tumors

EUS-RFA is rapidly emerging as a cutting-edge technique in the endoscopic community, offering a minimally invasive solution applicable to a variety of pancreatic conditions. The best indications for the technique are still being studied, as are the characteristics of the ideal patient. The developing indications, characteristics of enrolled patients in the current literature, and mean lesion sizes are summarized in Table 1.

The most encouraging results come from the small (maximum size 20 mm) pNETs, particularly from the secerning variant. In contrast, the application of EUS-RFA in PCLs and PDAC is still at an early stage of study. As the field is continuing to evolve, the following section will delve into the different types of pancreatic lesions, solid and cystic, where EUS-RFA is gaining increasing attention for its potential application.

Table 1. Summary of developing indications, patient's characteristics (considering MDT discussion), and mean lesion size reported in the available literature *.

	Indications	Characteristics of Patients	Mean Lesion Size (mm)
pNETs	Treatment for F-pNETs (insulinoma)	Elderly, unfit, or refusing surgery	13.8
	Treatment for NF-pNETs (G1/G2 grading)	Elderly, unfit, or refusing surgery/surveillance	15.2
	Combined treatment (surgery + EUS-RFA) in multifocal pNETs in MEN	MDT discussion	-
PCLs	Treatment for PCLs	Elderly, unfit, or refusing surgery	
	Ablation of mural nodules in IPMNs and MCNs	Elderly, unfit, or refusing surgery	34.2
	Cytovolumetric reduction in symptoms of compression	Elderly, unfit, or refusing surgery	
PDAC	Local treatment for cytovolumetric reduction in combination or not with CT	Locally advanced PDAC, unfit for surgery or with local progression after the first line of CT, or unfit for CT Metastatic PDAC	39.5
PMs	Local treatment for oligometastatic disease with PM	Stable oligometastatic disease, elderly, unfit, or refusing surgery	17.5

* The average size values correspond to the weighted average of the values given in Tables 2–6. CT: chemotherapy; IPMNs: intraductal papillary mucinous neoplasms; MCNs: mucinous cystic neoplasms; MDT: multidisciplinary team; MEN: multiple endocrine neoplasia; PCLs: pancreatic cystic lesions; PDAC: pancreatic ductal adenocarcinoma; PM: pancreatic metastasis; pNETs: pancreatic neuroendoscrine tumors.

4.1. EUS-RFA in pNETs

pNETs can be both functional and non-functional. Functional pNETs (F-pNETs) are marked by a clinical syndrome related to abnormal levels of biologically activated hormones secreted by the tumor mass. On the other hand, non-functional pNETs (NF-pNETs) secrete hormone variants that are inactive or at low levels, and hence they are not associated with symptoms.

4.1.1. F-pNETs

The most common digestive functional NETs are insulinomas and gastrinomas; the first is almost exclusively pancreatic, with an incidence of up to 32 cases 10^6 of inhabitants/year and malignant in less than 10% of cases, while the latter is pancreatic in 25% of the cases, with an overall incidence of up to 21 cases 10^6 of inhabitants/year and malignant in 60–90% of cases [29,30].

Currently, the treatment of choice for localized pancreatic insulinomas and gastrinomas is surgical resection. The knowledge of EUS-RFA on gastrinomas is limited to very few reports and with questionable clinical success, so its use should be limited to a trial setting. Otherwise, for insulinomas, the European Neuroendocrine Tumor Society (ENETS) has recently published a paper in which EUS-RFA is indicated as a possible treatment for insulinomas ≤2 cm in patients unfit for surgery in experienced centers, although with a low grade of recommendation [31].

Most of the available literature (reported in Table 2) on EUS-RFA in F-pNETs is related to case reports and case series with a small number of treated lesions. The first experience with EUSRA™ is that of Lakhtakia et al. [12], with a published case series of three symptomatic insulinomas successfully treated in a single session of EUS-RFA (mean size 17.3 mm) and with a mean number of applications of five. No post-procedural adverse events occurred, and in all three cases, a rapid improvement of hypoglycemia was observed, with glycemic values settling into a normal range within 24 h after the treatment.

In the same year, Waung et al. [32] also published a case report of an insulinoma (tumor size 18 mm) successfully treated with Habib™ EUS RFA following three sessions of RFA. Choi et al. in 2018 published a prospective study on EUS-RFA treatment of PCLs and pNETs, where a 12 mm insulinoma of the pancreatic head was successfully treated at 13 months of follow-up; however, in a 2020 study update, the same patient had experienced a recurrence at month 19 of follow-up [13,27]. To our knowledge, the largest case series is that presented by Crinò et al. [25] in a retrospective multicenter analysis collecting data from 89 patients with insulinoma who underwent EUS-RFA. In this study, the EUS-guided technique was feasible and safe, with a much lower rate of adverse events (AEs) compared to the control group undergoing surgery (procedure-related AEs: 18% vs. 61.8%). Of 89 patients, 16.9% experienced a recurrence of symptoms within one year after the procedure, and yet most of them were effectively treated with a new session of thermoablation (see Figure 2).

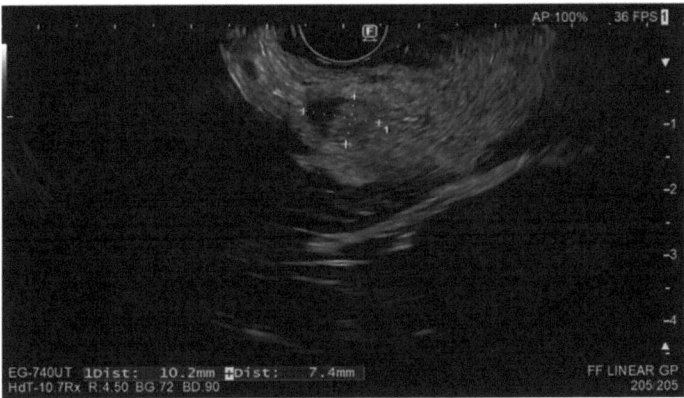

Figure 2. Six-month follow-up in an asymptomatic patient after EUS-RFA on an insulinoma of the uncinate: oval-shaped area with blurred margins and inhomogeneous hypo- and hyperechogenic structure.

When comparing the papers, we found that most of the adverse effects related to EUS-RFA were mild to moderate (see Section 5). The only reported case of post-EUS-RFA death was that of a 97-year-old patient with multiple comorbidities, who developed an infected retrogastric collection; the patient refused further invasive interventions, so the collection was not drained and the patient died despite the best supportive care [33].

EUS-RFA is feasible and safe; it could represent a breakthrough in the treatment of F-pNETs, and promising data are reported in the literature. A recently published systematic review and meta-analysis that analyzed the results of nineteen studies with 101 F-pNETs showed a clinical success rate of 95.1%, with an overall AE rate of 17.8% [34]. Nevertheless, prospective randomized controlled trials with longer follow-ups are needed to confirm these records and to assess whether refinement of the endoscopic technique over the years will result in a reduction in the number of recurrences.

Table 2. Results from studies reporting EUS-RFA on F-pNETs *.

Author, Year	Study Design	N. of Patients/N. of F-pNET	Tumor Size (Mean, mm) and Location **	Device	N. of RFA Sessions/ Lesion **	Mean Time of Application (s)/Mean N. of Applications **	Technical Success (%) **	Follow-Up (Months) **	Clinical Success (%) **
Lesmana [35], 2024	Case series	3/3	27.7 Head: 2 Body: 1	EUSRA™, TaeWoong (30–40 W)	NR	10–50/15	100	6–12	100
Biermann [36], 2024	Case series	3/3	14 Head: 2 Tail: 1	EUSRA™, TaeWoong (20 W)	1	NR/6.7	100	12.7	100
Napoléon [23], 2023	Retrospective, multicenter	16/16	15 NR	EUSRA™, TaeWoong (50 W)	1.12	25/3	97	13	87.5
Crinò [25], 2023	Retrospective, multicenter	89/89	13.4 Head: 34 Body: 39 Tail: 16	EUSRA™, TaeWoong (10–50 W)	1.12	NR/3.2	100	23	95.5
Borrelli de Andreis [28], 2023	Retrospective, monocenter	10/10	11.9 Head: 3 Body: 3 Tail: 4	EUSRA™, TaeWoong (25–50 W)	1.1	10/6.6	100	19.5	100
Gugger [37], 2023	Case report	1/1 (somatostatinoma)	9 Tail	EUSRA™, TaeWoong (10 W)	1	NR/3	100	10	100
Rizzatti [38], 2023	Prospective, multicenter	30/30	12.1 Head: 15 Body: 10 Tail: 5	EUSRA™, TaeWoong (50 W)	1.16	NR	100	12	100
Figueiredo Ferreira [39], 2022	Prospective, multicenter	13/13	14.4 NR	EUSRA™, TaeWoong (50 W)	1	NR/3	100	12	100
Marx [33], 2022	Prospective, multicenter	7/7	13.3 Head: 1 Body: 6	EUSRA™, TaeWoong (50 W)	1	NR/4	100	21	85.7
Chang [40], 2022	Case report	1/1	12 Head	EUSRA™, TaeWoong (50 W)	1	10/2	100	18	100
Rossi [41], 2022	Prospective, monocenter	3/3	16 Head: 3 Body: 3 Tail: 4	EUSRA™, TaeWoong (30 W)	1	11.8/3.3	100	22	100
Younis [42], 2022	Prospective, monocenter	1/1	8 Tail	EUSRA™, TaeWoong (50 W)	1	NR/6	100	7	100
Nabi [43], 2022	Retrospective, monocenter	12/15	17 Head: 6 Body: 8 Tail: 1	EUSRA™, TaeWoong	NR	NR	100	41	100
De Nucci [44], 2020	Prospective, monocenter	5/5	12.8 Body: 3 Tail: 2	EUSRA™, TaeWoong (20 W)	1	15–25/2.2	100	12	100
Lakhtakia [45], 2020	Prospective, monocenter	10/13	11.5 NR	EUSRA™, TaeWoong	NR	NR	100	10–64	100
Kluz [46], 2020	Case report	1/1	9 Head	EUSRA™, TaeWoong (50 W)	1	10/3	100	NR	NR
Furnica [47], 2020	Retrospective, monocenter	4/4	12 Head: 2 Body: 1 Tail: 1	EUSRA™, TaeWoong (50 W)	1	NR/2	100	22	100
Jonica [48], 2020	Case report	1/1	22 Body	EUSRA™, TaeWoong (30 W)	1	20/5	100	6	100
Borwn [49], 2020	Case report	1/1	18 Head	EUSRA™, TaeWoong (20 W)	1	15/NR	100	8	100
Oleinikov [50], 2019	Retrospective, multicenter	7/9	14.8 Head: 7 Body: 2	EUSRA™, TaeWoong (10–50 W)	0.78	5–12/3–10	100	9.7	100

Table 2. *Cont.*

Author, Year	Study Design	N. of Patients/N. of F-pNET	Tumor Size (Mean, mm) and Location **	Device	N. of RFA Sessions/ Lesion **	Mean Time of Application (s)/Mean N. of Applications **	Technical Success (%) **	Follow-Up (Months) **	Clinical Success (%) **
Kandula [51], 2019	Case report	1/1	17 Head	NR	1	NR	100	6	100
Choi [13], 2018	Prospective, monocenter	1/1	12 Head	EUSRA™, TaeWoong (50 W)	1	NR/3	100	13	100
Gueneau de Mussy [52], 2018	Case report	1/1	12 Body	EUSRA™, TaeWoong	1	NR	100	2	100
Thosani [53], 2018	Retrospective, multicenter	3/3 (including 1 VIPoma)	23 NR	NR	1.6	NR/4.6	100	5	100
Goyal [54], 2017	Case series	1/1	7.5 Body	Habib™ EUS RFA (10 W)	1	120/3–5	100	NR	100
Bas-Cutrina [15], 2017	Case report	1/1	10 Body	Habib™ EUS RFA (10 W)	1	120/3	100	10	100
Waung [32], 2016	Case report	1/1	18 Head	Habib™ EUS RFA (10 W)	3	93.6/8.3	100	10	100
Lakhtakia [12], 2016	Case series	3/3	17.3 Head: 3	EUSRA™, TaeWoong (50 W)	1	12.5/5	100	12	100

* Table legend: N. of RFA sessions/lesion expresses the ratio of the number of total procedures to the total number of pancreatic lesions. If equal to 1, the number of procedures is equal to the number of lesions; if >1, it indicates that some lesions are subjected to more than one session; if <1, it indicates that more lesions in the same patient are treated in the same session. Mean time of application (s) indicates the mean time per single application, expressed in seconds, to achieve the desired effect from ablation. Mean N. of applications indicates the mean number of applications needed to obtain complete treatment of the mass. NR: not reported. ** In studies involving more than one type of pancreatic lesion, the overall data were reported when it was not possible to extract the specific data per lesion group.

4.1.2. NF-pNETs

The majority of pNETs, ranging from 60% to 90%, are non-functional [30]. Compared to their functional counterparts, NF-pNETs locate more frequently at the level of the pancreatic head and appear larger at diagnosis, with a more aggressive histopathology and more advanced stage of disease (like lymph node involvement or liver metastases) [55]. The gold standard for treatment is once again surgery, but with a non-negligible complication rate.

Due to the technological advancement of imaging techniques, the incidental diagnosis of pNETs is becoming increasingly frequent. These lesions are not biologically homogeneous; indeed, small and well differentiated ones often have an indolent behavior, with a low risk of malignant progression. While for NF-pNETs ≥ 2 cm, surgery represents the first-choice treatment [56], the best approach for NF-pNETs ≤ 2 cm remains controversial, as it is increasingly challenging to justify the risks of major surgery in these cases, with practitioners leaning towards active surveillance [57]. In this context, EUS-RFA could have a role as an alternative treatment; however, studies in the literature are scarce, restricted to a small number of patients, and not randomized. Another limitation is the difficult comparability of the results, due to different interpretations of the concept of a 'radiological response' among authors: univocally CR corresponds to 100% disappearance/necrosis of the lesion, demonstrated by an imaging technique; however, the definitions of a 'Partial Response' (PR) and 'No Response' (NoR) are variable. According to Barthet et al. [17,21], Figueiredo Ferreira et al. [39], and Younis et al. [42], a reduction of between 50% and

100% in the maximum diameter corresponds to a PR and a reduction <50% refers to NoR; according to Napoléon et al. [23], a PR corresponds to a reduction in the lesion volume of between 75% and 95% and NoR to a reduction <75%. Other authors, such as Marx et al. [58] and Choi et al. [13,27], do not give a quantitative definition of the radiological response, referring generally to the absence or persistence of enhancing tissue on the tumor site. This limitation is also found in studies on PCLs and PDAC. Among the most relevant papers, the multicenter prospective study by Marx et al. achieved a 92.6% CR in 27 NF-G1-pNETs at 15.7 months of follow-up, with two patients requiring more than one session to obtain this result; four patients developed acute post-procedural pancreatitis, requiring endoscopic or surgical maneuvers in three cases (see paragraph 8) [58]. Rizzatti et al. [38] published data on 32 NF-pNETs (median size 16.8 mm) successfully treated with single or multiple sessions of EUS-RFA with a 100% CR one year after the procedure and reported only mild AEs. In the retrospective analysis by Napoléon et al. [23], a CR of 71.7% was reported for 48 NF-pNETs (mostly graded G1) at 13 months of follow-up.

The longest follow-up was reported by Barthet et al. (45.6 months on average), where 12 of 14 NF-pNETs went on to reach CR at the 1-year follow-up, although 1 of these had a late recurrence at the 3-year follow-up. The other 2 of 14 experienced NoR at the 1-year follow-up: one evolved into metastatic disease, while the other had disappeared on both a CT scan and EUS at the 53-month follow-up. Thus, at 3 years, 85.6% achieved a CR (12 of 14 lesions) [17,21].

The literature data on EUS-RFA of NF-pNETs are summarized in Table 3.

Table 3. Results from studies reporting EUS-RFA on NF-pNETs *.

Author, Year	Study Design	N. of Patients/N. of NF-pNET	Tumor Size (Mean, mm) and Location **	Device	N. of RFA Sessions/ Lesion **	Mean Time of Application (s)/Mean N. of Applications **	Technical Success (%) **	Follow-Up (Months) **	Radiologic Response
Napoléon [23], 2023	Retrospective, multicenter	NR/48	15 NR	EUSRA™, TaeWoong (50 W)	1.12	25/3	97	13	CR: 33/48 (71.7%) PR: 12/48 (26.1%) NoR: 1/48 (2.2%) Missing data 2
Rizzatti [38], 2023	Prospective, multicenter	32/32	16.8 Head: 8 Body: 15 Tail: 9	EUSRA™, TaeWoong (50 W)	1.25	NR	100	12	CR: 24/24 (100%) Missing data 8
Figueiredo Ferreira [39], 2022	Prospective, multicenter	9/10	14.4 NR	EUSRA™, TaeWoong (50 W)	0.86	NR/3	100	9.6	CR: 6/11 (54.6%) PR: 3/11 (27.2%) NoR 2/11 (18.2%) Results F-pNET+ NF-pNET
Marx [58], 2022	Prospective, multicenter	27/27	14 Head: 8 Body: 8 Tail: 11	EUSRA™, TaeWoong (30–50 W)	1.15	10–12/1–5	100	15.7	CR: 25/27 (92.6%) NoR: 2/27 (7.4%)
Younis [42], 2022	Prospective, monocenter	6/6	8.9 Head: 2 Body: 4	EUSRA™, TaeWoong (50 W)	1	NR/2.7	100	7	CR: 4/6 (66.7%) NoR: 2/6 (33.3%)
Lesmana [59], 2022–2024	Case report	1/1	35 Head	EUSRA™, TaeWoong	1	NR	100	36	CR of the solid part, non-significant shrinkage of the cystic part

Table 3. Cont.

Author, Year	Study Design	N. of Patients/N. of NF-pNET	Tumor Size (Mean, mm) and Location **	Device	N. of RFA Sessions/ Lesion **	Mean Time of Application (s)/Mean N. of Applications **	Technical Success (%) **	Follow-Up (Months) **	Radiologic Response
De Nucci [44], 2020	Prospective, monocenter	5/6	16 Head: 3 Body: 2 Tail: 2	EUSRA™, TaeWoong (20 W)	0.83	15–25/2.4	100	12	CR: 5/5 (100%)
Barthet [17,21], 2019–2021	Prospective, multicenter	12/14	13.4 Head: 3 Body: 6 Tail: 5	EUSRA™, TaeWoong (50 W)	NR	20–45/NR	100	45.6	CR: 12/14 (85.7%) NoR: 2/14 (14.3%) Including 1 late recurrence
Oleinikov [50], 2019	Retrospective, multicenter	11/16	14.2 Head: 8 Body: 6 Tail: 2	EUSRA™, TaeWoong (10–50 W)	0.69	5–12/3–10	100	8.9	CR: 8/11 (72.7%) PR: 1/11 (9.1%) Missing data: 2
Choi [13,27], 2018 and 2020	Prospective, monocenter	13/13	18.1 Head: 5 Body: 7 Tail: 1	EUSRA™, TaeWoong (50 W)	1.69	NR/4.77	100	28	CR: 9/13 (69.2%) PR: 3/13 (23.1%) NoR: 1/13 (7.7%)
Pai [11], 2015	Prospective, multicenter	2/2	27.5 Head Body	Habib™ EUS RFA (5–25 W)	1.5	90–120/5	100	3–6	NR Change in vascularity
Armellini [60], 2015	Case report	1/1	20 Tail	EUSRA™, TaeWoong	1	NR	100	NR	CR
Rossi [10], 2014	Prospective, monocenter	1/1	9 Head	Habib™ EUS RFA (10–15 W)	1	360/1	100	34	CR

* Table legend: N. of RFA sessions/lesion expresses the ratio of the number of total procedures to the total number of pancreatic lesions. If equal to 1, the number of procedures is equal to the number of lesions; if >1, it indicates that some lesions are subjected to more than one session; if <1, it indicates that more lesions in the same patient are treated in the same session. Mean time of application (s) indicates the mean time per single application, expressed in seconds, to achieve the desired effect from ablation. Mean N. of applications indicates the mean number of applications needed to obtain complete treatment of the mass. CR: complete response; NoR: no response; NR: not reported; PR: partial response. ** In studies involving more than one type of pancreatic lesion, the overall data were reported when it was not possible to extract the specific data per lesion group.

4.2. EUS-RFA in PCLs

The detection of PCLs is increasingly common, mostly in completely asymptomatic individuals, due to the spread of cross-sectional imaging techniques and the aging population [61]. PCLs are heterogeneous, with different biochemical and histopathological features, and are classified as serous cystic neoplasms (SCNs), mucinous cystic neoplasms (MCNs), intraductal papillary mucinous neoplasms (IPMNs), and solid pseudopapillary tumors (SPTs). The risk of malignancy is widely variable in cystic panels: the evolutionary potential is considered negligible in SCNs, while it becomes moderate–high for SPTs and MCNs; namely, the probability of finding high-grade dysplasia (HGD) or invasive carcinoma (IC) in mucinous masses is associated with cyst-related factors such as a large size, presence of an enhanced solid component, duct dilatation, and patient-related factors such as the presence of symptoms and CA19-9 elevation [62]. These hazard attributes are also encountered in the risk stratification of IPMNs, classified as high-risk stigmata (HRS) and worrisome features (WFs). IPMNs have the widest variability in malignant evolution, ranging from the lowest risk of finding HGD/IC in brunch duct IPMNs (BD-IPMNs) without HRS and WF, to the highest risk in main duct IPMNs (MD-IPMNs), as demonstrated by histopathological samples [63].

The dramatic increase in diagnoses in comparison to the relative low degree of malignant transformation highlights the importance of an accurate characterization of cystic lesions to find a risk–benefit compromise between surveillance and treatment. In recent years, efforts have been made to find alternatives to surgery, such as less invasive local therapies for PCLs bearing a high risk potential for malignancy or that are symptomatic, ranging from EUS-guided ethanol ablation to EUS-RFA and EUS-fine needle injection (FNI). Despite its clinical relevance, only a few studies of EUS-RFA on PCLs are available, mainly case reports and small case series (literature data reported in Table 4), with different criteria for defining a radiological response, which limits the comparability of the results, as already mentioned for non-functional pNETs. The experience of Barthet et al. [17,21] was reported on 16 IPMNs and 1 MCN, with a total of 12 mural nodules undergoing RFA with EUSRA™: 40% and 26.7% of the subjects achieved CR and PR, respectively, with a mean follow-up of 42.6 months and all 12 mural nodules having disappeared. The most severe AE was perforation of a jejunal loop, which was managed surgically. Younis et al. and Napoléon et al. reported similar results on 11 and 5 PCLs, with a CR in around 60% and average follow-up of 13 months [23,42].

Conversely, none of the 13 SCNs reported by Oh et al. [26] reached a CR at the end of the follow-up, and five patients had NoR (defined as a reduction of less than 30% in longest diameter). An assumption is that the microcystic, honeycomb appearance of serous neoplasms may have hampered heat diffusion during ablation, thus affecting the outcome.

Rigorous studies and longer follow-ups are needed to understand the best indication of this minimally invasive technique in the context of pancreatic cystic lesions. For example, it is at least debatable that some studies have included SCNs, given their negligible malignant potential. Accordingly, so far, the only possible indication in this group of lesions is obtaining a sufficient cytovolumetric reduction in large cystic masses causing compression, with the aim of regressing symptoms and avoiding surgery, though existing studies have not focused on clinical aspects. Furthermore, the role of EUS-RFA is still vague for lesions with a higher risk of malignancy, such as MCNs, solid pseudopapillary tumors (SPTs), or IPMNs with worrisome features and high-risk stigmata; despite encouraging results on the ablation of mural nodules, solid data on late recurrences in CR and disease progression in PR are lacking.

Table 4. Results from studies reporting EUS-RFA on PCLs *.

Author, Year	Study Design	N. of Patients and Types of PCLs	Tumor Size (Mean, mm) and Location **	Device	N. of RFA Sessions/Lesion **	Mean Time of Application (s)/Mean N. of Applications **	Technical Success (%) **	Follow-Up (Months) **	Radiologic Response
Napoléon [23], 2023	Retrospective, multicenter	11 - 10 IPMNs with mural nodules - 1 SPT	29 (IPMN) 9 (SPT) NR	EUSRA™, TaeWoong (50 W)	1.12	25/3	97	13	CR: 5/10 (62.5%) PR: 3/10 (37.5%) Missing data: 1
Younis [42], 2022	Prospective, monocenter	5 - 4 IPMNs with worrisome features/mural nodules - 1 MCN	36 Head: 3 Body: 2	EUSRA™, TaeWoong (50 W)	1.6	NR/4	100	13	CR: 3/5 (60%) PR: 1/5 (20%) NoR: 1/5 (20%)

Table 4. Cont.

Author, Year	Study Design	N. of Patients and Types of PCLs	Tumor Size (Mean, mm) and Location **	Device	N. of RFA Sessions/ Lesion **	Mean Time of Application (s)/Mean N. of Applications **	Technical Success (%) **	Follow-Up (Months) **	Radiologic Response
Oh [26], 2021	Retrospective, monocenter	13 SCNs	50 Head: 5 Body/Tail: 8	EUSRA™, TaeWoong	1.5	NR	100	9.21	CR: 0/13 (0%) PR: 8/13 (61.5%) NoR: 5/13 (38.5%)
Barthet [17,21], 2019–2021	Prospective, multicenter	17 - 16 IPMNs - 1 MCN with 12 mural nodules	29.1 Head: 10 Body: 4 Tail: 3	EUSRA™, TaeWoong (50 W)	1.12	20–45/NR	100	42.6	CR: 6/15 (40%) PR: 4/15 (26.7%) NoR: 5/15 (33.3%) 100% disappearance of mural nodules
Choi [13], 2018	Prospective, monocenter	2 SPNs	21.5 Head: 1 Tail: 1	EUSRA™, TaeWoong (50 W)	1	NR/4	100	13	CR: 1 (50%) PR: 1 (50%)
Feng [16], 2018	Case report	1 SCN	35 Tail	Habib™ EUS RFA + lauromacrogol injection after 2 months	1	120/3	100	3	NoR after 2 months, CR with combined therapy
Thosani [53], 2018	Retrospective, multicenter	1 SCN	23 NR	EUSRA™, TaeWoong	1.6	NR/4.6	100	5	NR
Goyal [54], 2017	Case series	2 MCNs	20.5 Body: 1 Tail: 1	Habib™ EUS RFA (10 W)	1	120/3–5	100	NR	NR
Pai [11], 2015	Prospective, multicenter	6 - 4 MCNs - 1 IPMN - 1 Microcystic SCN	36.5 NR	Habib™ EUS RFA (5–25 W)	1	90–120/4.2	100	3–6	CR: 2/6 (33.3%) PR: 3/6 (50%) NoR: 1/6 (16.7%)

* Table legend: N. of RFA sessions/lesion expresses the ratio of the number of total procedures to the total number of pancreatic lesions. If equal to 1, the number of procedures is equal to the number of lesions; if >1, it indicates that some lesions are subjected to more than one session; if <1, it indicates that more lesions in the same patient are treated in the same session. Mean time of application (s) indicates the mean time per single application, expressed in seconds, to achieve the desired effect from ablation. Mean N. of applications indicates the mean number of applications needed to obtain complete treatment of the mass. CR: complete response; NoR: no response; NR: not reported; PR: partial response. ** In studies involving more than one type of pancreatic lesion, the overall data were reported when it was not possible to extract the specific data per lesion group.

4.3. EUS-RFA in PDAC

PDAC is the most frequent histotype of pancreatic cancer (over 80% of cases) and statistics report an increasing incidence trend in both males and females. Moreover, PDAC still holds primacy in terms of aggressiveness, with a 5-year relative survival rate of 13% [64]. The gold-standard treatment with curative intent is surgical resection plus perioperative chemotherapy, but less than 20% of lesions are resectable at diagnosis [65].

As with other solid tumors, in recent years, interest has arisen in local PDAC therapy in the context of a multimodal therapeutic strategy, with the aim of locally controlling the disease, reducing symptoms, and increasing survival. EUS-RFA has been proposed as a local ablative approach to decelerate tumor progression by promoting antitumor immunity and facilitating the penetration of chemotherapeutic drugs.

The first evidence of the application of EUS-RFA on PDAC in vivo is the Italian–German feasibility study [19] conducted on 22 individuals with locally advanced PDAC, using a prototype of the Hybrid-Therm® Probe HTP (ERBE, Germany). The technical success of EUS-RFA was 72.8%, as stable probe insertion was not possible in six patients due to the stiffness of the tumor tissue and an infiltrated gastrointestinal wall. No survival benefit was observed (see Table 5). A randomized controlled phase II trial [20] compared the efficacy of ablative treatment with Hybrid-Therm® Probe in combination with chemotherapy versus chemotherapy alone in the management of patients with locally advanced and borderline resectable PDAC; however, both due to the restricted inclusion criteria and the manufacturer's withdrawal of the HTP probe, enrolment was difficult and the trial had to be stopped early: an intention-to-treat analysis was performed on 17 patients for the study group and on 20 for the control group. Progression-free survival (PFS) and volumetric reduction of the tumor mass at 6 months were slightly better for the study group, although without statistical significance; no relevant differences emerged in either surgical resection rate or OS. Oh et al. [66] reported the results of 22 patients with locally advanced and metastatic PDAC who underwent EUS-RFA in combination with gemcitabine-based chemotherapy before and after ablation: OS was 24.03 months with a PFS of 16.37 months, and when analyzing the subgroup of metastatic patients, the OS was reduced to 15.05 months. These results appear encouraging compared to what has been reported in previous studies; this could be explained by the fact that the EUS-RFA procedure was performed repeatedly if deemed unsatisfactory, for a total of 107 RFA sessions (a mean of 5 per patient), and the number of sessions correlated with PFS.

Currently, the literature on EUS-RFA in pancreatic cancer is rather scarce, most of the papers are small feasibility studies, data on the impact of this treatment on patient survival are often lacking, and those collected so far are not encouraging, with rare exceptions. Randomized controlled, multicenter trials are needed to establish whether EUS-RFA can really play a role in the multimodal treatment of PDAC and which patient groups can really benefit from it; currently, the involvement of patients with metastases is at least disputable.

Table 5. Results from studies reporting EUS-RFA on PDAC *.

Author, Year	Study Design	N. of Patients	Tumor Size (Mean, mm) and Location **	Device	N. of RFA Sessions/Lesion **	Mean Time of Application (s)/Mean N. of Applications **	Technical Success (%) **	Median Post-RFA Survival (Months)	Follow-Up (Months) **
Robles-Medandra [67], in press	Retrospective, monocenter	26 locally advanced and metastatic PDAC	39.5 Head: 22 Body: 3 Tail: 1	EUSRA™, TaeWoong (50 W)	1.27	5–10/NR	100	7	16.5
Napoléon [23], 2023	Retrospective, multicenter	6 PDAC	27 NR	EUSRA™, TaeWoong (50 W)	1.12	25/3	97	NR	13
Kongkam [68], 2023	Prospective, monocenter	14 locally advanced and metastatic PDAC	59.7 NR	EUSRA™, TaeWoong (50 W)	2.5	NR/5.6	100	NR	6
Figueiredo Ferreira [39], 2022	Prospective, multicenter	1 PDAC	14.4 NR	EUSRA™, TaeWoong (50 W)	0.86	NR/3	100	NR	9.5
Oh [66], 2022	Retrospective, monocenter	22 locally advanced and metastatic PDAC	38 Head: 14 Body: 4 Tail: 3	EUSRA™, TaeWoong (50 W)	5	NR	100	Overall survival 24.03	21.23

Table 5. Cont.

Author, Year	Study Design	N. of Patients	Tumor Size (Mean, mm) and Location **	Device	N. of RFA Sessions/Lesion **	Mean Time of Application (s)/Mean N. of Applications **	Technical Success (%) **	Median Post-RFA Survival (Months)	Follow-Up (Months) **
Thosani [69], 2022	Prospective, monocenter	10 locally advanced and metastatic PDAC	39.2 Head: 4 Body: 4 Tail: 2	Habib™ EUS RFA (10–15 W)	2.2	NR	100	13.4	>30
Testoni [70], 2022	Retrospective, monocenter	13 locally advanced PDAC	42.3 Head: 8 Body/Tail: 5	HTP® Probe, ERBE (18 W, 650 psi)	>1	125/NR	100	7	NR
Lawerence [71], 2022	Case series	2 locally advanced PDAC	NR	Habib™ EUS RFA (10 W)	3	120/NR	100	NR	NR
Testoni [20], 2021	Randomized controlled trial, Phase II	17 locally advanced and borderline resectable PDAC	47.1 Head: 10 Body/Tail: 7	HTP® Probe, ERBE (18 W, 650 psi)	1	NR	94.1	13	45.4
Jiang [72], 2021	Prospective, monocenter	8 locally advanced PDAC	46.9 Head: 5 Body: 2 Tail: 1	Habib™ EUS RFA (5 W)	1	95.3/2.4	100	10.7	NR
Wang [73], 2021	Retrospective, monocenter	11 locally advanced and metastatic PDAC	28 Head: 4 Body: 6 Tail: 1	Habib™ EUS RFA (5–10 W)	2.36	NR/3	100	5.2	12
Ligresti [74], 2019	Case report	1 resectable PDAC (unfit for surgery)	15 Body	EUSRA™, TaeWoong (20 W)	1	NR/2	100	NR	12
Crinò [7], 2018	Retrospective, monocenter	7 locally advanced PDAC	36 Head: 4 Body: 3	EUSRA™, TaeWoong (30 W)	1	58/1.5	100	NR	4.3
Scopelliti [8], 2018	Prospective, monocenter	10 locally advanced PDAC	49.2 Head: 4 Body: 6	EUSRA™, TaeWoong (20–30 W)	1	270/1.4	100	NR	1
Thosani [53], 2018	Retrospective, multicenter	10	23 NR	NR	1.6	NR/4.6	100	NR	5
Goyal [54], 2017	Case series	2	26.5 Head: 2	Habib™ EUS RFA (10 W)	1	120/3–5	100	NR	NR
Song [14], 2016	Prospective, monocenter	6 locally advanced and metastatic PDAC	38 Head: 4 Body: 2	EUSRA™, TaeWoong (20–50 W)	1.33	10	100	NR	4.2
Wang [75], 2013	Case series	3	37.3	Habib™ EUS RFA (10–15 W)	1.67	120/NR	100	NR	1.6
Arcidiacono [19], 2012	Prospective, multicenter	22 locally advanced PDAC	35.7 Head: 13 Body: 9	HTP® Probe, ERBE (18 W, 650 psi)	1	107/NR	72.8	6	NR

* Table legend: N. of RFA sessions/lesion expresses the ratio of the number of total procedures to the total number of pancreatic lesions. If equal to 1, the number of procedures is equal to the number of lesions; if >1, it indicates that some lesions are subjected to more than one session; if <1, it indicates that more lesions in the same patient are treated in the same session. Mean time of application (s) indicates the mean time per single application, expressed in seconds, to achieve the desired effect from ablation. Mean N. of applications indicates the mean number of applications needed to obtain complete treatment of the mass. NR: not reported. ** In studies involving more than one type of pancreatic lesion, the overall data were reported when it was not possible to extract the specific data per lesion group.

4.4. EUS-RFA in Pancreatic Metastases from Renal Cell Carcinoma (mRCC) and Other Pancreatic Metastases (PMs)

The pancreas is rarely the site of metastatic localization of primary tumors of other origin. Clear-cell renal cell carcinoma is the neoplasm that most frequently metastasizes to the pancreas; the most frequent sites of secondarism for RCC are the lungs, bones, lymph nodes, and brain, although it may infrequently associate with glandular metastases (pancreas, breast, thyroid, and parathyroid). The literature suggests that glandular metastases, especially pancreatic metastases, have a more favorable prognosis than other localization sites [76,77]. Focal treatment is the treatment of choice in oligometastatic diseases, and surgery is the gold standard for pancreatic metastases.

A number of studies have proposed the use of EUS-RFA in pancreatic metastases as an alternative to surgery; however, data are still rather limited and the results are conflicting (see Table 6). Biasutto et al. [78] published the results of four pancreatic metastases from RCC undergoing EUS-RFA, showing that the procedure was feasible and safe in all three patients involved. At imaging control, an area of necrosis was confirmed in the treated sites; however, no clear data on the radiological response were given. Later, Chanez et al. [79] published one of the most relevant reports of EUS-RFA applied to pancreatic metastases from RCC: 21 lesions underwent 26 sessions of EUS-RFA. Two patients developed severe adverse events, which were managed with hospitalization and intervention; at the end of follow-up (mean follow-up of 27.7 months), all patients were alive. At radiological follow-up at 12 months, a complete response and a partial response (defined as regression of 30% or more of the tumor contrast uptake) were obtained in 40% and 33.3% of lesions, respectively. Similar findings were also reported by Napoléon et al. [23] out of 23 pancreatic metastases submitted to EUS-RFA. On the contrary, Figueiredo Ferreira et al. [39] showed completely different results in nine mRCC lesions and one metastatic lesion from lung cancer. In this case, there was failure in all renal metastases, and the only CR was seen in the lesion of lung origin. The authors speculated that such different results may be explained by both the different criteria used in defining the disease response and by the different disease stages and uses of systemic therapy.

Table 6. Results from studies reporting EUS-RFA on PMs *.

Author, Year	Study Design	N. of Patients/N. of PMs	Tumor size (Mean, mm) and Location **	Device	N. of RFA Sessions/ Lesion **	Mean Time of Application (s)/Mean N. of Applications **	Technical Success (%) **	Follow-Up (Months) **	Radiological Response
Vohra [80], 2023	Case report	1/1 mRCC invading duodenal wall	34 Head	EUSRA™, TaeWoong (50 W)	3	NR	100	3	NR
Napoléon [23], 2023	Retrospective, multicenter	NR/23 mRCC and other PM	17 NR	EUSRA™, TaeWoong (50 W)	1.12	25/3	97	13	CR: 7/23 (30.4%) PR: 10/23 (43.5%) NoR: 6/23 (26.1%)
Figueiredo Ferreira [39], 2022	Prospective, multicenter	NR/10 mRCC and PM of lung cancer	14.4 NR	EUSRA™, TaeWoong (50 W)	0.86	NR/3	100	9.5	CR: 1/9 (11.1%) NoR: 8/9 (88.9%) Missing data: 1

Table 6. Cont.

Author, Year	Study Design	N. of Patients/N. of PMs	Tumor size (Mean, mm) and Location **	Device	N. of RFA Sessions/ Lesion **	Mean Time of Application (s)/Mean N. of Applications **	Technical Success (%) **	Follow-Up (Months) **	Radiological Response
Chanez [79], 2021	Prospective, monocenter	12/21 mRCC	17 Head: 11 Body: 6 Tail: 4	EUSRA™, TaeWoong (50 W)	1.24	30–60/1–3	100	27.7	CR: 6/15 (40%) PR: 5/15 (33.3%) NoR: 4/15 (26.7%) Missing data: 6
Biasutto [78], 2020	Prospective, monocenter	3/4 mRCC	26 Head: 3 Body /Tail: 1	EUSRA™, TaeWoong (30 W)	NR	NR	100	3	NR
Crinò [7], 2018	Retrospective, monocenter	1/1 mRCC	22 Head	EUSRA™, TaeWoong (30 W)	1	55/1	100	3	PR

* Table legend: N. of RFA sessions/lesion expresses the ratio of the number of total procedures in relation to the total number of pancreatic lesions. If equal to 1, the number of procedures is equal to the number of lesions; if >1, it indicates that some lesions are subjected to more than one session; if <1, it indicates that more lesions in the same patient are treated in the same session. Mean time of application (s) indicates the mean time per single application, expressed in seconds, to achieve the desired effect from ablation. Mean N. of applications indicates the mean number of applications needed to obtain complete treatment of the mass. CR: complete response; NoR: no response; NR: not reported; PR: partial response. ** In studies involving more than one type of pancreatic lesion, the overall data were reported when it was not possible to extract the specific data per lesion group.

5. AEs in EUS-RFA

The pancreas is a highly thermosensitive organ, and for many years, this has limited the application of radiofrequency ablation techniques in pancreatic lesions due to the risk of thermal damage of pancreatic tissue and nearby anatomical structures (wall of the GI tract, common bile duct, blood vessels). The few available studies on intraoperative radiofrequency ablation do not show reassuring results in terms of safety, with high rates of complications and post-procedural mortality [81,82]. The advent of EUS has opened a new door for radiofrequency ablation of pancreatic neoplasms, as real-time visualization of the lesion potentially minimizes the risk of thermal damage to healthy pancreatic tissue and adjacent structures.

After pooling the data from the studies presented above, the AEs were compiled (Table 7) and divided into classes of severity according to the Classification for Adverse Events GastRointEstinal Endoscopy (AGREE) [83]. AGREE classes I and II refer to mild–moderate adverse events that result in a prolonged hospitalization of the patient with conservative therapeutic management (e.g., administration of drugs such as antiemetics, antipyretics, analgesics, antibiotics, and antithrombotics, blood transfusion or blood products). AGREE classes III and IV refer to severe AEs requiring endoscopic or surgical intervention or admission of the patient to the intensive care unit. Class V implies the patient's death.

We have data on post-treatment AEs, with EUS-RFA in 206 lesions of F-pNETs and 109 lesions of NF-pNETs, and with a mean number of sessions/lesion of 1.1 equal to the weighted value (w.v.), for a total of 325.9 sessions of EUS-RFA in 315 pNETs. Data from three papers [23,39,53] were excluded, as it is not possible to determine in which patients the reported AEs occurred (in the table, shown as Not specified). In 325.9 EUS-RFA sessions, 58 adverse events occurred, with a total AE rate of 17.8%; the most frequent AEs were abdominal pain managed with analgesics and acute post-RFA pancreatitis, which was managed conservatively in the majority of cases (22 out of 28 cases). The rate of severe AEs was 3.1%, and there were six cases of severe acute pancreatitis managed pharmacologically and endoscopically (only in one case, the patient underwent distal splenopancreasectomy for acute pancreatitis with pancreatic fistula, in which pancreatic stent placement failed) [58], one case of MPD injury, and two cases of MPD stenosis treated with pancreatic stent placement (and in one case, also biliary stent placement). Furthermore, Marx et al. [33] reported a single case of death of a 97-year-old patient, who developed fever and abdominal pain two weeks after the procedure and was subsequently diagnosed with retrogastric collection; the patient refused to undergo interventional maneuvers and died after two weeks despite supportive care.

Of 46 PCNs treated with EUS-RFA, the mean number of sessions/lesion was 1.03 (1.3 w.v.) for a total of 47.38 sessions (59.8 w.v.) (again, data from two studies were not taken into account due to the above-mentioned limitations [23,53]). The total number of AEs was 11 (total AE rate of 23.2%, 18.4% w.v.), with a single severe adverse event (2.1%, se usi ponderata 1.7%), namely a perforation of a jejunal loop that was treated surgically. The patient had been treated for an 18 mm IPMN of the uncinate process [17].

Of 153 PDAC lesions treated with EUS-RFA, the total number of sessions was 275.4 (306 w.v.), and the mean number of sessions/lesion was 1.8 (2.0 w.v.). The total number of adverse events was forty-eight (total AEs rate of 17.4% or, 15.7% w.v.), with six severe adverse events (2.2%, or 2.0% w.v.), namely, six cases of jaundice treated with endoscopic biliary prosthesis placement. In addition to the studies already mentioned, data from Testoni et al. [70] and Jiang et al. [72] were also excluded as they did not report data on complications.

With regard to patients with PMs, in particular, from clear-cell renal cell carcinoma, the available data are limited; Chanez et al. [79] reported two severe AEs in the only two patients treated with tyrosine kinase inhibitors (TKIs) at the time as EUS-RFA. In the first case, they reported the development of a duodenal abscess, and in the second case, in a patient with a biliary stent, the development of a hepatic abscess.

Table 7. Pooled data on AEs in EUS-RFA.

	AGREE I/II % of AEs (n)	AGREE III/IV/V % of AEs (n)
pNETs 325.9 EUS-RFA sessions *	5.8% abdominal pain (19) 6.8% acute pancreatitis (22) 0.6% post-procedural bleeding or upper GI ulcer (2) 0.6% spleen/gastric wall/peripancreatic hematoma (2) 0.3% diabetes (1) 0.6% other than GI AEs– fever (2) Total mild-moderate AEs 14.7%	1.8% acute pancreatitis (6) 0.3% abdominal collections (1, death) 0.3% MPD injury (1) 0.6% MPD stenosis (2) Total severe AEs 3.1%
PCLs 47.38 EUS-RFA sessions *	19.0% abdominal pain (9) 2.1% acute pancreatitis (1) Total mild-moderate AEs 21.1%	2.1% small bowel perforation or stricture (1) Total severe AEs 2.1%
PDAC 275.4 EUS-RFA sessions *	9.8% abdominal pain (27) 1.5% acute pancreatitis (4) 0.7% peripancreatic effusion (2) 0.7% ascites (2) 0.7% abdominal collections (2) 0.4% peritonitis (1) 0.4% spenoportal axis thrombosis (1) 0.4% post-procedural bleeding or upper GI ulcer (1) 0.4% small bowel perforation or stricture (1) 0.4% other than GI AEs– fever (1) Total mild-moderate AEs 15.3%	2.2% jaundice (6) Total severe AEs 2.2%
PMs 21.88 EUS-RFA sessions *	4.6% abdominal pain (1) Total mild-moderate AEs 4.6%	9.1% abdominal abscess (2) Total severe AEs 9.1%
Not Specified [23,39,53] ^ 180 EUS-RFA sessions *	6.7% abdominal pain (12) 6.7% acute pancreatitis (12) 1.1% MPD injury (2) 2.2% MPD stenosis (4) 0.6% post-procedural bleeding or upper GI ulcer (1) 0.6% spleen/gastric wall/peripancreatic hematoma (1) 1.7% other than GI AEs—atrial fibrillation (1), fever (1), acute urine retention post-anesthesia (1) Total mild-moderate AEs 19.4%	1.1% acute pancreatitis (2) 0.6% MPD injury (1) Total severe AEs 1.7%

* In studies not reporting the N. of RFA sessions/lesion (NR), it was considered as 1. ^ Pooled data of three studies' data in which AEs by lesion type cannot be derived.

6. Conclusions

In conclusion, the advent of EUS has opened up new local therapeutic options for pancreatic lesions, and among these, radiofrequency ablation is one of those on which experts' interest is focused. The EUS-RFA technique is feasible, repeatable, and safe, and the adverse events reported are mild in most cases, or, in cases of severe complications, they have almost always been successfully managed with endoscopic or surgical intervention. A standardized protocol for the EUS-RFA technique is not yet defined in relation to the device and the type of tissue and lesion to be treated. Furthermore, the literature data are confined to studies with small sample sizes and short follow-ups; the most encouraging data concern the application of EUS-RFA in pNETs, particularly in F-pNETs where it is aimed to be curative. The role of EUS-RFA still remains nebulous in PCLs, PDAC, and PMs, and prospective, randomized controlled studies are needed to answer the open questions on this topic.

Author Contributions: C.B., C.C. and S.C. were responsible for conceptualization, literature acquisition, and preparation of the manuscript. S.C., C.C., P.G., G.R., V.D.G., S.F. and C.F. critically revised the manuscript. All authors have read and agreed to the published version of the manuscript.

Funding: This research received no external funding.

Conflicts of Interest: The following authors disclose financial relationships: C.C.: Speaker for Steris. C.B.: Speaker for Steris, Fujifilm, Boston Scientific, and Q3 Medical. C.F.: Consultant for Boston Scientific; speaker for Steris and Q3 Medical.

References

1. Schuh, F.; Mihaljevic, A.L.; Probst, P.; Trudeau, M.T.; Müller, P.C.; Marchegiani, G.; Besselink, M.G.; Uzunoglu, F.; Izbicki, J.R.; Falconi, M.; et al. A Simple Classification of Pancreatic Duct Size and Texture Predicts Postoperative Pancreatic Fistula: A Classification of the International Study Group of Pancreatic Surgery. *Ann. Surg.* **2023**, *277*, e597–e608. [CrossRef] [PubMed]
2. Bassi, C.; Marchegiani, G.; Dervenis, C.; Sarr, M.; Abu Hilal, M.; Adham, M.; Allen, P.; Andersson, R.; Asbun, H.J.; Besselink, M.G.; et al. The 2016 Update of the International Study Group (ISGPS) Definition and Grading of Postoperative Pancreatic Fistula: 11 Years After. *Surgery* **2017**, *161*, 584–591. [CrossRef] [PubMed]
3. Bazeed, A.Y.; Day, C.M.; Garg, S. Pancreatic Cancer: Challenges and Opportunities in Locoregional Therapies. *Cancers* **2022**, *14*, 4257. [CrossRef]
4. Wu, J.; Zhou, Z.; Huang, Y.; Deng, X.; Zheng, S.; He, S.; Huang, G.; Hu, B.; Shi, M.; Liao, W.; et al. Radiofrequency Ablation: Mechanisms and Clinical Applications. *MedComm* **2024**, *5*, e746. [CrossRef] [PubMed]
5. Faraoni, E.Y.; O'Brien, B.J.; Strickland, L.N.; Osborn, B.K.; Mota, V.; Chaney, J.; Atkins, C.L.; Cen, P.; Rowe, J.; Cardenas, J.; et al. Radiofrequency Ablation Remodels the Tumor Microenvironment and Promotes Neutrophil-Mediated Abscopal Immunomodulation in Pancreatic Cancer. *Cancer Immunol. Res.* **2023**, *11*, 4–12. [CrossRef]
6. Goldberg, S.N.; Mallery, S.; Gazelle, G.S.; Brugge, W.R. EUS-Guided Radiofrequency Ablation in the Pancreas: Results in a Porcine Model. *Gastrointest. Endosc.* **1999**, *50*, 392–401. [CrossRef]
7. Crinò, S.F.; D'Onofrio, M.; Bernardoni, L.; Frulloni, L.; Iannelli, M.; Malleo, G.; Paiella, S.; Larghi, A.; Gabbrielli, A. EUS-Guided Radiofrequency Ablation (EUS-RFA) of Solid Pancreatic Neoplasm Using an 18-Gauge Needle Electrode: Feasibility, Safety, and Technical Success. *J. Gastrointest. Liver Dis. JGLD* **2018**, *27*, 67–72. [CrossRef]
8. Scopelliti, F.; Pea, A.; Conigliaro, R.; Butturini, G.; Frigerio, I.; Regi, P.; Giardino, A.; Bertani, H.; Paini, M.; Pederzoli, P.; et al. Technique, Safety, and Feasibility of EUS-Guided Radiofrequency Ablation in Unresectable Pancreatic Cancer. *Surg. Endosc.* **2018**, *32*, 4022–4028. [CrossRef]
9. Barret, M.; Leblanc, S.; Rouquette, A.; Chaussade, S.; Terris, B.; Prat, F. EUS-Guided Pancreatic Radiofrequency Ablation: Preclinical Comparison of Two Currently Available Devices in a Pig Model. *Endosc. Int. Open* **2019**, *7*, E138–E143. [CrossRef]
10. Rossi, S.; Viera, F.T.; Ghittoni, G.; Cobianchi, L.; Rosa, L.L.; Siciliani, L.; Bortolotto, C.; Veronese, L.; Vercelli, A.; Gallotti, A.; et al. Radiofrequency Ablation of Pancreatic Neuroendocrine Tumors: A Pilot Study of Feasibility, Efficacy, and Safety. *Pancreas* **2014**, *43*, 938. [CrossRef]
11. Pai, M.; Habib, N.; Senturk, H.; Lakhtakia, S.; Reddy, N.; Cicinnati, V.R.; Kaba, I.; Beckebaum, S.; Drymousis, P.; Kahaleh, M.; et al. Endoscopic Ultrasound Guided Radiofrequency Ablation, for Pancreatic Cystic Neoplasms and Neuroendocrine Tumors. *World J. Gastrointest. Surg.* **2015**, *7*, 52–59. [CrossRef] [PubMed]

12. Lakhtakia, S.; Ramchandani, M.; Galasso, D.; Gupta, R.; Venugopal, S.; Kalpala, R.; Reddy, D.N. EUS-Guided Radiofrequency Ablation for Management of Pancreatic Insulinoma by Using a Novel Needle Electrode (with Videos). *Gastrointest. Endosc.* **2016**, *83*, 234–239. [CrossRef] [PubMed]
13. Choi, J.-H.; Seo, D.-W.; Song, T.J.; Park, D.H.; Lee, S.S.; Lee, S.K.; Kim, M.-H. Endoscopic Ultrasound-Guided Radiofrequency Ablation for Management of Benign Solid Pancreatic Tumors. *Endoscopy* **2018**, *50*, 1099–1104. [CrossRef] [PubMed]
14. Song, T.J.; Seo, D.W.; Lakhtakia, S.; Reddy, N.; Oh, D.W.; Park, D.H.; Lee, S.S.; Lee, S.K.; Kim, M.-H. Initial Experience of EUS-Guided Radiofrequency Ablation of Unresectable Pancreatic Cancer. *Gastrointest. Endosc.* **2016**, *83*, 440–443. [CrossRef]
15. Bas-Cutrina, F.; Bargalló, D.; Gornals, J.B. Small Pancreatic Insulinoma: Successful Endoscopic Ultrasound-Guided Radiofrequency Ablation in a Single Session Using a 22-G Fine Needle. *Dig. Endosc.* **2017**, *29*, 636–638. [CrossRef]
16. Feng, X.; Linghu, E.; Chai, N.; Li, H. New Treatment of the Pancreatic Cystic Neoplasm: Endoscopic Ultrasonography-Guided Radiofrequency Ablation Combined with Lauromacrogol Ablation. *Turk. J. Gastroenterol.* **2018**, *29*, 101–104. [CrossRef]
17. Barthet, M.; Giovannini, M.; Lesavre, N.; Boustiere, C.; Napoleon, B.; Koch, S.; Gasmi, M.; Vanbiervliet, G.; Gonzalez, J.-M. Endoscopic Ultrasound-Guided Radiofrequency Ablation for Pancreatic Neuroendocrine Tumors and Pancreatic Cystic Neoplasms: A Prospective Multicenter Study. *Endoscopy* **2019**, *51*, 836–842. [CrossRef]
18. Rossi, G.; Petrone, M.C.; Schiavo Lena, M.; Albarello, L.; Palumbo, D.; Testoni, S.G.G.; Archibugi, L.; Tacelli, M.; Zaccari, P.; Vanella, G.; et al. Ex-Vivo Investigation of Radiofrequency Ablation in Pancreatic Adenocarcinoma after Neoadjuvant Chemotherapy. *DEN Open* **2023**, *3*, e152. [CrossRef]
19. Arcidiacono, P.G.; Carrara, S.; Reni, M.; Petrone, M.C.; Cappio, S.; Balzano, G.; Boemo, C.; Cereda, S.; Nicoletti, R.; Enderle, M.D.; et al. Feasibility and Safety of EUS-Guided Cryothermal Ablation in Patients with Locally Advanced Pancreatic Cancer. *Gastrointest. Endosc.* **2012**, *76*, 1142–1151. [CrossRef]
20. Testoni, S.G.G.; Petrone, M.C.; Reni, M.; Rossi, G.; Barbera, M.; Nicoletti, V.; Gusmini, S.; Balzano, G.; Linzenbold, W.; Enderle, M.; et al. Efficacy of Endoscopic Ultrasound-Guided Ablation with the HybridTherm Probe in Locally Advanced or Borderline Resectable Pancreatic Cancer: A Phase II Randomized Controlled Trial. *Cancers* **2021**, *13*, 4512. [CrossRef]
21. Barthet, M.; Giovannini, M.; Gasmi, M.; Lesavre, N.; Boustière, C.; Napoleon, B.; LaQuiere, A.; Koch, S.; Vanbiervliet, G.; Gonzalez, J.-M. Long-Term Outcome after EUS-Guided Radiofrequency Ablation: Prospective Results in Pancreatic Neuroendocrine Tumors and Pancreatic Cystic Neoplasms. *Endosc. Int. Open* **2021**, *9*, E1178–E1185. [CrossRef] [PubMed]
22. Dumonceau, J.-M. ERCP-Related Adverse Events: European Society of Gastrointestinal Endoscopy (ESGE) Guideline | ESGE. Available online: https://www.esge.com/ercp-related-adverse-events-esge-guideline (accessed on 8 May 2024).
23. Napoléon, B.; Lisotti, A.; Caillol, F.; Gasmi, M.; Ah-Soune, P.; Belle, A.; Charachon, A.; Cholet, F.; Eyraud, P.-Y.; Grandval, P.; et al. Risk Factors for EUS-Guided Radiofrequency Ablation Adverse Events in Patients with Pancreatic Neoplasms: A Large National French Study (RAFPAN Study). *Gastrointest. Endosc.* **2023**, *98*, 392–399.e1. [CrossRef] [PubMed]
24. Kochar, B.; Akshintala, V.S.; Afghani, E.; Elmunzer, B.J.; Kim, K.J.; Lennon, A.M.; Khashab, M.A.; Kalloo, A.N.; Singh, V.K. Incidence, Severity, and Mortality of Post-ERCP Pancreatitis: A Systematic Review by Using Randomized, Controlled Trials. *Gastrointest. Endosc.* **2015**, *81*, 143–149.e9. [CrossRef] [PubMed]
25. Crinò, S.F.; Napoleon, B.; Facciorusso, A.; Lakhtakia, S.; Borbath, I.; Caillol, F.; Do-Cong Pham, K.; Rizzatti, G.; Forti, E.; Palazzo, L.; et al. Endoscopic Ultrasound-Guided Radiofrequency Ablation Versus Surgical Resection for Treatment of Pancreatic Insulinoma. *Clin. Gastroenterol. Hepatol.* **2023**, *21*, 2834–2843.e2. [CrossRef]
26. Oh, D.; Ko, S.W.; Seo, D.-W.; Hong, S.-M.; Kim, J.H.; Song, T.J.; Park, D.H.; Lee, S.K.; Kim, M.-H. Endoscopic Ultrasound-Guided Radiofrequency Ablation of Pancreatic Microcystic Serous Cystic Neoplasms: A Retrospective Study. *Endoscopy* **2021**, *53*, 739–743. [CrossRef]
27. Choi, J.-H.; Seo, D.-W.; Song, T.J.; Park, D.H.; Lee, S.S.; Lee, S.K.; Kim, M.-H. Utility of Contrast-Enhanced Harmonic Endoscopic Ultrasound for the Guidance and Monitoring of Endoscopic Radiofrequency Ablation. *Gut Liver* **2020**, *14*, 826–832. [CrossRef]
28. Borrelli de Andreis, F.; Boškoski, I.; Mascagni, P.; Schepis, T.; Bianchi, A.; Schinzari, G.; Annicchiarico, B.E.; Quero, G.; Tortora, G.; Alfieri, S.; et al. Safety and Efficacy of Endoscopic Ultrasound-Guided Radiofrequency Ablation for Pancreatic Insulinoma: A Single-Center Experience. *Pancreatology* **2023**, *23*, 543–549. [CrossRef]
29. Jensen, R.T.; Cadiot, G.; Brandi, M.L.; de Herder, W.W.; Kaltsas, G.; Komminoth, P.; Scoazec, J.-Y.; Salazar, R.; Sauvanet, A.; Kianmanesh, R.; et al. ENETS Consensus Guidelines for the Management of Patients with Digestive Neuroendocrine Neoplasms: Functional Pancreatic Endocrine Tumor Syndromes. *Neuroendocrinology* **2012**, *95*, 98–119. [CrossRef]
30. Falconi, M.; Eriksson, B.; Kaltsas, G.; Bartsch, D.K.; Capdevila, J.; Caplin, M.; Kos-Kudla, B.; Kwekkeboom, D.; Rindi, G.; Klöppel, G.; et al. ENETS Consensus Guidelines Update for the Management of Patients with Functional Pancreatic Neuroendocrine Tumors and Non-Functional Pancreatic Neuroendocrine Tumors. *Neuroendocrinology* **2016**, *103*, 153–171. [CrossRef]
31. Hofland, J.; Falconi, M.; Christ, E.; Castaño, J.P.; Faggiano, A.; Lamarca, A.; Perren, A.; Petrucci, S.; Prasad, V.; Ruszniewski, P.; et al. European Neuroendocrine Tumor Society 2023 Guidance Paper for Functioning Pancreatic Neuroendocrine Tumour Syndromes. *J. Neuroendocrinol.* **2023**, *35*, e13318. [CrossRef]

32. Waung, J.A.; Todd, J.F.; Keane, M.G.; Pereira, S.P. Successful Management of a Sporadic Pancreatic Insulinoma by Endoscopic Ultrasound-Guided Radiofrequency Ablation. *Endoscopy* **2016**, *48* (Suppl. 1), E144–E145. [CrossRef] [PubMed]
33. Marx, M.; Trosic-Ivanisevic, T.; Caillol, F.; Demartines, N.; Schoepfer, A.; Pesenti, C.; Ratone, J.-P.; Robert, M.; Giovannini, M.; Godat, S. EUS-Guided Radiofrequency Ablation for Pancreatic Insulinoma: Experience in 2 Tertiary Centers. *Gastrointest. Endosc.* **2022**, *95*, 1256–1263. [CrossRef] [PubMed]
34. Armellini, E.; Facciorusso, A.; Crinò, S.F. Efficacy and Safety of Endoscopic Ultrasound-Guided Radiofrequency Ablation for Pancreatic Neuroendocrine Tumors: A Systematic Review and Metanalysis. *Medicina* **2023**, *59*, 359. [CrossRef]
35. Lesmana, C.R.A. Endoscopic Loco-Regional Treatment in Controlling Pancreatic Neuroendocrine Tumors (PNETs) Behavior: A Case Series and Literature Review. *Clin. J. Gastroenterol.* **2024**, *17*, 754–759. [CrossRef]
36. Biermann, M.R.; Sundar, P.; Veeramachaneni, H.; Chawla, S.; Patel, V.; Orr, J.; Keilin, S.; Willingham, F.F. Radiofrequency ablation for the management of symptomatic pancreatic insulinomas. *VideoGIE* **2024**, *9*, 45–50. [CrossRef]
37. Gugger, A.S.; Fang, J.; Visrodia, K.H.; Page-Wilson, G. Cushing Syndrome Due to a Pancreatic Neuroendocrine Tumor Treated With Radiofrequency Ablation. *JCEM Case Rep.* **2023**, *1*, luad022. [CrossRef]
38. Rizzatti, G.; De Nucci, G.; Caillol, F.; Crinò, S.F.; Pham, K.; Palazzo, L.; Tripodi, G.; Gasbarrini, A.; Spada, C.; Larghi, A.; et al. Safety and Efficacy of Endoscopic Ultrasound-Guided Radiofrequency Ablation for the Treatment of Functional and Non-functional Pancreatic Neuroendocrine Neoplasms: Preliminary Results of a Multicentre Prospective Study. *Gastrointest. Endosc.* **2023**, *97*, AB805. [CrossRef]
39. Figueiredo Ferreira, M.; Garces-Duran, R.; Eisendrath, P.; Devière, J.; Deprez, P.; Monino, L.; Van Laethem, J.-L.; Borbath, I. EUS-Guided Radiofrequency Ablation of Pancreatic/Peripancreatic Tumors and Oligometastatic Disease: An Observational Prospective Multicenter Study. *Endosc. Int. Open* **2022**, *10*, E1380–E1385. [CrossRef]
40. Chang, J.Y.-C.; Woo, C.S.-L.; Lui, D.T.-W.; Fung, M.M.-H.; Lee, A.C.-H.; Leung, E.K.-H.; Woo, Y.-C.; Chow, W.-S.; Lam, K.S.-L.; Tan, K.C.-B.; et al. Case Report: Insulinoma Co-Existing With Type 2 Diabetes—Advantages and Challenges of Treatment With Endoscopic Ultrasound-Guided Radiofrequency Ablation. *Front. Endocrinol.* **2022**, *13*, 957369. [CrossRef]
41. Rossi, G.; Petrone, M.C.; Capurso, G.; Partelli, S.; Falconi, M.; Arcidiacono, P.G. Endoscopic Ultrasound Radiofrequency Ablation of Pancreatic Insulinoma in Elderly Patients: Three Case Reports. *World J. Clin. Cases* **2022**, *10*, 6514–6519. [CrossRef]
42. Younis, F.; Ben-Ami Shor, D.; Lubezky, N.; Geva, R.; Osher, E.; Shibolet, O.; Phillips, A.; Scapa, E. Endoscopic Ultrasound-Guided Radiofrequency Ablation of Premalignant Pancreatic-Cystic Neoplasms and Neuroendocrine Tumors: Prospective Study. *Eur. J. Gastroenterol. Hepatol.* **2022**, *34*, 1111–1115. [CrossRef] [PubMed]
43. Long-Term Outcomes of EUS Guided RFA in Pancreatic Neuroendocrine Tumors: A Tertiary Care Centre Experience. Available online: https://ueg.eu/library/long-term-outcomes-of-eus-guided-rfa-in-pancreatic-neuroendocrine-tumors-a-tertiary-care-centre-experience/3e277f12-9363-11ed-a167-0242ac140004 (accessed on 11 April 2024).
44. de Nucci, G.; Imperatore, N.; Mandelli, E.D.; di Nuovo, F.; d'Urbano, C.; Manes, G. Endoscopic Ultrasound-Guided Radiofrequency Ablation of Pancreatic Neuroendocrine Tumors: A Case Series. *Endosc. Int. Open* **2020**, *8*, E1754–E1758. [CrossRef]
45. Lakhtakia, S.; Memon, S.F.F.; Medarapalem, J.B.; Chavan, R.; Nabi, Z.; Ramchandani, M.K.; Gupta, R.; Duvvur, N.R. 99 SUSTAINED CLINICAL RESPONSE WITH EUS GUIDED RFA OF PANCREATIC INSULINOMA. *Gastrointest. Endosc.* **2020**, *91*, AB14. [CrossRef]
46. Kluz, M.; Staroń, R.; Krupa, Ł.; Partyka, M.; Polkowski, M.; Gutkowski, K. Successful Endoscopic Ultrasound-Guided Radiofrequency Ablation of a Pancreatic Insulinoma. *Pol. Arch. Intern. Med.* **2020**, *130*, 145–146. [CrossRef]
47. Furnica, R.M.; Deprez, P.; Maiter, D.; Vandeleene, B.; Borbath, I. Endoscopic Ultrasound-Guided Radiofrequency Ablation: An Effective and Safe Alternative for the Treatment of Benign Insulinoma. *Ann. Endocrinol.* **2020**, *81*, 567–571. [CrossRef]
48. Jonica, E.R.; Wagh, M.S. Endoscopic Treatment of Symptomatic Insulinoma with a New EUS-Guided Radiofrequency Ablation Device. *VideoGIE* **2020**, *5*, 483–485. [CrossRef] [PubMed]
49. Brown, N.G.; Patel, A.A.; Gonda, T.A. Immediate and Durable Therapeutic Response after EUS-Guided Radiofrequency Ablation of a Pancreatic Insulinoma. *VideoGIE* **2020**, *5*, 676–678. [CrossRef] [PubMed]
50. Oleinikov, K.; Dancour, A.; Epshtein, J.; Benson, A.; Mazeh, H.; Tal, I.; Matalon, S.; Benbassat, C.A.; Livovsky, D.M.; Goldin, E.; et al. Endoscopic Ultrasound-Guided Radiofrequency Ablation: A New Therapeutic Approach for Pancreatic Neuroendocrine Tumors. *J. Clin. Endocrinol. Metab.* **2019**, *104*, 2637–2647. [CrossRef]
51. Sehemby, M.; Lila, A.; Jadhav-Ramteke, S.; Patil, V.; Shah, N.; Bandgar, T. ESICON 2019 Abstracts. *Indian J. Endocrinol. Metab.* **2019**, *23*, S5–S83.
52. de Mussy, P.G.; Lamine, F.; Godat, S.; Marino, L.; Di, G.S.; Gonzalez, R.E.; Desmartines, N.; Pitteloud, N. A Case of Benign Insulinoma Successfully Treated with Endoscopic Ultrasound Guided Radiofrequency Ablation. In *Proceedings of the Endocrine Abstracts*; Bioscientifica: Bristol, 2018; Volume 56.
53. Thosani, N.; Sharma, N.R.; Raijman, I.; Thosani, A.J.; Kannadath, B.S.; Guider, J.C.; Raza, A.; Guha, S. 483 Safety and Efficacy of Endoscopic Ultrasound Guided Radiofrequency Ablation (EUS-RFA) in the Treatment of Pancreatic Lesions: A Multi-Center Experience. *Gastrointest. Endosc.* **2018**, *87*, AB84. [CrossRef]

54. Goyal, D.; Cen, P.; Wray, C.J.; Rowe, J.; Guha, S.; Singhal, S.; Rahimi, E.F.; Ertan, A.; Thosani, N. 1111 Feasibility, Safety, and Efficacy of Endoscopic Ultrasound (EUS) Guided Radiofrequency Ablation (RFA) of the Pancreatic Lesions: Single Center Us Experience. *Gastrointest. Endosc.* **2017**, *85*, AB144. [CrossRef]
55. Yang, Z.; Shi, G. Comparative Outcomes of Pancreatic Neuroendocrine Neoplasms: A Population-Based Analysis of the SEER Database. *Eur. J. Surg. Oncol.* **2022**, *48*, 2181–2187. [CrossRef] [PubMed]
56. Linee Guida Neoplasie Neuroendocrine. Available online: https://www.aiom.it/linee-guida-aiom-2021-neoplasie-neuroendocrine/ (accessed on 16 November 2024).
57. Kos-Kudła, B.; Castaño, J.P.; Denecke, T.; Grande, E.; Kjaer, A.; Koumarianou, A.; de Mestier, L.; Partelli, S.; Perren, A.; Stättner, S.; et al. European Neuroendocrine Tumour Society (ENETS) 2023 Guidance Paper for Nonfunctioning Pancreatic Neuroendocrine Tumours. *J. Neuroendocrinol.* **2023**, *35*, e13343. [CrossRef]
58. Marx, M.; Godat, S.; Caillol, F.; Poizat, F.; Ratone, J.-P.; Pesenti, C.; Schoepfer, A.; Hoibian, S.; Dahel, Y.; Giovannini, M. Management of Non-Functional Pancreatic Neuroendocrine Tumors by Endoscopic Ultrasound-Guided Radiofrequency Ablation: Retrospective Study in Two Tertiary Centers. *Dig. Endosc.* **2022**, *34*, 1207–1213. [CrossRef]
59. Lesmana, C.R.A.; Lirendra, M.; Inggriani, S.; Sudoyo, A.W.; Lesmana, L. Treatment Outcome of Endoscopic Ultrasound Radiofrequency Ablation for Incidentaloma Pancreatic Neuroendocrine Tumor in Young Female Patient: A 2-Year Follow-Up. *Case Rep. Gastroenterol.* **2022**, *16*, 583–587. [CrossRef]
60. Armellini, E.; Crinò, S.F.; Ballarè, M.; Occhipinti, P. Endoscopic Ultrasound-Guided Radiofrequency Ablation of a Pancreatic Neuroendocrine Tumor. *Endoscopy* **2015**, *47*, E600–E601. [CrossRef]
61. Kromrey, M.-L.; Bülow, R.; Hübner, J.; Paperlein, C.; Lerch, M.M.; Ittermann, T.; Völzke, H.; Mayerle, J.; Kühn, J.-P. Prospective Study on the Incidence, Prevalence and 5-Year Pancreatic-Related Mortality of Pancreatic Cysts in a Population-Based Study. *Gut* **2018**, *67*, 138–145. [CrossRef]
62. Kim, G.H.; Choi, K.; Paik, N.; Lee, K.T.; Lee, J.K.; Lee, K.H.; Han, I.W.; Kang, S.H.; Heo, J.S.; Park, J.K. Diagnostic Concordance and Preoperative Risk Factors for Malignancy in Pancreatic Mucinous Cystic Neoplasms. *Gut Liver* **2022**, *16*, 637–644. [CrossRef]
63. Ohtsuka, T.; Fernandez-Del Castillo, C.; Furukawa, T.; Hijioka, S.; Jang, J.-Y.; Lennon, A.M.; Miyasaka, Y.; Ohno, E.; Salvia, R.; Wolfgang, C.L.; et al. International Evidence-Based Kyoto Guidelines for the Management of Intraductal Papillary Mucinous Neoplasm of the Pancreas. *Pancreatology* **2024**, *24*, 255–270. [CrossRef]
64. Siegel, R.L.; Giaquinto, A.N.; Jemal, A. Cancer Statistics, 2024. *CA. Cancer J. Clin.* **2024**, *74*, 12–49. [CrossRef]
65. Bockhorn, M.; Uzunoglu, F.G.; Adham, M.; Imrie, C.; Milicevic, M.; Sandberg, A.A.; Asbun, H.J.; Bassi, C.; Büchler, M.; Charnley, R.M.; et al. Borderline Resectable Pancreatic Cancer: A Consensus Statement by the International Study Group of Pancreatic Surgery (ISGPS). *Surgery* **2014**, *155*, 977–988. [CrossRef] [PubMed]
66. Oh, D.; Seo, D.-W.; Song, T.J.; Park, D.H.; Lee, S.K.; Kim, M.-H. Clinical Outcomes of EUS-Guided Radiofrequency Ablation for Unresectable Pancreatic Cancer: A Prospective Observational Study. *Endosc. Ultrasound* **2022**, *11*, 68–74. [CrossRef] [PubMed]
67. Robles-Medranda, C.; Del Valle, R.; Puga-Tejada, M.; Arevalo-Mora, M.; Cunto, D.; Egas-Izquierdo, M.; Estrada-Guevara, L.; Bunces-Orellana, O.; Moreno-Zambrano, D.; Alcivar-Vasquez, J.; et al. Assessing Endoscopic Ultrasound-Guided Radiofrequency Ablation in Unresectable Pancreatic Ductal Adenocarcinoma: A Single-Center Historic Cohort Study. *Gastrointest. Endosc.* **2024**, *100*, 250–258. [CrossRef] [PubMed]
68. Kongkam, P.; Tiankanon, K.; Seo, D.W.; Luangsukrerk, T.; Sriuranpong, V.; Nantavithya, C.; Jantarattana, T.; Cañones, A.; Kerr, S.J.; Tantitanawat, K.; et al. EUS-Guided Radiofrequency Ablation plus Chemotherapy versus Chemotherapy Alone for Pancreatic Cancer (ERAP): An Observational Open-Label Pilot Study. *Endosc. Ultrasound* **2023**, *12*, 402–408. [CrossRef]
69. Thosani, N.; Cen, P.; Rowe, J.; Guha, S.; Bailey-Lundberg, J.M.; Bhakta, D.; Patil, P.; Wray, C.J. Endoscopic Ultrasound-Guided Radiofrequency Ablation (EUS-RFA) for Advanced Pancreatic and Periampullary Adenocarcinoma. *Sci. Rep.* **2022**, *12*, 16516. [CrossRef]
70. Testoni, S.G.G.; Petrone, M.C.; Reni, M.; Di Serio, C.; Rancoita, P.M.; Rossi, G.; Balzano, G.; Linzenbold, W.; Enderle, M.; Della-Torre, E.; et al. EUS-Guided Ablation with the HybridTherm Probe as Second-Line Treatment in Patients with Locally Advanced Pancreatic Ductal Adenocarcinoma: A Case-Control Study. *Endosc. Ultrasound* **2022**, *11*, 383–392. [CrossRef]
71. Lawrence, P.V.; Desai, K.; Wadsworth, C.; Mangal, N.; Kocher, H.M.; Habib, N.; Sadanandam, A.; Sodergren, M.H. A Case Report on Longitudinal Collection of Tumour Biopsies for Gene Expression-Based Tumour Microenvironment Analysis from Pancreatic Cancer Patients Treated with Endoscopic Ultrasound Guided Radiofrequency Ablation. *Curr. Oncol.* **2022**, *29*, 6754–6763. [CrossRef]
72. Jiang, J.; Lou, Q.; Yang, J.; Zhang, X. Feasibility and Safety of EUS-Guided Radiofrequency Ablation in Treatment of Locally Advanced, Unresectable Pancreatic Cancer. *Endosc. Ultrasound* **2021**, *10*, 398–399. [CrossRef]
73. Wang, J.; Wang, Y.; Zhao, Y.; Wu, X.; Zhang, M.; Hou, W.; Chen, Q.; Cheng, B. Endoscopic Ultrasound-Guided Radiofrequency Ablation of Unresectable Pancreatic Cancer with Low Ablation Power and Multiple Applications: A Preliminary Study of 11 Patients. *Ann. Palliat. Med.* **2021**, *10*, 1842–1850. [CrossRef]

74. Ligresti, D.; Amata, M.; Barresi, L.; Traina, M.; Tarantino, I. EUS-Guided Radiofrequency Ablation of Small Pancreatic Adenocarcinoma: A New Therapeutic Option for Patients Unfit for Surgery. *VideoGIE* **2019**, *4*, 29–31. [CrossRef]
75. Wang, D.; Jin, Z.; Lei, W.; Leung, J.W.; Li, Z. Mo1524 Endoscopic Ultrasound Guided Radiofrequency Ablation for the Treatment of Advanced Pancreatic Carcinoma. *Gastrointest. Endosc.* **2013**, *77*, AB414. [CrossRef]
76. Gravis, G.; Chanez, B.; Derosa, L.; Beuselinck, B.; Barthelemy, P.; Laguerre, B.; Brachet, P.-E.; Joly, F.; Escudier, B.; Harrison, D.J.; et al. Effect of Glandular Metastases on Overall Survival of Patients with Metastatic Clear Cell Renal Cell Carcinoma in the Antiangiogenic Therapy Era. *Urol. Oncol. Semin. Orig. Investig.* **2016**, *34*, e17–e167. [CrossRef] [PubMed]
77. Grassi, P.; Doucet, L.; Giglione, P.; Grünwald, V.; Melichar, B.; Galli, L.; De Giorgi, U.; Sabbatini, R.; Ortega, C.; Santoni, M.; et al. Outcome of Patients with Renal Cell Carcinoma and Multiple Glandular Metastases Treated with Targeted Agents. *Oncology* **2017**, *92*, 269–275. [CrossRef] [PubMed]
78. Biasutto, D.; Stigliano, S.; Matteo, F.M.D. Sa1441 endoscopic ultrasound-guided radiofrequency ablation of pancreatic metastases from renal cell cancer: Feasibility and safety. *Gastrointest. Endosc.* **2020**, *91*, AB191–AB192. [CrossRef]
79. Chanez, B.; Caillol, F.; Ratone, J.-P.; Pesenti, C.; Rochigneux, P.; Pignot, G.; Thomassin, J.; Brunelle, S.; Walz, J.; Salem, N.; et al. Endoscopic Ultrasound-Guided Radiofrequency Ablation as an Future Alternative to Pancreatectomy for Pancreatic Metastases from Renal Cell Carcinoma: A Prospective Study. *Cancers* **2021**, *13*, 5267. [CrossRef]
80. Vohra, M.; Goyal, H.; Cen, P.; Joseph-Talreja, M.; Thosani, N. A Novel Case of EUS–Guided Targeted Radiofrequency Ablation of Metastatic Duodenal Renal Cell Carcinoma. *Endosc. Ultrasound* **2023**, *12*, 433. [CrossRef]
81. Wu, Y.; Tang, Z.; Fang, H.; Gao, S.; Chen, J.; Wang, Y.; Yan, H. High Operative Risk of Cool-Tip Radiofrequency Ablation for Unresectable Pancreatic Head Cancer. *J. Surg. Oncol.* **2006**, *94*, 392–395. [CrossRef]
82. Girelli, R.; Frigerio, I.; Salvia, R.; Barbi, E.; Tinazzi Martini, P.; Bassi, C. Feasibility and Safety of Radiofrequency Ablation for Locally Advanced Pancreatic Cancer. *Br. J. Surg.* **2010**, *97*, 220–225. [CrossRef]
83. Nass, K.J.; Zwager, L.W.; van der Vlugt, M.; Dekker, E.; Bossuyt, P.M.M.; Ravindran, S.; Thomas-Gibson, S.; Fockens, P. Novel Classification for Adverse Events in GI Endoscopy: The AGREE Classification. *Gastrointest. Endosc.* **2022**, *95*, 1078–1085.e8. [CrossRef]

Disclaimer/Publisher's Note: The statements, opinions and data contained in all publications are solely those of the individual author(s) and contributor(s) and not of MDPI and/or the editor(s). MDPI and/or the editor(s) disclaim responsibility for any injury to people or property resulting from any ideas, methods, instructions or products referred to in the content.

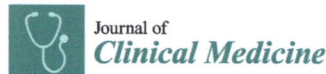 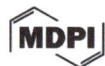

Review

Endoscopic Management of Benign Pancreaticobiliary Disorders

Amar Vedamurthy [1], Rajesh Krishnamoorthi [1], Shayan Irani [1] and Richard Kozarek [1,2,*]

[1] Division of Gastroenterology and Hepatology, Center for Digestive Health, Virginia Mason, Franciscan Health, Seattle, WA 98101, USA
[2] Center for Interventional Immunology, Benaroya Research Institute, Virginia Mason, Franciscan Health, 1100 9th Avenue, G-250B, Seattle, WA 98101, USA
* Correspondence: richard.kozarek@commonspirit.org; Tel.: +1-206-515-5397

Abstract: Endoscopic management of benign pancreaticobiliary disorders encompasses a range of procedures designed to address complications in gallstone disease, choledocholithiasis, and pancreatic disorders. Acute cholecystitis is typically treated with cholecystectomy or percutaneous drainage (PT-GBD), but for high-risk or future surgical candidates, alternative decompression methods, such as endoscopic transpapillary gallbladder drainage (ETP-GBD), and endoscopic ultrasound (EUS)-guided gallbladder drainage (EUS-GBD), are effective. PT-GBD is associated with significant discomfort as well as variable adverse event rates. EUS-GBD leverages lumen-apposing metal stents (LAMS) for direct access to the gallbladder, providing the ability to treat an inflamed GB internally. Choledocholithiasis is primarily managed with ERCP, utilizing techniques to include balloon extraction, mechanical lithotripsy, or advanced methods such as electrohydraulic or laser lithotripsy in cases of complex stones. Altered anatomy from bariatric procedures like Roux-en-Y gastric bypass may necessitate specialized approaches, including balloon-assisted ERCP or EUS-directed transgastric ERCP (EDGE). Post-operative complications, including bile leaks and strictures, are managed endoscopically using sphincterotomy and stenting. Post-liver transplant anastomotic and non-anastomotic strictures often require repeated stent placements or advanced techniques like magnetic compression anastomosis in refractory cases. In chronic pancreatitis (CP), endoscopic approaches aim to relieve pain and address structural complications like pancreatic duct (PD) strictures and calculi. ERCP with sphincterotomy and stenting, along with extracorporeal shock wave lithotripsy (ESWL), achieves effective ductal clearance for PD stones. When traditional approaches are insufficient, direct visualization with peroral pancreatoscopy-assisted lithotripsy is utilized. EUS-guided interventions, such as cystgastrostomy, pancreaticogastrostomy, and celiac plexus blockade, offer alternative therapeutic options for pain management and drainage of peripancreatic fluid collections. EUS plays a diagnostic and therapeutic role in CP, with procedures tailored for high-risk patients or those with complex anatomy. As techniques evolve, endoscopic management provides minimally invasive alternatives for patients with complex benign pancreaticobiliary conditions, offering high clinical success and fewer complications.

Keywords: endoscopy; management; gallstones; cholecystitis; cholangitis; bile; leak; strictures; pancreatitis; necrosis; transplant; stents; calculi

Academic Editors: Saburo Matsubara and Morihisa Hirota

Received: 27 November 2024
Revised: 9 January 2025
Accepted: 9 January 2025
Published: 14 January 2025

Citation: Vedamurthy, A.; Krishnamoorthi, R.; Irani, S.; Kozarek, R. Endoscopic Management of Benign Pancreaticobiliary Disorders. *J. Clin. Med.* **2025**, *14*, 494. https://doi.org/10.3390/jcm14020494

Copyright: © 2025 by the authors. Licensee MDPI, Basel, Switzerland. This article is an open access article distributed under the terms and conditions of the Creative Commons Attribution (CC BY) license (https://creativecommons.org/licenses/by/4.0/).

1. Introduction

Benign pancreaticobiliary disorders, which include a variety of gallbladder, bile duct, and pancreatic conditions, are a significant source of morbidity worldwide. For instance, gallstone disease and its complications, including cholecystitis, choledocholithiasis, and acute pancreatitis account for a million emergency visits, 625,000 hospital discharges, and 2000 deaths annually [1]. Traditionally, these conditions have been managed with surgical interventions; however, many now benefit from endoscopic techniques that provide comparable outcomes with reduced invasiveness and faster recovery. Advances in endoscopic retrograde cholangiopancreatography (ERCP), endoscopic ultrasound (EUS)-guided interventions, and stent technologies have broadened the therapeutic options available. These innovations are instrumental in addressing challenges ranging from acute cholecystitis to complications related to the bile duct and pancreatic duct. They are especially valuable for patients with complex or altered anatomy, as well as for those who cannot undergo surgery [2]. This narrative review provides an overview of the endoscopic procedures available for managing benign pancreaticobiliary diseases. It places particular emphasis on the endoscopic management of acute cholecystitis, bile duct disorders in patients with both normal and variant anatomy, and complications associated with acute and chronic pancreatitis. While it offers a broad perspective for general practitioners, the manuscript also aims to serve as a focused resource for gastroenterologists and surgeons looking to integrate advanced endoscopic techniques into their practice.

2. Methods

This narrative review examines the literature on benign pancreaticobiliary disorders treated with endoscopic therapies. We conducted searches on PubMed and Google Scholar to identify relevant articles using titles or keywords such as "Cholecystitis", "Choledocholithiasis", "Post-hepatobiliary surgery complications", "Bile leak", "Biliary stricture", "post-liver transplant biliary strictures", "Recurrent acute pancreatitis", "Pancreatic fluid collections", and "Endoscopic ultrasound directed therapies". Articles in languages other than English or those lacking full text availability were excluded. Systematic reviews, meta-analyses, and randomized controlled trials were prioritized for inclusion. Ultimately, a total of 80 articles were included in the final review.

3. Discussion

3.1. Gallstone Disease

Gallstones are the commonest cause of emergency room presentation in patients with abdominal pain. Asymptomatic gallstones do not need treatment. In symptomatic patients, they can result in complications as a consequence of cystic or common bile duct blockage.

3.2. Acute Cholecystitis

Acute cholecystitis is caused by the obstruction of the cystic duct, leading to inflammation of the gallbladder (GB). The diagnosis is typically made with US or CT, which shows pericholecystic fluid collection, wall thickening, or distension. Cholecystectomy remains the standard of care. In cases where surgery is deemed high risk, decompression should be considered to prevent complications such as perforation, gangrene, or fistulization into the bowel. The most common technique for decompression is percutaneous drainage (PT-GBD), along with antibiotic therapy. PT-GBD can be cumbersome to manage due to the presence of an external drain and a drainage bag. The availability of procedural expertise and recommendations from extensive studies led to the rise in the use of PT-GBD. Multicenter studies have shown that PT-GBD is associated with higher post-procedure pain scores and high adverse events at 30 days and 1 year [3–5]. The external catheter must remain in place until the tract matures and becomes potentially longer. There are two endoscopic treatment options available for the management of acute cholecystitis, specifically in patients with high co-morbidities or deemed unfit for surgery. Decompression can be performed in one of two ways: internal drainage can be performed by placing a transpapillary stent into the gallbladder; or lumen through ERCP or transmurally by placement of a metal stent from the stomach or the duodenum.

3.3. Transpapillary Gallbladder Drainage (ETP-GBD)

The technique was first described by Kozarek in 1984 [6]. This involves the following: deep bile duct cannulation using ERCP techniques, visualization of the cystic duct by cholangiography, the passage of a hydrophilic guidewire in the cystic duct to curl in the gallbladder and insertion of a long 7 Fr double pigtail stent, leaving one pigtail in the gallbladder and the other in the duodenum (refer to Figure 1). Endoscopic transpapillary GB drainage is an effective procedure in patients with ascites, severe coagulopathy, and inaccessible gallbladder with EUS. It can be technically challenging due to the tortuous nature of the cyst duct and whether the cystic duct has inflammatory changes from the extension of gallbladder inflammation. Cystic duct obstruction and the inability to identify the cystic duct on cholangiography are additional challenges. Special designs of stents have also been developed specifically for ETP-GBD. Glessing et al. described the use of a Johlin pancreatic wedge stent compared to a standard pigtail [7]. Some case series have reported the use of direct cholangioscopy to identify the cystic duct take-off and guide the placement of a wire into the gallbladder. However, cannulating the cystic duct with ERCP can be challenging, and there is a risk of perforation during attempts to pass the guidewire [8,9]. A sphincterotomy may be advanced deep into the bile duct and withdrawn slowly; the tip may catch the cystic duct opening [10]. Transpapillary GB drainage is an important option for patients with higher comorbidities. This technique can also lead to a potential surgical option should the patient's condition improve. The surgeon simply removes the stent from the gallbladder at the time of cholecystectomy. In the series by Irani et al., most transpapillary drainage cases proceeded to cholecystectomy. Patients with ascites have difficulty with tract maturation. Some experts recommend performing a small-volume paracentesis prior to the attempt. Significant ascites lead to inadequate apposition of the GB to the luminal tract (EUS-GBD) or skin (PT-GBD) which could result in bile leak. Hence, these patients should be considered for transpapillary drainage before attempts at EUS-guided drainage. Kjaer et al. [11] showed that technical success improves with experience, demonstrating an improvement from 50% to 89% after 4–5 years of adopting the technique. An international multicenter study comparing transpapillary versus EUS versus percutaneous (PCT) drainage found significantly lower technical and clinical success rates in the ETP-GBD [12]. Reported adverse events of this technique include cystic duct perforation, cholangitis, and sepsis, as well as the inherent risks of ERCP, such as post-ERCP pancreatitis (PEP) and sphincterotomy-related bleeding (PSB). Refer to Table 1 for a summary of outcomes associated with ETP-GBD.

Table 1. Selected studies on technical and clinical outcomes of transpapillary gallbladder drainage (ETP-GBD).

Study	No. of Patients	Technical Success (%)	Clinical Success (%)	Adverse Events (%)	Need for Recurrent Intervention (%)
Oh et al. [12]	96	86.6	86	19.3	10.4
Higa et al. [13]	38	87.2	76.3	9.4	15.8
Siddiqui et al. [14]	124	87.9	79.8	7.3	11.4
Inoue et al. [15]	90	78.6	74.4	21.1	Not reported

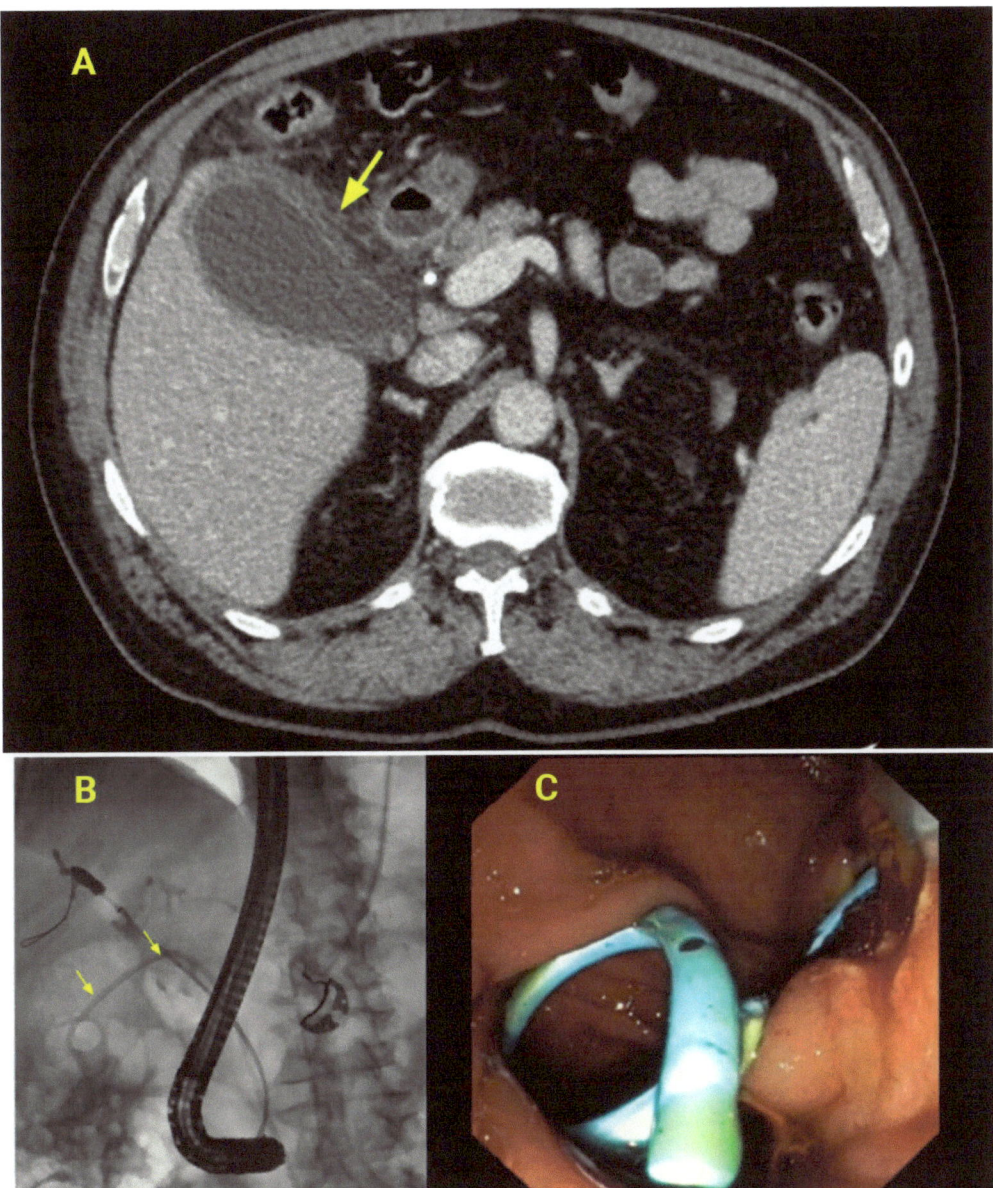

Figure 1. (**A**): CT scan demonstrating gallbladder wall thickening with pericholecystic fluid. The patient was on anticoagulation at the time of presentation (**Top**). Arrow shows thickened gallbladder wall with pericholecystic fluid. (**B**): ERCP with the placement of transpapillary double pigtail stent for acute cholecystitis (**Left**). Arrows demonstrated the pigtail of the stent within the gallbladder lumen. (**C**): Endoscopic view of transpapillary gallbladder stent placement (**Right**).

3.4. Endoscopic Ultrasound-Guided Gallbladder Drainage (EUS-GBD)

The second technique of gallbladder decompression includes the use of endoscopic ultrasound (EUS). Initial attempts with EUS drainage included the use of a 19G needle to puncture the gastric or duodenal wall to enter the gallbladder lumen. A guidewire is then coiled within. The tract is then serially dilated with a graded dilation catheter or a dilating balloon. The procedure was initially performed using 7 Fr pigtail stents or biliary fully covered metal stents. These were prone to migration. The technique has evolved since the advent of lumen-apposing metal stents (LAMS). Refer to Figure 2. LAMS are available in different sizes and are fully covered. A 10 mm × 10 mm LAMS is usually the preferred size for gallbladder drainage. A LAMS is dumbbell-shaped, deployed under EUS guidance, and the flanges hold the layers of the gallbladder wall and gastrointestinal lumen in apposition, thereby preventing bile leak. The procedure involves the insertion of a LAMS between the gallbladder and the stomach or duodenum [16]. EUS-GBD has very high technical and clinical success rates ranging from 90% to 98% and 89 to 98.4% in expert hands. Non-surgical candidates can be treated endoscopically with EUS-guided gallbladder drainage. This method avoids the risk of PEP. Secondly, it provides access to the gallbladder lumen for treatment of gallstones using lithotripsy. This technique is technically not feasible in patients with ascites due to the risk of bile leak and inability to form a fistulous tract.

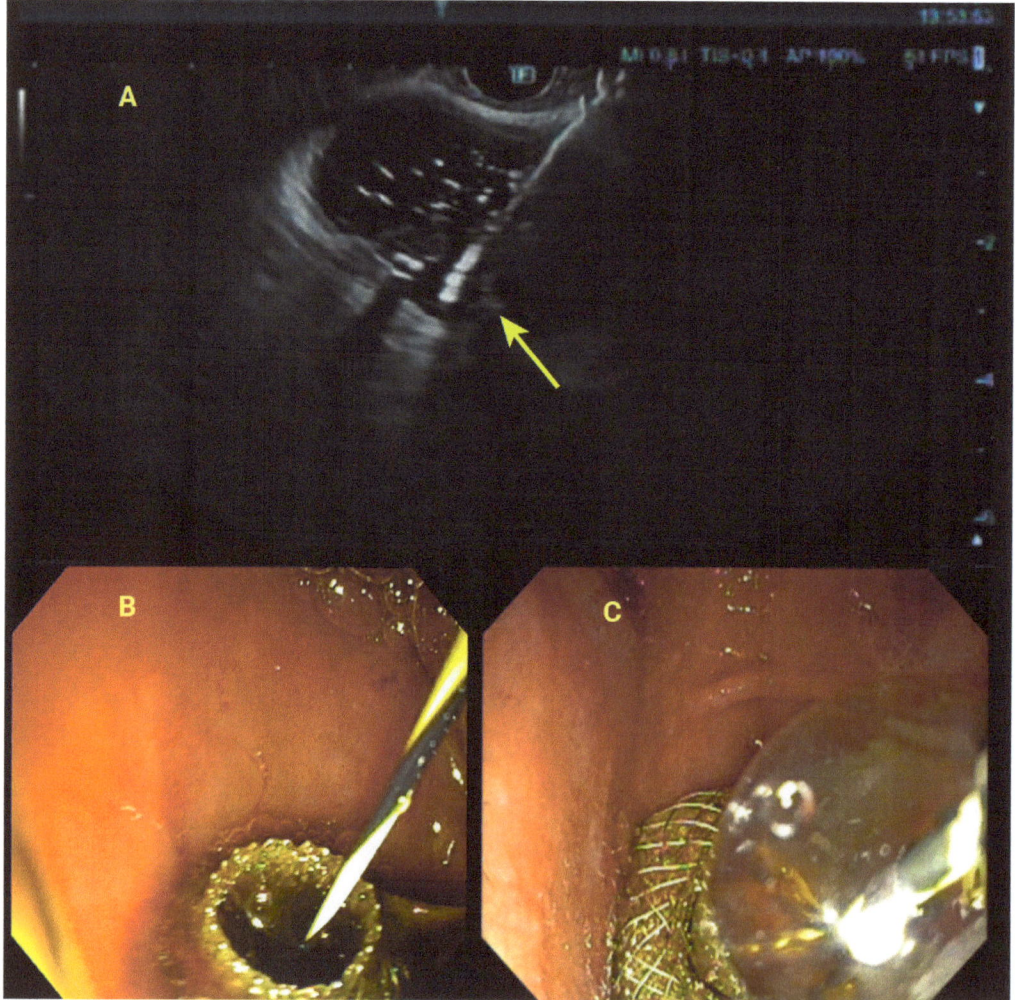

Figure 2. (**A**): Deployment of distal flange (yellow arrow of the lumen-apposing metal stent into the gallbladder lumen). (**B**): View of the lumen-apposing metal stent from the duodenum. (**C**): Balloon dilation of the lumen-apposing metal stent to allow drainage of bile.

The creation of a cholecystoduodenal or cholecystogastric fistula may affect future candidacy for surgery. A multicenter international study [17] showed a shorter surgical procedure, shorter length of stay, and shorter time to cholecystectomy when compared to PT-GBD. The operative adverse events were similar between the PT-GBD and EUS-GBD groups. However, the rate of open conversion was higher in the EUS-GBD but failed to reach statistical significance [18] and reported three cases of failed robotic or laparoscopic cholecystectomy due to the presence of adhesions and fistula. See Figure 3 for a suggested algorithm for endoscopic management of acute cholecystitis.

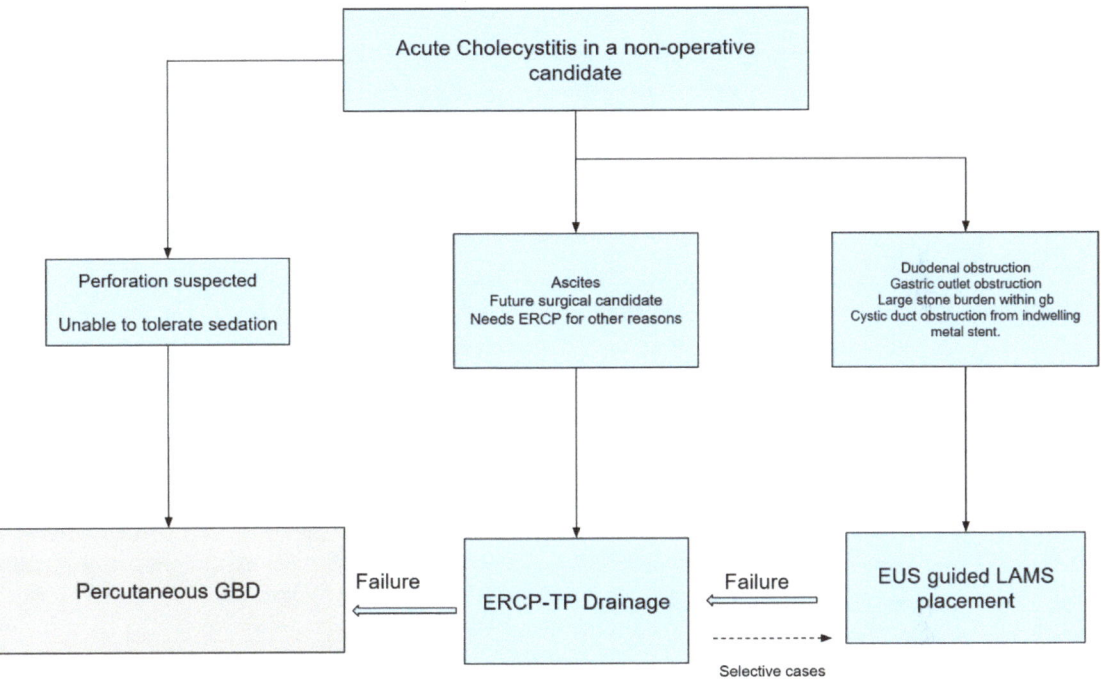

Figure 3. Suggested algorithm for endoscopic management of acute cholecystitis.

Compared to PCT, there is no inconvenience or discomfort in maintaining an external drain. The LAMS will often allow complete stone clearance. Once the gallbladder is cleared, exchanging the LAMS for plastic pigtail stents helps to maintain the cholecystointestinal fistula and potentially reduce the risks of an indwelling LAMS. Percutaneous drainage serves as a bridge to future cholecystectomy. However, in patients who were deemed fit for surgery due to acute illnesses precluding surgical options, resulting in long-term external GB drainage, conversion to internal EUS-GBD can be considered. A study by Law et al. [19] suggests that internalization of PT-GBD catheters using EUS GBD and LAMS placement as a conversion strategy is feasible and was performed successfully in seven patients without adverse events. In transmural drainage with EUS-GBD, there is the risk of bile leak or gallbladder perforation from stent misdeployment, bleeding, and occlusion of stents by food material. However, adverse event rates are similar to percutaneous drains placed by interventional Radiology. See Table 2 for procedural outcomes of EUS-GBD.

Table 2. Technical success rates of endoscopic ultrasound-guided gallbladder drainage.

Study	N	Technical Success %	Clinical Success %	Adverse Events %	Need for Recurrent Interventions %
Tyberg et al. [20]	42	95.2	95.2	21.4	11.9
Irani et al. [3]	45	97.8	95.6	17.8	24.4
Teoh et al. [4]	39	97.4	92.3	12.8	2.6
Jang et al. [5]	30	96.7	96.7	6.7	-
Oh et al. [12]	76	99.3	99.3	7.1	3.9
Higa et al. [13]	40	97.5	95	17.9	17.9
Siddiqui et al. [14]	102	94.1	90.2	11.8	0
Inoue et al. [15]	90	96.7	88.9	12.2	-

3.5. Choledocholithiasis

Choledocholithiasis refers to the presence of stones within the extrahepatic biliary system. It can be primary or secondary. Secondary stones originate within the gallbladder and migrate into the CBD via the cystic duct. The diagnosis is based on abnormal bilirubin, alkaline phosphatase, or GGT. The biochemical tests progressively increase with the duration and severity of biliary obstruction. Transabdominal US has a relatively poor sensitivity (22–55%) for detecting CBD stones but a higher sensitivity for CBD dilation (77–87%) [21]. Helical CT has shown a sensitivity of 88% and specificity of 97%. MR has 85–92% sensitivity and 93–97% specificity for choledocholithiasis detection. However, the sensitivity of MRCP seems to diminish in the setting of small (<6 mm) stones, and sensitivity is reduced to 33–71% in this subset [22]. Intraoperative cholangiography [IOC] is performed in the setting of cholecystectomy and can be successfully done in 88–100% of patients. A sensitivity of 59–100% and specificity of 93–199% for choledocholithiasis has been reported. It requires an additional 10–15 min during a laparoscopic cholecystectomy [23]. EUS is the most sensitive test for the detection of choledocholithiasis, with a sensitivity greater than 95% and 100% specificity [23,24].

3.6. Endoscopic Retrograde Cholangiopancreatography (ERCP)

The majority of patients with CBD stones are treated with biliary sphincterotomy and an extraction balloon or a retrieval basket. This technique works for the majority of stones smaller than 10 mm. With larger stones, dilation-assisted stone extraction can be performed (DASE). The latter is the combination of two techniques: endoscopic papillary large balloon dilation and a limited sphincterotomy. In some cases of large, irregularly shaped, or boxcar stones, mechanical lithotripsy and cholangioscopy-guided techniques such as electrohydraulic lithotripsy or laser lithotripsy can be performed (see Figure 4). A meta-analysis concluded that biliary sphincterotomy plus balloon sphincteroplasty was associated with fewer complications than biliary sphincterotomy alone [25]. Mechanical lithotripsy involves the use of a cranking mechanism attached to a stone retrieval basket. Single operator cholangioscopy with laser lithotripsy or EHL has been reported to have a stone clearance of 88%, with some reports reaching 100% with repeated sessions. Because of cost issues, many endoscopists employ DASE or mechanical lithotripsy prior to resorting to SOC. However, in a network meta-analysis, SOC resulted in statistically significantly higher rates of complete stone removal than mechanical lithotripsy. (RR of 1.5, $p < 0.04$). EHL systems work through a bipolar probe and charge generator. The tip of the probe generates a spark, leading to the expansion of surrounding fluid, creating an oscillating shock wave of pressure that fragments the stone [26]. LL works by focusing laser light of a high-power density on the surface of a stone. The concentrated high power creates a plasma composed of a gaseous collection of ions and free electrons that oscillates and induces waves breaking the stone. EHL equipment is relatively inexpensive compared to LL. However, the risk of perforation is higher in EHL than in LL [26].

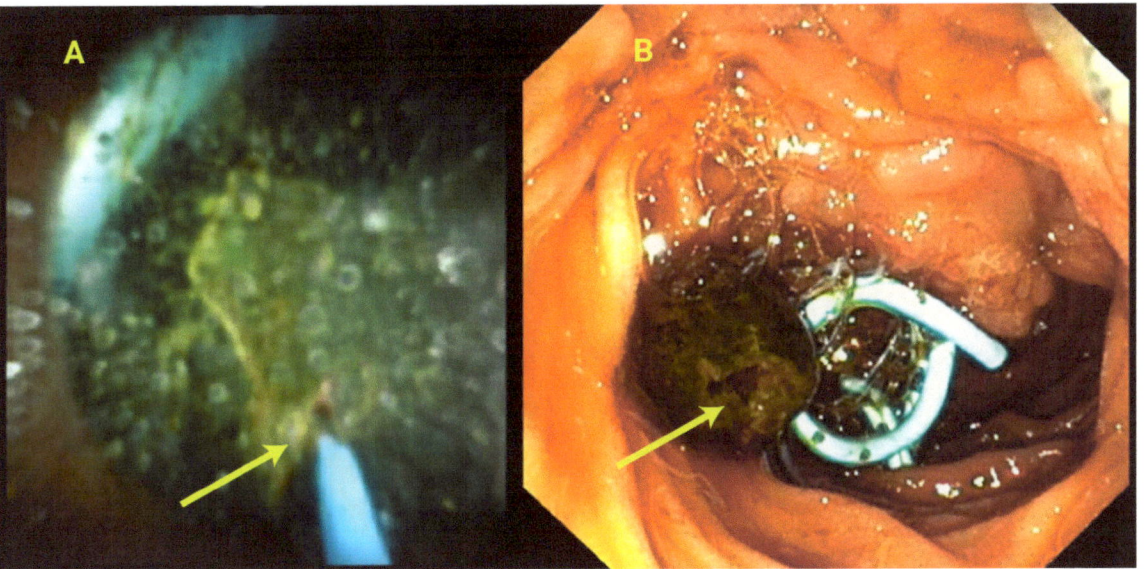

Figure 4. (**A**): A large, impacted stone leading to multiple failed attempts with extraction balloon, mechanical lithotripsy; stone was fragmented using a laser lithotripter (yellow arrow) and could be removed with extraction balloon after fragmentation. (**B**): Shows the effect of laser lithotriptor on the stone. A plastic double pigtail stent is placed in the bile duct to prevent cholangitis from impaction of stone fragments.

In a systematic review and meta-analysis, LL had a higher rate of ductal clearance (95%) than EHL (75.5%) and ESWL (89.3%). The post-procedure complication rates were higher for patients treated with EHL (13%) compared to ESWL (8.4%) or LL (9.6%) [27]. Anecdotally, plastic biliary stent placement alone can fragment residual stones over time, making subsequent stone extraction easier.

3.7. Altered Anatomy

Roux-en-Y gastric bypass (RYGB) is one of the most common bariatric procedures worldwide. The altered anatomy requires traversing a significant length of the alimentary and biliopancreatic limbs to reach the papilla. This led to the development of balloon-assisted ERCP (BE-ERCP). The use of a single balloon or double balloon-assisted enteroscope facilitates the ability to reach the papilla and perform biliary interventions. A multicenter study of ERCPs performed using a short DBE in 39 RYGB patients noted an 82% success rate for reaching the papilla and a 90% cannulation rate. The complication rate was 5%. However, BE ERCP can be challenging due to the following factors: the absence of an elevator, using a forward viewing scope, and limited accessories. In failed cases, we can resort to laparoscopic-assisted ERCP (LA ERCP). However, LA ERCP is associated with longer hospital stays, an increase in costs, higher complications, and the need to involve both surgery and interventional endoscopy teams. Endoscopic ultrasound-directed transgastric ERCP (EDGE) was first described by Kedia et al. [28]. EDGE-ERCP uses a

LAMS to create agastrogastrostomy or gastrojejunostomy connecting the gastric pouch or the proximal jejunum to the excluded stomach. See Figure 5. This enables the usage of a duodenoscope to perform the ERCP [29]. Based on a meta-analysis, the pooled rate of technical success of EDGE in RYGB was similar to LA-ERCP and was superior to BE ERCP. The most commonly reported adverse event is the failure of gastro-gastric fistula closure, requiring the need for over-the-scope clips or endoscopic suturing. See Figure 6 for a suggested algorithm in the management of choledocholithiasis in RYGB patients.

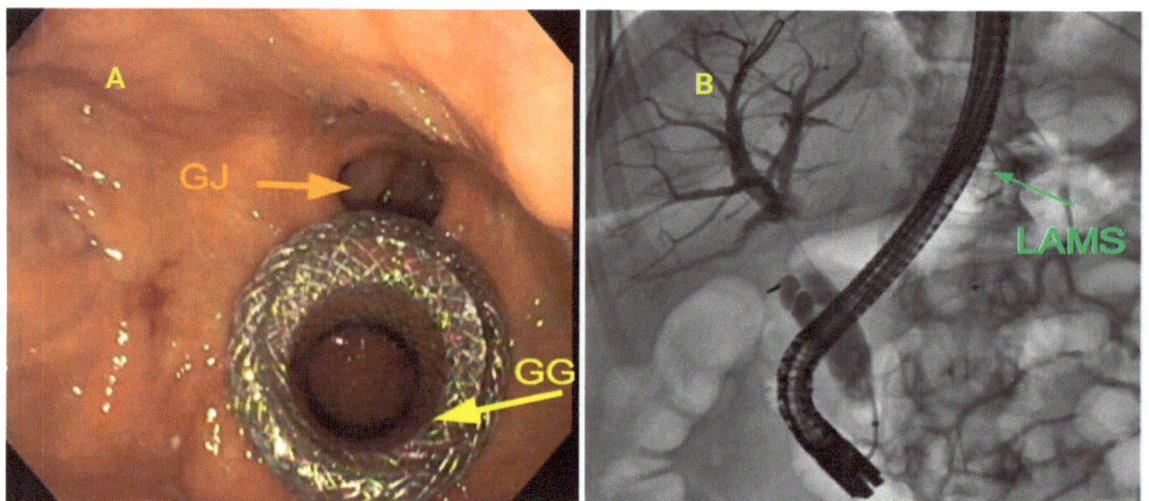

Figure 5. (A): Patient with RYGB gastric bypass, presents with choledocholithiasis, undergoes EDGE procedure to enable ERCP through the excluded stomach. GG—gastrogastrostomy, GJ—gastrojejunostomy. LAMS—lumen-apposing metal stent. (B): Shows the passage of duodenoscope through the LAMS into the descending duodenum to perform ERCP.

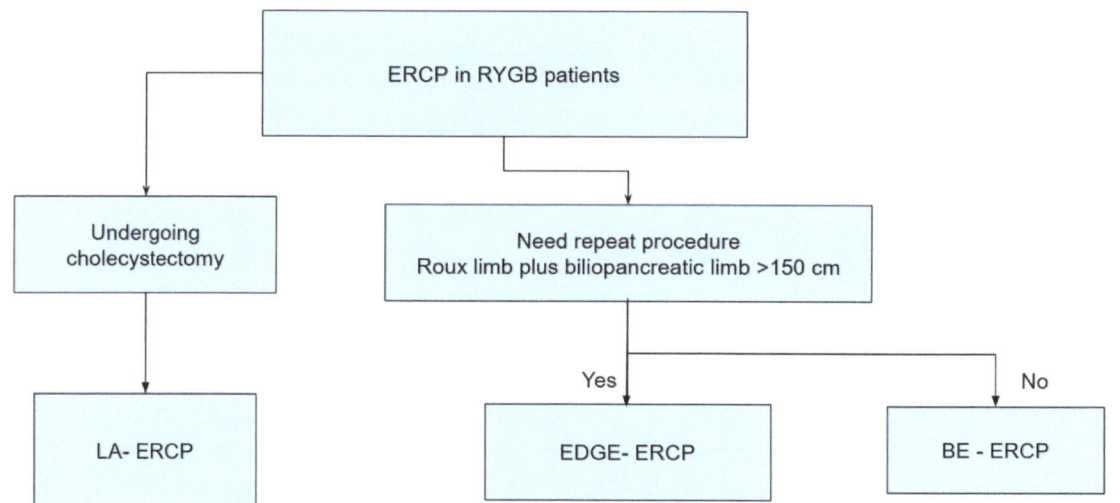

Figure 6. Suggested algorithm for endoscopic management of choledocholithiasis in Roux-en-Y gastric bypass patients.

3.8. Post-Operative Complications

Bile leaks most commonly occur in the setting of severe acute cholecystitis and often are associated with incomplete cholecystectomy. Likewise, loss of tissue planes from severe cholecystitis or an intrahepatic gall bladder may result in inadvertent and unrecognized laceration, transection, or clip placement on the common bile duct, the latter sometimes presenting months or even years later with jaundice, elevated liver functions, or stone formation proximal to the clip.

3.9. Bile Leak and Strictures

Bile leaks continue to be a persistent challenge following liver and biliary tract surgeries. Post cholecystectomy, bile leaks occur in 0.3–2.7% of patients, and post-hepatectomy leaks range from 3–20%. The risk factors for the probability of a bile leak after surgery include choledocholithiasis, gangrenous cholecystitis, or severe inflammation, which makes the surgery complex. Cystic duct stump leakage occurs from misplaced or displaced clipping, electrosurgical injury to the cystic duct, or from excessive traction. More commonly, the impaction of a stone in the ampulla leads to dehiscence of the cystic duct stump. Ducts of Luschka can also be severed, leading to a bile leak. The first line for management of biliary leaks has been the endoscopic approach using ERCP. Sandha et al. classified post-lap-cholecystectomy (LC) bile leak into low-grade and high-grade. Low-grade leaks are identified after intrahepatic opacification, and high-grade leaks occur before intrahepatic opacification. The study reported a 91% success rate with biliary sphincterotomy alone with low-grade leaks and 100% in high-grade leaks when stents were used. High-grade bile leaks occur due to a tear in the CBD wall or one of the biliary branches that form the main hepatic confluence. A stent placement benefits this in two ways: to reduce the transpapillary pressure and bypass the leak, thereby diverting bile flow into the duodenum. Stent placement also prevents secondary stricture formation at the site of injury. The stents are left in place for a minimum of 4 weeks. The success rate of endoscopic therapy remains high. The treatment aims to reduce ampullary resistance, thereby facilitating transpapillary bile flow and reducing leakage. During ERCP, there are options for sphincterotomy with or without stent placement. Sphincterotomy alone could be considered in the presence of choledocholithiasis, which causes a small leak. Sphincterotomy, in addition to plastic or fully covered metal stents, can be considered for high-grade or complex leaks. The use of multiple plastic stents or fully covered metal stents can be considered in refractory leaks [30–33].

Bergman et al. classified bile duct injuries into four categories [34]: A—cystic duct leak from aberrant or hepatic radicles (minor lesions), B—major bile duct leaks with or without concomitant strictures, C—bile duct strictures without leakage, and D—Complete transection of the duct with or without excision of a portion of the biliary tree. Post-operative bile duct strictures occur in 0.2–0.5% of patients following LC [35]. They are often due to direct surgical trauma from partial or complete transection by clipping or ligation of the bile duct. The stricture can also occur due to an ischemic insult to the biliary tree during dissection or cauterization [36]. The outcome of endotherapy depends on factors such as early identification and referral. Only 10% of post-operative strictures are identified within the first week after LC, and nearly 70% within the first six months [37]. Occasionally, the diagnosis can be delayed for several years. Such patients present with cholangitis or choledocholithiasis. The endoscopic approach remains the first line for the management of post-operative strictures.

Endotherapy, albeit requiring multiple sessions, is often successful except in certain cases of complete transection of the bile duct. Plastic stents of 10–12 Fr placement/replacement every 3–4 months, along with balloon dilation for a period of 12 months, are associated with the disappearance of stricture [38] Costamagna et al. showed that multiple stent placement resulted in stricture resolution in 97% of cases, with a recurrence rate of 9.4% after a mean follow-up of 11.2 years. Patients who received more than four plastic stents had a reduced recurrence rate, supporting the need for an aggressive approach. A randomized controlled trial with 31 patients compared multiple plastic stents (MPS) (>4) versus partially covered SEMS (PCSEMS) (8–10 mm) to treat post-surgery biliary strictures showed a higher adverse event in the MPS group compared with PCSEMS [39]. See Figure 7 for a case of high-grade bile leak treated with multiple plastic stents. Biliary patency was higher in the PCSEMS group. In LC patients, the biliary strictures are closer to the hepatic hilum [40]; hence, placement of SEMS is technically challenging due to the risk of side branch occlusion. The use of an FCSEMS for post-cholecystectomy bile duct strictures is currently off-label [41]. A recently published study by [42] Jang et al. showed that magnetic compression devices can be used for complete biliary obstruction post LC. The recent advances in endoscopic treatment with stents for the treatment of major bile duct injuries and strictures are at least as effective as surgical treatment. However, endoscopic management and surgical therapies are complementary and should be considered on a case-by-case basis based on complexity.

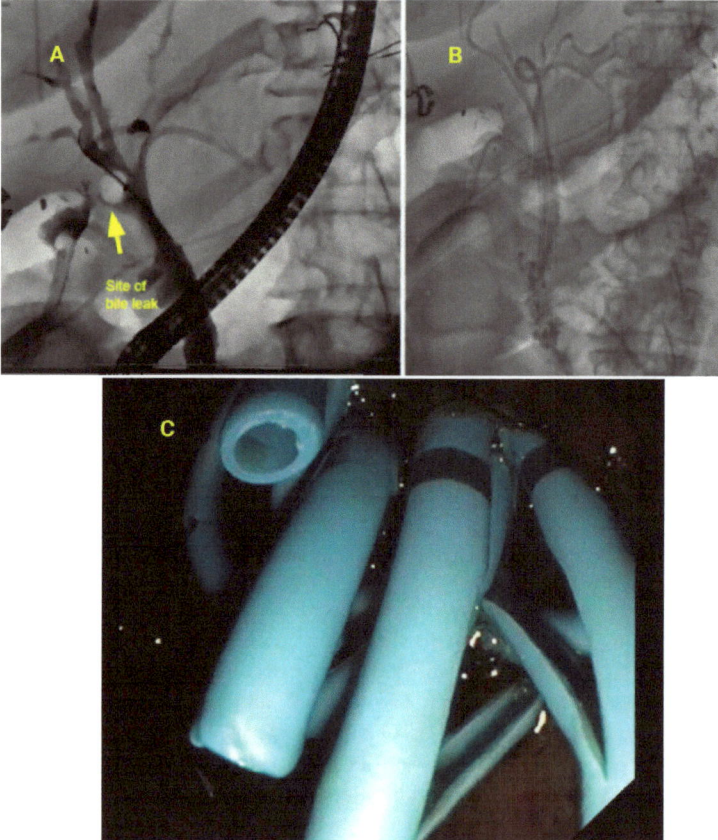

Figure 7. (**A**): High-grade bile leak noted at the common hepatic duct, treated with multiple plastic stents draining different segments, diverting bile from the site of leak. (**B**): High-grade bile leak treated with multiple double pigtail plastic stents (**C**): Endoscopic view of the transpapillary plastic stents.

3.10. Post-Liver Transplant (LT) Biliary Strictures

Post-transplant biliary strictures are classified as anastomotic and non-anastomotic. Most centers perform a biliary duct-to-duct anastomosis at the time of liver transplant, as it allows access for future endoscopic interventions and retains the sphincter functions. Anastomotic biliary strictures are known to be more common in living donor LT than in deceased donor LT, with rates similar to a Roux-en Y choledochojejunostomy. Bile leaks post LT occur in the first month and mostly at the anastomotic site [43]. Bile leaks post LT are treated similarly to post-LC leaks. Plastic biliary stents (10–11.5 Fr), with or without biliary sphincterotomy placed across the leak, have a success rate of 90–95% [44]. However, the stents are left in place for 6–8 weeks due to the delayed healing that occurs as a consequence of immunosuppression [45,46].

In a systematic review of 200 patients by Kao et al., structures associated with LT resolved after placement of multiple plastic stents at 12 months (94–100%), comparable to resolution rates of 80–95% for SEMS left in place for 3 months or longer. However, the overall migration rate was 16% in the SEMS group [47]. Plastic stent distal migration occurs in 5–10% of cases in single stent placement compared to multiple stent placement. The steps involved in the management of an anastomotic stricture start by traversing the stricture with a guidewire. This maneuver is more challenging in post-operative strictures than malignant strictures. The narrow and often angulated lumen is cannulated with hydrophilic guidewires measuring 0.021 or 0.018 inches with a straight or angled tip. Secondly, dilation of the stricture using a hydrostatic balloon facilitates stent placement. Lastly, stent placement keeps the stricture open for an extended period, leading to remodeling. The majority of anastomotic strictures occur within the first year after liver transplantation. A thin narrowing occurs in the area of biliary anastomosis, which becomes apparent after the resolution of post-operative edema and inflammation. Biliary strictures occurring at or greater than 5 mm proximal to the anastomosis are considered non-anastomotic (NAS) biliary strictures caused by ischemia secondary to hepatic artery stenosis or thrombosis. This stricture mostly occurs at the hilum but can also involve the intrahepatic ducts. Endoscopic therapy is not as effective for NAS, with an estimated success rate of 40–82% [48,49]. Such strictures often require repeated dilations and prolonged stenting [50]

Newer devices, such as magnetic compression anastomosis, are available in certain centers to treat anastomotic strictures refractory to conventional procedures. Two tracts are required to deliver the magnets above and below the strictures. This can lead to new fistula formation and is similar to a surgical anastomosis [51]. After 6 weeks, the magnets are removed, and an FCSEMS is placed for 6 months. This technique, however, lacks long-term study data and clinical trials to support routine use. Refer to Table 3 for procedural outcomes of anastomotic strictures treated with plastic stents.

Table 3. Outcomes in liver transplant anastomotic strictures using plastic stents.

	N	Technical Success	Stricture Resolution	Stricture Recurrence Rate
Rerknimitr et al. [52]	43	100	100	0
J.Morelli et al. [53]	25	96	88	9
Alazmi et al. [54]	148	97	89	18
Pasha et al. [55]	25	100	72	22
Holt et al. [56]	53	92	64	3
G Morelli et al. [57]	38	100	89	15
Tabibian et al. [58]	69	100	94	3

3.11. Benign Pancreatic Disorders

There are myriad benign pancreatic disorders for which EUS and ERCP are used, to include defining the characteristics of pancreatic cysts and strictures to assure that they are benign. Therapeutically these techniques have been integrated into endoscopic practice in pancreaticobiliary referral centers. Although not an exhaustive list, the following are the most common applications of endoscopic therapies currently used.

3.12. Recurrent Acute Pancreatitis

Recurrent acute pancreatitis (RAP) is defined as two or more episodes of acute pancreatitis (AP) with clinical and radiologic remission between episodes. The term idiopathic RAP is used when the cause remains unidentified based on history, exam, biochemical tests, and imaging. Common causes include biliary microlithiasis caused by rapid weight loss, critical illness, and in organ transplant recipients. Stones < 3 mm that are not visible on routine imaging impact at the ampulla of Vater leading to inflammation and fibrosis. This results in ampullary stenosis thereby causing biliary pancreatitis. Historically, experts have resorted to empiric cholecystectomy even if there is an insignificant stone burden or sludge. ERCP with ES is an effective alternative treatment, as it allows crystals and small stones to pass without causing pancreatic duct obstructions. Pancreatic divisum is the nonunion of the ventral and dorsal ducts resulting in the majority of drainage occurring through the minor papilla. This can be a cause of RAP. However, the decision to intervene should be carefully assessed. Multiple observational studies have shown the benefit of minor papillotomy or transpapillary dilation in reducing attacks of pancreatitis. The aim of this therapy in symptomatic patients with pancreatic divisum is to relieve outflow obstruction at the level of minor papilla. A randomized controlled clinical trial shows patients with minor papilla stents had fewer episodes of pancreatitis and hospitalizations [59]. The current practice is minor papilla sphincterotomy (miES) with stenting of the dorsal duct. This practice remains to be validated by randomized studies. The SHARP trial is a randomized controlled trial that will determine whether ERCP with minor papilla ES benefits patients with idiopathic RAP and pancreas divisum [60].

3.13. Pancreatic Fluid Collection and Duct Leak

Pancreatic duct (PD) leaks occur in the setting of acute pancreatitis causing ductal disruption. Low-grade leaks often are asymptomatic or can result in mild symptoms. High-grade leaks are associated with peripancreatic fluid collections (PFC), abdominal fluid collections such as pancreatic ascites, or high amylase pleural effusions. Endoscopic therapy is warranted if large asymptomatic fluid collections persist despite conservative management, as well as those that cause symptoms secondary to compression of contiguous organs, sepsis, fistulization, or persistent pain. Pseudocysts are the most common presentation of a PD leak. The acute collections tend to encapsulate after 4 weeks or more. These collections persist in 30–50% of acute fluid collections. A mature collection can cause gastric or duodenal outlet obstruction. Treatment entails the creation of a fistulous tract between the PFC and the gastrointestinal lumen by the placement of stents. Drainage of PFCs has historically been performed without EUS using a needle knife or cystotome to access the cyst cavity, followed by dilation of the tract and placement of double pigtail stents. A randomized prospective trial [61] showed higher technical success for EUS-guided access (94% vs. 72%) and its utility in cases where there is a lack of bulging in the gastric wall [62] performed a meta-analysis of randomized trials and prospective studies involving 229 patients and confirmed the higher technical success rate of pseudocyst drainage. Since the development of lumen-apposing metal stents (LAMS) by Binmoeller in 2011 [63], their application has revolutionized the management of PFCs. Refer to Figure 8.

The large diameter (10–20 mm) which ensures the apposition of two walls and delivery of electrocautery to create a fistulous tract makes it an effective option for drainage of various PFC including pseudocysts and walled-off necrosis (WON). A LAMS needs to be removed in 4 weeks to minimize the risk of bleeding. In contrast, plastic stents can be left indefinitely. Common practice is to replace the LAMS with pigtail stents before the cavity collapses. It is hypothesized that the conformation of the intracavitary flange of the Hot Axios with rigid spikes can lead to trauma of the back wall of the cavity as it shrinks. The advent of another LAMS in 2016, the Spaxus stent which has rounded edges and flanges that fold back, theoretically reduces this risk of bleeding. This prosthesis is not available in the United States. A propensity-matched study showed that bleeding requiring transfusion occurred more commonly in the Hot Axios group than in the Spaxus group. (6.8% vs. 1.5%) [64]. The lumen of the LAMS is enlarged to allow the endoscope to perform necrosectomy. A LAMS with a diameter of 15 or 20 mm is preferred for placement into walled-off necroses. Repeat endoscopies are needed to debride the necrotic material within the cavity. Accessories such as snares, forceps, and Roth nets have been traditionally used for direct endoscopic necrosectomy [65]. A novel device known as EndoRotor (Microtech) allows for non-thermal debridement, combining the functions of suction, irrigation, and tissue dissection for symptomatic WON [66].

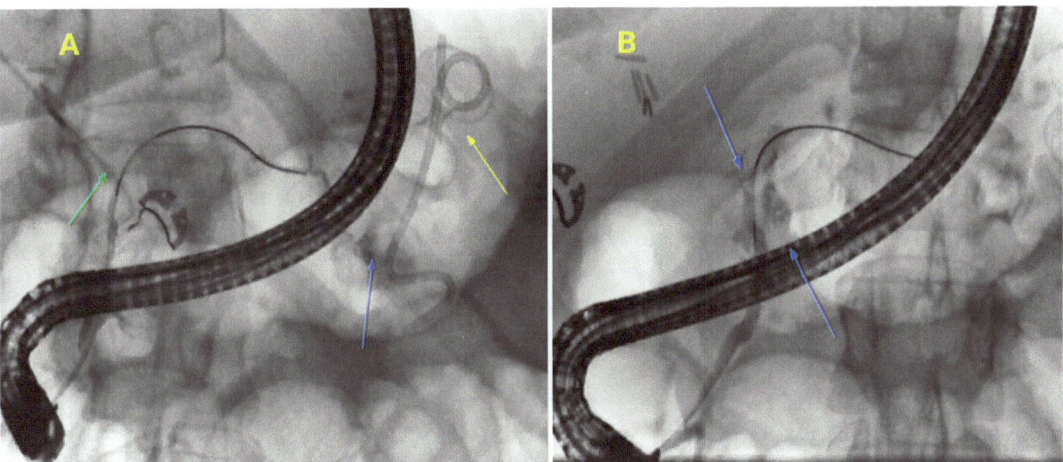

Figure 8. (**A**): Peripancreatic fluid collection treated with LAMS cystogastrostomy as well as ERCP with transpapillary PD stent. Disrupted duct in the tail of the pancreas leading into the pseudocyst cavity. (Green arrow—post cholecystectomy abdominal drain, blue arrow—extravasation of contrast from the tail of PD into the cyst cavity, yellow arrow—Cystgastrostomy using LAMS). (**B**): A tail leak and multiple side branches leaking on pancreatogram concerning disrupted duct (Blue arrows—indicate leakage from multiple side branches).

3.14. Chronic Pancreatitis

Abdominal pain is the most common symptom experienced by patients with chronic pancreatitis (CP). The causes of this pain are complex and often related to factors such as strictures, gallstones, or fluid collections around the pancreas. The primary goal of endotherapy is to manage pain and address complications associated with CP. Traditionally, computed tomography (CT) and magnetic resonance imaging (MRI) have been used for diagnosing CP, along with clinical evaluations. However, endoscopic ultrasound (EUS) is increasingly utilized because it provides detailed structural information about pancreatic tissue and helps evaluate ductal issues. Endoscopic management of chronic pancreatitis involves decompressing the pancreatic duct by dilating strictures or performing lithotripsy to reduce the stone burden. Assessing both the stone burden and the location of the calculi, whether they are intraductal or within the pancreatic tissue, can aid in selecting the appropriate treatment approach. Endoscopic retrograde pancreatography (ERP) with PD stenting may be offered for patients with pancreatic duct (PD) strictures. Removing PD stones can alleviate pain in symptomatic patients and may potentially help to preserve gland function in asymptomatic patients; however, the latter is not routinely recommended due to insufficient clinical data. Patients with multifocal strictures or extensive parenchymal calcifications may need to be referred for surgical management. Most patients with CP are treated using an initial trial of endotherapy prior to referral for surgery. However, three randomized trials from Europe showed greater improvement in pain in the early surgery group compared to endoscopic management [67–69]. Despite the available evidence, endotherapy remains the initial approach in most centers given its less invasive nature and the perception of lower risk compared with surgery. It is a reasonable alternative to surgery in candidates with significant comorbidities. An ideal candidate for endotherapy is those with single dominant stricture or an obstructive calculus in the head.

3.15. Endoscopic Management of PD Calculi and Strictures

ERCP can be attempted to clear stones using an extraction balloon or stone basket. The success of clearance depends on the size of the stone, the presence of strictures, and the degree of impaction within the duct. A small pancreatic sphincterotomy is performed to allow the removal of stones and to improve drainage. Various anatomical variations of the main PD such as ansa pancreaticus or partial ansa loops can make passage of ERCP accessories challenging. Extracorporeal shock wave lithotripsy (ESWL) is recommended for stones larger than 5 mm to achieve fragmentation. ESWL can be used to fragment large stones or those adjacent to a stricture, followed by ERCP to achieve ductal clearance. Refer to Figure 9. ESWL monotherapy may provide pain relief for selected patients suffering from painful chronic pancreatitis with main pancreatic duct (PD) obstruction [70]. A meta-analysis of 22 studies found that complete ductal clearance was achieved in 70% of cases, and pain relief was reported in 64%. Stone fragmentation occurred in 86% of the patients. However, adverse events, including pancreatitis and cholangitis, were noted in 4% of the cases [71].

ESWL is contraindicated for patients with coagulopathy or calcified blood vessels in the path of the shock waves. An effective alternative treatment is peroral pancreatoscopy-assisted electrohydrolithitripsy (POP EHL) or laser lithotripsy (LL). A study by Atwell et al., involving 46 patients with PD calculi, demonstrated complete ductal clearance in 70% of participants [72]. Furthermore, a systematic review of 10 studies on POP with lithotripsy indicated that the pooled technical success rate was 92%, with a fragmentation success rate of 86% [73]. The potential advantages of POP-guided lithotripsy include direct visualization and targeting of stones. Adverse events include PEP (7%), perforation, or hemorrhage (3–4%) [74].

In cases with PD stricture, an EUS should be performed to exclude pancreatic malignancy. The views during EUS can be challenging due to the shadowing of calculi. Additional imaging, such as pancreas protocol CT or MRCP, can also be performed. Endoscopic treatment of PD strictures involves performing a pancreatic sphincterotomy and dilation of the stricture using a balloon or a dilating catheter. One or more stents are placed routinely and replaced every 4–6 months. Endotherapy should be performed every 12 months for stricture remodeling. Refractory strictures can be treated with multiple plastic stents or FCSEMS [75,76]. Adverse events reported are worsening of pain, stent migration, pancreatitis, or cholangitis. Pain is associated with the placement of larger stents over 8 mm in diameter [77].

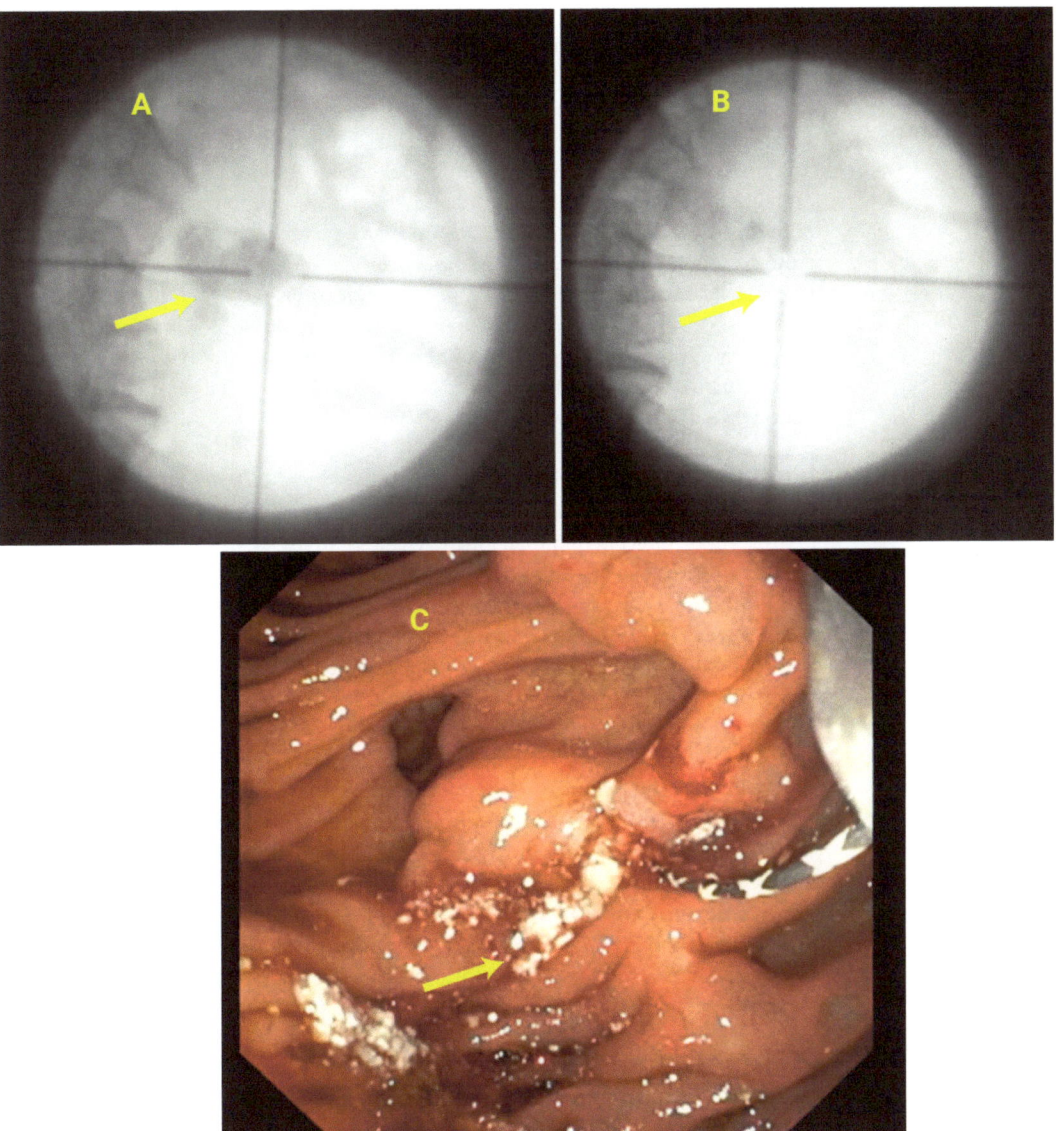

Figure 9. (**A**): Extracorporeal shock wave lithotripsy, 5000 shock waves performed targeting the stone. (**B**): Fragmentation of the radiopaque stone. (**C**): ERCP with stone retrieval. Arrow—fragmented stones.

Biliary strictures develop in 10–15% of patients with CP [78]. Similar to other strictures, treatment with multiple plastic stents or SEMS should be considered. In a long-term follow-up study, 62% of patients were stent-free after an FCSEMS after 5 years. However, severe CP and a longer length of stricture are associated with stricture recurrence [79].

3.16. Role of EUS in the Management of CP

EUS is an important diagnostic and therapeutic tool in the management of CP. Peripancreatic fluid collections occur in patients with CP. EUS-guided drainage is preferable with or without concomitant transpapillary PD stent placement if an active ductal leak can be bridged with the prosthesis. When drainage of the PD cannot be achieved by other methods, EUS-guided pancreaticogastrostomy can be performed in patients who are poor candidates for surgery or with post-surgical anatomy [80]. Celiac plexus blockade can be considered for pain management. The celiac ganglia are located anterolateral to the aorta, with the right ganglion positioned 6 mm inferior and the left ganglion 9 mm inferior to the origin of the celiac artery. It is important to note that the celiac ganglion may not be visible as a distinct structure during EUS. Celiac plexus blockade involves the injection of a local anesthetic and corticosteroids adjacent to and anterior to the lateral aspect of the aorta under direct visualization. The most serious adverse event associated with this procedure is the accidental injection into the spinal artery, which can lead to paraplegia. This risk is primarily associated with classic or posterior approach block techniques performed percutaneously [81]. Additionally, there is a risk of pneumothorax if there is a transverse entry through the diaphragm, a situation that can occur with the posterior approach. It is also worth noting that diarrhea has been reported as well as a mild decrease in mean blood pressure.

4. Conclusions

Endoscopic management has become a cornerstone in treating benign pancreaticobiliary disorders, offering minimally invasive alternatives for patients who are poor surgical candidates or present with complex anatomical challenges. Techniques such as ERCP, ETP-GBD, EUS-GBD, and advanced lithotripsy methods allow for effective intervention in conditions like acute cholecystitis, choledocholithiasis, chronic pancreatitis, and postoperative bile duct strictures and bile leaks. Innovations in stent technology, including lumen-apposing metal stents (LAMS) and fully covered self-expanding metal stents (FC-SEMS), have improved technical success and clinical outcomes while minimizing risks. Additionally, EUS plays a pivotal role in diagnostics and therapeutic interventions. The minimally invasive nature of these endoscopic techniques provides patients with reduced recovery times and lower complication rates compared to surgery. However, these approaches demand procedural expertise and individualized assessment. As technology and techniques advance, endoscopic management continues to expand the range of safe, effective treatment options which may include magnetic compression anastomoses, the integration of artificial intelligence, and robotic-assisted endoscopy, further underscoring its value as an essential therapeutic approach in benign pancreaticobiliary diseases.

Author Contributions: Conceptualization, A.V., R.K. (Rajesh Krishnamoorthi), R.K. (Richard Kozarek) and S.I.; methodology, A.V., R.K. (Rajesh Krishnamoorthi), R.K. (Richard Kozarek) and S.I.; software, not applicable; validation, A.V., R.K. (Rajesh Krishnamoorthi), R.K. (Richard Kozarek) and S.I.; formal analysis A.V., R.K. (Rajesh Krishnamoorthi), R.K. (Richard Kozarek) and S.I.; investigation, A.V., R.K. (Rajesh Krishnamoorthi), R.K. (Richard Kozarek) and S.I.; resources, A.V., R.K. (Rajesh Krishnamoorthi), R.K. (Richard Kozarek) and S.I.; data curation, A.V., R.K. (Rajesh Krishnamoorthi), R.K. (Richard Kozarek) and S.I.; writing–original draft preparation, A.V. and R.K. (Rajesh Krishnamoorthi); visualization, A.V., R.K. (Rajesh Krishnamoorthi), R.K. (Richard Kozarek) and S.I.; supervision, R.K. (Rajesh Krishnamoorthi), R.K. (Richard Kozarek) and S.I.; project administration A.V. and R.K. (Rajesh Krishnamoorthi); funding acquisition, not applicable. All authors have read and agreed to the published version of the manuscript.

Funding: All authors have no financial disclosure or support to report. There were no external sources of funding for this manuscript.

Institutional Review Board Statement: Not applicable.

Informed Consent statement: Not applicable.

Data Availability Statement: Not applicable.

Acknowledgments: The authors would also like to thank Terri Davis Smith from the Center for Digestive Health at Virginia Mason Franciscan Health (Seattle, WA, USA) for her assistance in the coordination and submission of the manuscript.

Conflicts of Interest: The authors declare no conflicts of interest. No conflicts of interest exist for all authors in this manuscript. All authors have no financial disclosure or support to report. This manuscript has not been previously published and is not currently under consideration elsewhere for publication.

References

1. Unalp-Arida, A.; Ruhl, C.E. Burden of gallstone disease in the United States population: Prepandemic rates and trends. *World J. Gastrointest. Surg.* **2024**, *16*, 1130–1148. [CrossRef] [PubMed]
2. ASGE Standards of Practice Committee; Pawa, S.; Marya, N.B.; Thiruvengadam, N.R.; Ngamruengphong, S.; Baron, T.H.; Bun Teoh, A.Y.; Bent, C.K.; Abidi, W.; Alipour, O.; et al. American Society for Gastrointestinal Endoscopy guideline on the role of therapeutic EUS in the management of biliary tract disorders: Summary and recommendations. *Gastrointest. Endosc.* **2024**, *100*, 967–979. [CrossRef] [PubMed]
3. Irani, S.; Ngamruengphong, S.; Teoh, A.; Will, U.; Nieto, J.; Dayyeh, B.K.A.; Gan, S.I.; Larsen, M.; Yip, H.C.; Topazian, M.D.; et al. Similar efficacies of endoscopic ultrasound gallbladder drainage with a lumen-apposing metal Stent versus percutaneous transhepatic gallbladder drainage for acute cholecystitis. *Clin. Gastroenterol. Hepatol.* **2017**, *15*, 738–745. [CrossRef] [PubMed]
4. Teoh, A.Y.B.; Kitano, M.; Itoi, T.; Pérez-Miranda, M.; Ogura, T.; Chan, S.M.; Serna-Higuera, C.; Omoto, S.; Torres-Yuste, R.; Tsuichiya, T.; et al. Endosonography-guided gallbladder drainage versus percutaneous cholecystostomy in very high-risk surgical patients with acute cholecystitis: An international randomised multicentre controlled superiority trial (DRAC 1). *Gut* **2020**, *69*, 1085–1091. [CrossRef]
5. Jang, J.W.; Lee, S.S.; Song, T.J.; Hyun, Y.S.; Park, D.H.; Seo, D.-W.; Lee, S.-K.; Kim, M.-H.; Yun, S.-C. Endoscopic ultrasound-guided transmural and percutaneous transhepatic gallbladder drainage are comparable for acute cholecystitis. *J. Dig. Endosc.* **2013**, *04*, 140–142.
6. Kozarek, R.A. Selective cannulation of the cystic duct at time of ERCP. *J. Clin. Gastroenterol.* **1984**, *6*, 37–40.
7. Glessing, B.R.; Attam, R.; Amateau, S.K.; Tiewala, M.; Bakman, Y.; Nemat, H.; Freeman, M.L.; Arain, M.A. Novel use of long, large-caliber, fenestrated stents for endoscopic transpapillary gallbladder stenting for therapy of symptomatic gallbladder disease. *Dig. Dis. Sci.* **2015**, *60*, 3817–3822. [CrossRef]
8. Itoi, T.; Sofuni, A.; Itokawa, F.; Tsuchiya, T.; Kurihara, T.; Ishii, K.; Tsuji, S.; Ikeuchi, N.; Tsukamoto, S.; Takeuchi, M.; et al. Endoscopic transpapillary gallbladder drainage in patients with acute cholecystitis in whom percutaneous transhepatic approach is contraindicated or anatomically impossible (with video). *Gastrointest. Endosc.* **2008**, *68*, 455–460. [CrossRef]
9. Nakahara, K.; Michikawa, Y.; Morita, R.; Suetani, K.; Morita, N.; Sato, J.; Tsuji, K.; Ikeda, H.; Matsunaga, K.; Watanabe, T.; et al. Endoscopic transpapillary gallbladder stenting using a newly designed plastic stent for acute cholecystitis. *Endosc. Int. Open* **2019**, *7*, E1105–E1114. [CrossRef]
10. Hasan, M.K.; Itoi, T.; Varadarajulu, S. Endoscopic management of acute cholecystitis. *Gastrointest. Endosc. Clin. N. Am.* **2013**, *23*, 453–459. [CrossRef]
11. Kjaer, D.W.; Kruse, A.; Funch-Jensen, P. Endoscopic gallbladder drainage of patients with acute cholecystitis. *Endoscopy* **2007**, *39*, 304–308. [CrossRef] [PubMed]
12. Oh, D.; Song, T.J.; Cho, D.H.; Park, D.H.; Seo, D.-W.; Lee, S.K.; Kim, M.-H.; Lee, S.S. EUS-guided cholecystostomy versus endoscopic transpapillary cholecystostomy for acute cholecystitis in high-risk surgical patients. *Gastrointest. Endosc.* **2019**, *89*, 289–298. [CrossRef] [PubMed]
13. Higa, J.T.; Sahar, N.; Kozarek, R.A.; La Selva, D.; Larsen, M.C.; Gan, S.-I.; Ross, A.S.; Irani, S.S. EUS-guided gallbladder drainage with a lumen-apposing metal stent versus endoscopic transpapillary gallbladder drainage for the treatment of acute cholecystitis (with videos). *Gastrointest. Endosc.* **2019**, *90*, 483–492. [CrossRef] [PubMed]
14. Siddiqui, A.; Kunda, R.; Tyberg, A.; Arain, M.A.; Noor, A.; Mumtaz, T.; Iqbal, U.; Loren, D.E.; Kowalski, T.E.; Adler, D.G.; et al. Three-way comparative study of endoscopic ultrasound-guided transmural gallbladder drainage using lumen-apposing metal stents versus endoscopic transpapillary drainage versus percutaneous cholecystostomy for gallbladder drainage in high-risk surgical patients with acute cholecystitis: Clinical outcomes and success in an International, Multicenter Study. *Surg. Endosc.* **2019**, *33*, 1260–1270. [PubMed]
15. Inoue, T.; Yoshida, M.; Suzuki, Y.; Kitano, R.; Urakabe, K.; Haneda, K.; Okumura, F.; Naitoh, I. Comparison of the long-term outcomes of EUS-guided gallbladder drainage and endoscopic transpapillary gallbladder drainage for calculous cholecystitis in poor surgical candidates: A multicenter propensity score-matched analysis. *Gastrointest. Endosc.* **2023**, *98*, 362–370. [CrossRef]

16. Irani, S.S.; Sharzehi, K.; Siddiqui, U.D. AGA Clinical Practice Update on Role of EUS-Guided Gallbladder Drainage in Acute Cholecystitis: Commentary. *Clin. Gastroenterol. Hepatol.* **2023**, *21*, 1141–1147. [CrossRef]
17. Tyberg, A.; Duarte-Chavez, R.; Shahid, H.M.; Sarkar, A.; Simon, A.; Shah-Khan, S.M.; Gaidhane, M.; Mohammad, T.F.; Nosher, J.; Wise, S.S.; et al. Endoscopic ultrasound-guided gallbladder drainage versus percutaneous drainage in patients with acute cholecystitis undergoing elective cholecystectomy. *Clin. Transl. Gastroenterol.* **2023**, *14*, e00593. [CrossRef]
18. Bang, J.Y.; Arnoletti, J.P.; Wagner, A.; Varadarajulu, S. EUS-guided gallbladder drainage in acute cholecystitis: Long-term problems with surgical approach. *Gut* **2024**, *73*, 395–397. [CrossRef]
19. Law, R.; Grimm, I.S.; Stavas, J.M.; Baron, T.H. Conversion of percutaneous cholecystostomy to internal transmural gallbladder drainage using an endoscopic ultrasound-guided, lumen-apposing metal Stent. *Clin. Gastroenterol. Hepatol.* **2016**, *14*, 476–480. [CrossRef]
20. Tyberg, A.; Saumoy, M.; Sequeiros, E.V.; Giovannini, M.; Artifon, E.; Teoh, A.; Nieto, J.; Desai, A.; Kumta, N.; Gaidhane, M.; et al. EUS-guided versus percutaneous gallbladder drainage: Isn't it time to convert? *J. Clin. Gastroenterol.* **2018**, *52*, 79–84. [CrossRef]
21. Gurusamy, K.S.; Giljaca, V.; Takwoingi, Y.; Higgie, D.; Poropat, G.; Štimac, D.; Davidson, B.R.; Cochrane Hepato-Biliary Group. Ultrasound versus liver function tests for diagnosis of common bile duct stones. *Cochrane Database Syst. Rev.* **2015**, *2015*, CD011548. [CrossRef] [PubMed]
22. Sonnenberg, A.; Enestvedt, B.K.; Bakis, G. Management of suspected choledocholithiasis: A decision analysis for choosing the optimal imaging modality. *Dig. Dis. Sci.* **2016**, *61*, 603–609. [CrossRef] [PubMed]
23. Luthra, A.K.; Aggarwal, V.; Mishra, G.; Conway, J.; Evans, J.A. A prospective blinded study evaluating the role of endoscopic ultrasound before endoscopic retrograde cholangiopancreatography in the setting of 'positive' intraoperative cholangiogram during cholecystectomy. *Am. Surg.* **2016**, *82*, 343–347. [CrossRef] [PubMed]
24. ASGE Standards of Practice Committee; Maple, J.T.; Ben-Menachem, T.; Anderson, M.A.; Appalaneni, V.; Banerjee, S.; Cash, B.D.; Fisher, L.; Harrison, M.E.; Fanelli, R.D.; et al. The role of endoscopy in the evaluation of suspected choledocholithiasis. *Gastrointest. Endosc.* **2010**, *71*, 1–9. [CrossRef]
25. Yang, X.-M.; Hu, B. Endoscopic sphincterotomy plus large-balloon dilation vs endoscopic sphincterotomy for choledocholithiasis: A meta-analysis. *World J. Gastroenterol.* **2013**, *19*, 9453–9460. [CrossRef]
26. ASGE Technology Committee; DiSario, J.; Chuttani, R.; Croffie, J.; Liu, J.; Mishkin, D.; Shah, R.; Somogyi, L.; Tierney, W.; Song, L.M.W.K.; et al. Biliary and pancreatic lithotripsy devices. *VideoGIE* **2018**, *3*, 329–338. [CrossRef]
27. Veld, J.V.; van Huijgevoort, N.C.M.; Boermeester, M.A.; Besselink, M.G.; van Delden, O.M.; Fockens, P.; van Hooft, J.E. A systematic review of advanced endoscopy-assisted lithotripsy for retained biliary tract stones: Laser, electrohydraulic or extracorporeal shock wave. *Endoscopy* **2018**, *50*, 896–909. [CrossRef]
28. Kedia, P.; Sharaiha, R.Z.; Kumta, N.A.; Kahaleh, M. Internal EUS-directed transgastric ERCP (EDGE): Game over. *Gastroenterology* **2014**, *147*, 566–568. [CrossRef]
29. Dhindsa, B.S.; Dhaliwal, A.; Mohan, B.P.; Mashiana, H.S.; Girotra, M.; Singh, S.; Ohning, G.; Bhat, I.; Adler, D.G. EDGE in Roux-en-Y gastric bypass: How does it compare to laparoscopy-assisted and balloon enteroscopy ERCP: A systematic review and meta-analysis. *Endosc. Int. Open* **2020**, *8*, E163–E171. [CrossRef]
30. Adler, D.G.; Papachristou, G.I.; Taylor, L.J.; McVay, T.; Birch, M.; Francis, G.; Zabolotsky, A.; Laique, S.N.; Hayat, U.; Zhan, T.; et al. Clinical outcomes in patients with bile leaks treated via ERCP with regard to the timing of ERCP: A large multicenter study. *Gastrointest. Endosc.* **2017**, *85*, 766–772. [CrossRef]
31. Wang, A.Y.; Ellen, K.; Berg, C.L.; Schmitt, T.M.; Kahaleh, M. Fully covered self-expandable metallic stents in the management of complex biliary leaks: Preliminary data—A case series. *Endoscopy* **2009**, *41*, 781–786. [CrossRef] [PubMed]
32. Lalezari, D.; Singh, I.; Reicher, S.; Eysselein, V.E. Evaluation of fully covered self-expanding metal stents in benign biliary strictures and bile leaks. *World J. Gastrointest. Endosc.* **2013**, *5*, 332–339. [CrossRef] [PubMed]
33. Ahmad, D.S.; Faulx, A. Management of postcholecystectomy biliary complications: A narrative review. *Am. J. Gastroenterol.* **2020**, *115*, 1191–1198. [CrossRef] [PubMed]
34. Bergman, J.J.; Brink, G.R.v.d.; A Rauws, E.; de Wit, L.; Obertop, H.; Huibregtse, K.; Tytgat, G.N.; Gouma, D.J. Treatment of bile duct lesions after laparoscopic cholecystectomy. *Gut* **1996**, *38*, 141–147. [CrossRef]
35. Vitale, G.C.; Tran, T.C.; Davis, B.R.; Vitale, M.; Vitale, D.; Larson, G. Endoscopic management of postcholecystectomy bile duct strictures. *J. Am. Coll. Surg.* **2008**, *206*, 918–923, discussion 924–925. [CrossRef]
36. Huibregtse, K.; Katon, R.M.; Tytgat, G.N. Endoscopic treatment of postoperative biliary strictures. *Endoscopy* **1986**, *18*, 133–137. [CrossRef]
37. Costamagna, G.; Shah, S.K.; Tringali, A. Current management of postoperative complications and benign biliary strictures. *Gastrointest. Endosc. Clin. N. Am.* **2003**, *13*, 635–648. [CrossRef]
38. Costamagna, G.; Tringali, A.; Perri, V. Endotherapy of postcholecystectomy biliary strictures with multiple plastic stents: Long term results in a large cohort of patients. *Gastrointest. Endosc.* **2020**, *91*, 81–89. [CrossRef]

39. Artifon, E.L.A.; Coelho, F.; Frazao, M.; Marques, S.; Paione, J.B.; Takada, J.; Boaventura, P.; Rebello, C.; Otoch, J.P. A prospective randomized study comparing partially covered metal stent versus plastic multistent in the endoscopic management of patients with postoperative benign bile duct strictures: A follow-up above 5 years. *Rev. Gastroenterol. Peru* **2012**, *32*, 26–31.
40. Sicklick, J.K.; Camp, M.S.; Lillemoe, K.D.; Melton, G.B.; Yeo, C.J.; Campbell, K.A.; Talamini, M.A.; Pitt, H.A.; Coleman, J.; Sauter, P.A.; et al. Surgical management of bile duct injuries sustained during laparoscopic cholecystectomy: Perioperative results in 200 patients. *Ann. Surg.* **2005**, *241*, 786–792, discussion 793–795. [CrossRef]
41. Bill, J.G.; Mullady, D.K. Stenting for benign and malignant biliary strictures. *Gastrointest. Endosc. Clin. N. Am.* **2019**, *29*, 215–235. [CrossRef] [PubMed]
42. Jang, S.I.; Choi, Y.; Kim, J.; Cho, J.H.; Joo, S.M.; Lee, K.H.; Chung, M.J.; Lee, D.K. Magnetic compression anastomosis for the treatment of complete biliary obstruction after cholecystectomy. *Gastrointest. Endosc.* **2024**, *100*, 1053–1060.e4. [CrossRef] [PubMed]
43. Oh, D.-W.; Lee, S.K.; Song, T.J.; Park, D.H.; Lee, S.S.; Seo, D.-W.; Kim, M.-H. Endoscopic management of bile leakage after liver transplantation. *Gut Liver* **2015**, *9*, 417–423. [CrossRef] [PubMed]
44. Morelli, J.; Mulcahy, H.E.; Willner, I.R. Endoscopic treatment of post-liver transplantation biliary leaks with stent placement across the leak site. *Gastrointest Endosc.* **2001**, *54*, 471–475. [CrossRef]
45. Londoño, M.-C.; Balderramo, D.; Cárdenas, A. Management of biliary complications after orthotopic liver transplantation: The role of endoscopy. *World J. Gastroenterol.* **2008**, *14*, 493–497. [CrossRef]
46. Verdonk, R.C.; Buis, C.I.; Porte, R.J.; van der Jagt, E.J.; Limburg, A.J.; Berg, A.P.v.D.; Slooff, M.J.; Peeters, P.M.; de Jong, K.P.; Kleibeuker, J.H.; et al. Anastomotic biliary strictures after liver transplantation: Causes and consequences. *Liver Transpl.* **2006**, *12*, 726–735. [CrossRef]
47. Kao, D.; Zepeda-Gomez, S.; Tandon, P.; Bain, V.G. Managing the post-liver transplantation anastomotic biliary stricture: Multiple plastic versus metal stents: A systematic review. *Gastrointest. Endosc.* **2013**, *77*, 679–691. [CrossRef]
48. Ryu, C.H.; Lee, S.K. Biliary strictures after liver transplantation. *Gut Liver* **2011**, *5*, 133–142. [CrossRef]
49. Chang, J.H.; Lee, I.S.; Choi, J.Y. Biliary stricture after adult rightlobe living-donor liver transplantation with duct-to-duct anastomosis: Long-term outcome and its related factors after endoscopic treatment. *Gut Liver* **2010**, *4*, 226–233. [CrossRef]
50. Ashat, M.; Berei, J.; El-Abiad, R.; Khashab, M.A. Benign biliary strictures: A comprehensive review. *Turk. J. Gastroenterol.* **2024**, *35*, 513–522.
51. Jang, S.I.; Cho, J.H.; Lee, D.K. Magnetic compression anastomosis for the treatment of post-transplant biliary stricture. *Clin. Endosc.* **2020**, *53*, 266–275. [CrossRef] [PubMed]
52. Rerknimitr, R.; Sherman, S.; Fogel, E.L.; Kalayci, C.; Lumeng, L.; Chalasani, N.; Kwo, P.; Lehman, G.A. Biliary tract complications after orthotopic liver transplantation with choledochocholedochostomy anastomosis: Endoscopic findings and results of therapy. *Gastrointest. Endosc.* **2002**, *55*, 224–231. [CrossRef] [PubMed]
53. Morelli, J.; Mulcahy, H.E.; Willner, I.R.; Cunningham, J.T.; Draganov, P. Long-term outcomes for patients with post-liver transplant anastomotic biliary strictures treated by endoscopic stent placement. *Gastrointest. Endosc.* **2003**, *58*, 374–379. [CrossRef] [PubMed]
54. Alazmi, W.M.; Fogel, E.L.; Watkins, J.L. Recurrence Rate of Anastomotic Biliary Strictures in Patients Who Have Had Previous Successful Endo Scopic Therapy for Anastomotic Narrowing after Orthotopic Liver Trans Plantation. *Endoscopy* **2006**, *38*, 571–574. [CrossRef]
55. Pasha, S.F.; Harrison, M.E.; Das, A. Endoscopic Treatment of Anasto Motic Biliary Strictures after Deceased Donor Liver Transplantation. *Gastrointest. Endosc.* **2007**, *66*, 44–51. [CrossRef]
56. Holt, A.P.; Thorburn, D.; Mirza, D.; Gunson, B.; Wong, T.; Haydon, G. A prospective study of standardized nonsurgical therapy in the management of biliary anastomotic strictures complicating liver transplantation. *Transplantation* **2007**, *84*, 857–863. [CrossRef]
57. Morelli, G.; Fazel, A.; Judah, J.; Pan, J.J.; Forsmark, C.; Draganov, P. Rapid-Sequence Endoscopic Manage Ment of Posttransplant Anastomotic Biliary Strictures. *Gastrointest. Endosc.* **2008**, *67*, 879–885. [CrossRef]
58. Tabibian, J.H.; Asham, E.H.; Han, S.; Saab, S.; Tong, M.J.; Goldstein, L.; Busuttil, R.W.; Durazo, F.A. Endoscopic treatment of postorthotopic liver transplantation anastomotic biliary strictures with maximal stent therapy (with video). *Gastrointest. Endosc.* **2010**, *71*, 505–512. [CrossRef]
59. Lans, J.I.; Geenen, J.E.; Johanson, J.F.; Hogan, W.J. Endoscopic therapy in patients with pancreas divisum and acute pancreatitis: A prospective, randomized, controlled clinical trial. *Gastrointest. Endosc.* **1992**, *38*, 430–434. [CrossRef]
60. Coté, G.A.; Durkalski-Mauldin, V.L.; Serrano, J.; Klintworth, E.; Williams, A.W.; Cruz-Monserrate, Z.; Arain, M.; Buxbaum, J.L.; Conwell, D.L.; Fogel, E.L.; et al. SpHincterotomy for Acute Recurrent Pancreatitis randomized trial: Rationale, methodology, and potential implications. *Pancreas* **2019**, *48*, 1061–1067. [CrossRef]
61. Park, D.H.; Lee, S.S.; Moon, S.H.; Choi, S.Y.; Jung, S.W.; Seo, D.W.; Kim, M.H. Endoscopic ultrasound-guided versus conventional transmural drainage for pancreatic pseudocysts: A prospective randomized trial. *Endoscopy* **2009**, *41*, 842–848. [CrossRef] [PubMed]

62. Panamonta, N.; Ngamruengphong, S.; Kijsirichareanchai, K.; Nugent, K.; Rakvit, A. Endoscopic ultrasound-guided versus conventional transmural techniques have comparable treatment outcomes in draining pancreatic pseudocysts. *Eur. J. Gastroenterol. Hepatol.* 2012, *24*, 1355–1362. [CrossRef] [PubMed]
63. Binmoeller, K.F.; Shah, J. A novel lumen-apposing stent for transluminal drainage of nonadherent extraintestinal fluid collections. *Endoscopy* 2011, *43*, 337–342. [CrossRef]
64. Mangiavillano, B.; Lakhtakia, S.; Samanta, J.; Auriemma, F.; Vargas-Madrigal, J.; Arcidiacono, P.G.; Barbera, C.; Ashhab, H.; Song, T.J.; Pham, K.D.-K.; et al. Lumen-apposing metal stents for the treatment of pancreatic and peripancreatic fluid collections and bleeding risk: A propensity matched study. *Endoscopy* 2024, *56*, 249–257.
65. Rerknimitr, R. Endoscopic transmural necrosectomy: Timing, indications, and methods. *Clin. Endosc.* 2020, *53*, 49–53. [CrossRef]
66. Mony, S.; Shrigiriwar, A.; Khashab, M.A. Direct endoscopic necrosectomy using the novel 5-mm powered endoscopic debridement device: The larger winner? *VideoGIE* 2023, *8*, 283–285. [CrossRef]
67. Díte, P.; Ruzicka, M.; Zboril, V.; Novotný, I. A prospective, randomized trial comparing endoscopic and surgical therapy for chronic pancreatitis. *Endoscopy* 2003, *35*, 553–558.
68. Cahen, D.L.; Gouma, D.J.; Laramée, P.; Nio, Y.; Rauws, E.A.; Boermeester, M.A.; Busch, O.R.; Fockens, P.; Kuipers, E.J.; Pereira, S.P.; et al. Long-term outcomes of endoscopic vs surgical drainage of the pancreatic duct in patients with chronic pancreatitis. *Gastroenterology* 2011, *141*, 1690–1695. [CrossRef]
69. Issa, Y.; Kempeneers, M.A.; Bruno, M.J.; Fockens, P.; Poley, J.W.; Ali, U.A.; Bollen, T.L.; Busch, O.R.; Dejong, C.H.; van Duijvendijk, P.; et al. Effect of early surgery vs endoscopy-first approach on pain in patients with chronic pancreatitis: The ESCAPE randomized clinical trial. *JAMA* 2020, *323*, 237–247. [CrossRef]
70. Dumonceau, J.M.; Costamagna, G.; Tringali, A.; Vahedi, K.; Delhaye, M.; Hittelet, A.; Spera, G.; Giostra, E.; Mutignani, M.; De Maertelaer, V. Treatment for painful calcified chronic pancreatitis: Extracorporeal shock wave lithotripsy versus endoscopic treatment: A randomised controlled trial. *Gut* 2007, *56*, 545–552. [CrossRef] [PubMed] [PubMed Central]
71. van Huijgevoort, N.C.M.; Veld, J.V.; Fockens, P.; Besselink, M.G.; Boermeester, M.A.; Arvanitakis, M.; van Hooft, J.E. Success of extracorporeal shock wave lithotripsy and ERCP in symptomatic pancreatic duct stones: A systematic review and meta-analysis. *Endosc. Int. Open.* 2020, *8*, E1070–E1085. [CrossRef] [PubMed] [PubMed Central]
72. Attwell, A.R.; Brauer, B.C.; Chen, Y.K.; Yen, R.D.; Fukami, N.; Shah, R.J. Endoscopic retrograde cholangiopancreatography with per oral pancreatoscopy for calcific chronic pancreatitis using endoscope and catheter-based pancreatoscopes: A 10-year single-center experience. *Pancreas* 2014, *43*, 268–274. [CrossRef] [PubMed]
73. McCarty, T.R.; Sobani, Z.; Rustagi, T. Per-oral pancreatoscopy with intraductal lithotripsy for difficult pancreatic duct stones: A systematic review and meta-analysis. *Endosc. Int. Open* 2020, *8*, E1460–E1470. [CrossRef]
74. Saghir, S.M.; Mashiana, H.S.; Mohan, B.P.; Dhindsa, B.S.; Dhaliwal, A.; Chandan, S.; Bhogal, N.; Bhat, I.; Singh, S.; Adler, D.G. Efficacy of pancreatoscopy for pancreatic duct stones: A systematic review and meta-analysis. *World J. Gastroenterol.* 2020, *26*, 5207–5219. [CrossRef]
75. Sharaiha, R.Z.; Novikov, A.; Weaver, K.; Marfatia, P.; Buscaglia, J.M.; DiMaio, C.J.; Diehl, D.; Gabr, M.M.; Gaidhane, M.; Siddiqui, A.; et al. Fully covered self-expanding metal stents for refractory pancreatic duct strictures in symptomatic chronic pancreatitis, US experience. *Endosc. Int. Open* 2019, *7*, E1419–E1423. [CrossRef]
76. Shen, Y.; Liu, M.; Chen, M.; Li, Y.; Lu, Y.; Zou, X. Covered metal stent or multiple plastic stents for refractory pancreatic ductal strictures in chronic pancreatitis: A systematic review. *Pancreatology* 2014, *14*, 87–90. [CrossRef]
77. Oh, D.; Lee, J.H.; Song, T.J.; Park, D.H.; Lee, S.K.; Kim, M.H.; Lee, S.S. Long-term outcomes of 6-mm diameter fully covered self-expandable metal stents in benign refractory pancreatic ductal stricture. *Dig. Endosc.* 2018, *30*, 508–515. [CrossRef]
78. Hu, B.; Sun, B.; Cai, Q.; Wong Lau, J.Y.; Ma, S.; Itoi, T.; Moon, J.H.; Yasuda, I.; Zhang, X.; Wang, H.P.; et al. Asia-Pacific consensus guidelines for endoscopic management of benign biliary strictures. *Gastrointest. Endosc.* 2017, *86*, 44–58. [CrossRef]
79. Lakhtakia, S.; Reddy, N.; Dolak, W.; Ponchon, T.; Bruno, M.J.; Bourke, M.J.; Neuhaus, H.; Roy, A.; González-Huix Lladó, F.; Kortan, P.P.; et al. Long-term outcomes after temporary placement of a self-expanding fully covered metal stent for benign biliary strictures secondary to chronic pancreatitis. *Gastrointest. Endosc.* 2020, *91*, 361–369.e3. [CrossRef]
80. Krafft, M.R.; Nasr, J.Y. Anterograde endoscopic ultrasound-guided pancreatic duct drainage: A technical review. *Dig. Dis. Sci.* 2019, *64*, 1770–1781. [CrossRef]
81. Wiersema, M.J.; Wiersema, L.M. Endosonography-guided celiac plexus neurolysis. *Gastrointest. Endosc.* 1996, *44*, 656–662. [CrossRef] [PubMed]

Disclaimer/Publisher's Note: The statements, opinions and data contained in all publications are solely those of the individual author(s) and contributor(s) and not of MDPI and/or the editor(s). MDPI and/or the editor(s) disclaim responsibility for any injury to people or property resulting from any ideas, methods, instructions or products referred to in the content.

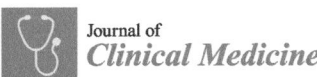

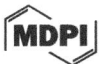

Review

Hereditary Pancreatic Cancer: Advances in Genetic Testing, Early Detection Strategies, and Personalized Management

Carmen Blanco Abad [1,2,*], Paula Gomila Pons [1,2], Sara Campos Ramírez [1], María Álvarez Alejandro [2,3], María Irene Torres Ramón [2,3], María Dolores Miramar Gallart [4], Silvia Izquierdo Álvarez [4], Eduardo Polo Marques [1,2] and Roberto Pazo Cid [1,3,5]

1. Medical Oncology Department, Hospital Universitario Miguel Servet, 50012 Zaragoza, Spain
2. Aragon Institute of Health Sciences (IIS-A), 50012 Zaragoza, Spain
3. Medical Oncology Department, Hospital Clinico Universitario Lozano Blesa, 50009 Zaragoza, Spain
4. Genetics Unit, Biochemistry Department, Hospital Universitario Miguel Servet, 50012 Zaragoza, Spain
5. Department of Medicine, Psychiatry and Dermatology, Faculty of Medicine, Zaragoza University, 50009 Zaragoza, Spain
* Correspondence: cblancoa@salud.aragon.es

Academic Editor: Cosimo Sperti

Received: 14 November 2024
Revised: 29 December 2024
Accepted: 4 January 2025
Published: 9 January 2025

Citation: Blanco Abad, C.; Gomila Pons, P.; Campos Ramírez, S.; Álvarez Alejandro, M.; Torres Ramón, M.I.; Miramar Gallart, M.D.; Izquierdo Álvarez, S.; Polo Marques, E.; Pazo Cid, R. Hereditary Pancreatic Cancer: Advances in Genetic Testing, Early Detection Strategies, and Personalized Management. *J. Clin. Med.* 2025, 14, 367. https://doi.org/10.3390/jcm14020367

Copyright: © 2025 by the authors. Licensee MDPI, Basel, Switzerland. This article is an open access article distributed under the terms and conditions of the Creative Commons Attribution (CC BY) license (https://creativecommons.org/licenses/by/4.0/).

Abstract: Background: Pancreatic ductal adenocarcinoma (PDAC) is a highly lethal malignancy with a five-year survival rate of approximately 13% for advanced stages. While the majority of PDAC cases are sporadic, a significant subset is attributable to hereditary and familial predispositions, accounting for approximately 25% of cases. This article synthesizes recent advancements in the understanding, detection, and management of hereditary pancreatic cancer (PC). **Results**: Our review highlights the critical role of genetic testing (GT) in identifying high-risk individuals (HRIs), with germline pathogenic variants (PVs) found in up to 20% of hereditary PDAC cases. Since the implementation of next-generation sequencing (NGS) panels in 2014, detection capabilities have been significantly enhanced. HRIs can be included in screening programs that facilitate the early detection of PDAC. Early detection strategies, including the use of microribonucleic acid (miRNAs) signatures and novel imaging techniques like hyperpolarized 13C-magnetic resonance spectroscopy (MRS) have shown promising results. The identification of germline pathogenic variants (PVs) or mutations in homologous recombination (HR) genes plays a predictive role in the response to various treatments, prolonging patient survival. **Discussion**: Universal germline testing for PDAC, as recommended by the National Comprehensive Cancer Network (NCCN), is now a standard practice, facilitating the identification of at-risk individuals and enabling targeted surveillance and intervention. Multidisciplinary management, integrating genetic counseling, imaging, and gastrointestinal services, is essential for optimizing outcomes. **Conclusions**: Advances in genetic testing and biomarker research are transforming the landscape of hereditary PC management. Early detection and personalized treatment strategies are pivotal in improving survival rates. Ongoing multi-institutional research efforts are crucial for validating biomarkers and developing preventive measures, ultimately aiming to reduce the burden of this aggressive cancer.

Keywords: pancreatic ductal adenocarcinoma; hereditary cancer; genetic testing; biomarkers; early detection; miRNA; hyperpolarized 13C-MRS; multidisciplinary management

1. Introduction

PDAC is a significant health burden. Its incidence is projected to increase, making it the second leading cause of cancer-related deaths by 2030 [1]. Early detection is crucial, as surgery represents the only curative treatment option, while the prognosis of patients diagnosed at stage IV remains poor [1,2]. However, most PDAC tumors are diagnosed at an advanced or locally advanced stage [2].

Given that typical risk factors, such as age or personal and familial history of cancer, are not reliable predictors of hereditary PC, GT has been recommended for all patients diagnosed with PDAC since 2019 [3]. Despite these recommendations, GT remains underutilized [1]. As a result, various strategies are being explored to increase the number of patients undergoing GT.

Identifying families carrying germline mutations in genes predisposing to PDAC and families meeting the criteria for familial pancreatic cancer (FPC) enables the identification of HRIs predisposed to developing PDAC. FPC criteria are defined as at least two first-degree relatives affected by PDAC without an identifiable hereditary syndrome [4–6]. Identifying these HRIs provides an opportunity to enroll them in screening programs. However, the selection of HRIs who may benefit from screening programs and surveillance strategies remains a challenge.

This review aims to summarize the evidence on mutations associated with hereditary PC and FPC, the current recommendations for GT in PDAC, the available evidence on PC screening in hereditary PC and methods to enhance its efficacy, as well as the prognostic and predictive implications of homologous recombination deficiency (HRD) mutations. Herein, for the purpose of this review, we will focus specifically on PDAC, which accounts for 95% of PC [6]. Other rarer pancreatic malignancies, such as squamous carcinoma, neuroendocrine tumors, and colloid carcinoma, are beyond the scope of this review.

2. Results

2.1. Risk Factors for PDAC

Risk factors can be divided into modifiable and non-modifiable risk factors.

2.1.1. Non-Modifiable Risk Factors

- Non-hereditary risk factors

PDAC incidence increases significantly with age and is frequently diagnosed in patients between 60 and 80 years of age. This age-related increase may be explained by mitochondrial electron transport chain dysfunction, which leads to the accumulation of oxygen radicals that damage cellular components [7].

The influence of sex on PDAC risk is also notable. The incidence of PDAC is higher in men, potentially due to a greater prevalence of exposure to modifiable risk factors [7].

Emerging evidence suggests that height and blood group may also influence PDAC risk; however, the exact mechanisms remain unclear [7].

- Genetic Mutations Linked to Hereditary PDAC

In patients diagnosed with "sporadic" PDAC, the incidence of germline mutations ranges from 3.9% to 19.8%, according to various studies [8–13]. Notably, higher incidences of germline PVs have been observed in certain ethnic groups. For example, Ashkenazi Jewish individuals show a *BRCA1/2* mutation prevalence of up to 15%, while African Americans exhibit a slightly lower, yet still significant, incidence of *BRCA* mutations, ranging from 7% to 13% [8].

Younger patients appear to harbor more germline mutations. Among those diagnosed before the age of 60, germline PVs are found in 21.2% of cases [9], emphasizing the importance of GT in this population, regardless of family history.

Genes identified in hereditary PDAC play a crucial role in the development of the disease. These genes may serve as prognostic factors of disease progression and help identify patients who are candidates for specific oncological treatments [10].

A wide variety of genes have been implicated in hereditary PDAC. In this section, we will review the most common genetic mutations associated with hereditary PDAC.

a. *BRCA1/2*

These tumor suppressor genes are associated with a variety of carcinomas, including breast, ovarian, prostate, and PDAC [11]. The incidence of PVs in these genes in the germline ranges from 5% to 9% [12]. Carriers of these mutations have an increased relative risk of developing PDAC, with a relative risk of 2.26 for *BRCA1* mutation carriers and 3.5–10 for *BRCA2* mutation carriers [10].

Patients with *BRCA1/2* PVs differ from patients with sporadic forms of PDAC [13]. The median age of diagnosis is 62.9 years, which is a decade younger than the median age of diagnosis in the general population, as reported in the Surveillance, Epidemiology, and End Results database [14]. There is conflicting evidence regarding whether the presence of germline *BRCA1/2* mutations has an impact on prognosis [13].

A cohort study that included 71 *BRCA*-positive PDAC patients found that *BRCA*-mutant patients had a better prognosis than the general PDAC population [14]. The authors suggested that this improvement may be related to the younger age of patients with PDAC carrying a germline mutation [14]. Therefore, the detection of PDAC at earlier stages is crucial, and new treatment strategies targeting this specific population need to be considered, as discussed further in this article [15,16].

b. Lynch Syndrome-associated Genes

Lynch Syndrome (LS) is an autosomal dominant disease produced by germline mutations in mismatch repair (MMR) genes (such as *MLH1, PMS2, MSH2,* and *MSH6*) or germline mutations in epithelial cell adhesion molecules (*EPCAM*) [17]. All these alterations cause microsatellite instability (MSI) due to a reduced capacity to produce MMR proteins and an inability of cells to correct nucleotide mismatches during deoxyribonucleic acid (DNA) replication [18].

Clinically, PDAC occurs in patients with LS type II. The incidence of PDAC in LS patients ranges from 1.3% to 4% [18]. The age of presentation does not significantly differ from sporadic PDAC, but it does vary from other tumors associated with LS. The reason for this finding is not well understood [18–20]. The majority of LS patients have a medical history of multiple cancers [19].

In general, MSI is a better prognostic factor for PDAC, potentially due to the stronger anti-tumoral response of the immune system in these patients [20]. Increased lymphocyte infiltration and PD-1 and PD-L1 expression are observed in PDAC tumors with MSI compared to those without MSI [21]. The implications of this finding for treatment selection will be discussed in more detail later in this article. Patients with MSI-PDAC tend to be less responsive to fluorouracil and gemcitabine but show greater responsiveness to FOLFIRINOX [20,21].

c. Other germline PVs: *CDKN2A, APC, STK11, TP53, ATM, PALB2, PRSS1,* and *CFTR*

Other less frequent germline mutations (<1–5%) are associated with an increased risk of PDAC, including *CDKN2A, APC, STK11, TP53, ATM, PALB2, PRSS1,* and *CFTR*. Each of these mutations causes a clinical hereditary syndrome that is associated with other clinical characteristics. A summary of these characteristics is provided in Table 1. Figure 1 presents the incidence of germline mutations in PDAC patients and the lifetime risk (%) of developing PDAC in individuals carrying these genetic mutations.

Table 1. Less frequent germline mutations associated with familial PDAC.

PV	Clinical Syndrome	Pattern of Inheritance	Risk of PDAC	Other Characteristics	References
CDKN2A	Familial atypical multiple melanoma syndrome FAMMM)	Autosomal dominant	Cumulative risk of 17% and relative risk of 13–39	Increased risk of melanoma in 70%	[10,22–24]
APC	Adenomatous polyposis syndrome	Autosomal dominant	Relative risk of 4.46; cumulative risk of 2%	Hundreds to thousands of adenomatous polyps, increased risk of colorectal cancer in 100% of carriers.	[10,24,25]
STK11	Peutz–Jeghers syndrome	Autosomal dominant	Cumulative risk of 11–36%, relative risk of 76.3	Mucocutaneous pigment macules and hamartomatous GI polyps, mean age of onset of PDAC is 40.8 years	[10,22]
TP53	Li–Fraumeni syndrome	Autosomal dominant	Cumulative risk of 1.1–9.5%, relative risk 2.41–6.5.	Ataxia, telangiectasias, immunosuppression, and an increased risk for leukemia and lymphoma, breast, ovarian, prostate, and other cancers	[10,22–24,26]
PALB2		Autosomal recessive	Cumulative risk of 2–3%, relative risk of 2.37	Monoallelic mutations predispose to breast, ovarian, and pancreatic familial cancers; increased sensitivity to platinum agents.	[10,22,23]
ATM	Ataxia–telangiectasia	Autosomal recessive	Relative risk of 2.41	Increased risk of breast, ovarian, and prostate cancer; reduced sensitivity to gemcitabine	[10,22,24,27,28]
PRSS1/SPINK1/CFTR	Hereditary pancreatitis	Autosomal dominant	PRSS1 and SPINK1: lifetime risk ranged between 18.8% and 53.3% CFTR: relative risk of 2.9–4.5	Linked to acute and chronic pancreatitis	[10,22,29,30]

Less frequent gene PVs and their different characteristics, including risk of PDAC, pattern of inheritance, and other clinical characteristics, are presented. GI: gastro-intestinal.

- Familial pancreatic cancer

FPC is defined as a familial cluster of PDAC with at least two first-degree relatives without a known hereditary syndrome [10]. Among patients who meet the criteria for FPC, germline PVs are found in only 10–20% of cases [32], suggesting that there are still undiscovered genes related to hereditary predisposition to PDAC.

Individuals who meet the criteria of FPC have a 9.0-fold higher (95% CI, 4.5–16.1) risk of developing PDAC [33]. The risk is especially high in those with three or more first-degree relatives affected, with a 32.0-fold increase in risk (95% CI, 10.4–74.7) [32]. Smoking significantly increases the risk of PDAC in families with FPC [33]. In addition, having a relative diagnosed with PDAC at an early age (<50 years) further increases the risk of developing PDAC [34]. The cumulative risk of developing PDAC by the age of 80 years is 15.7% in individuals with one or two relatives diagnosed at age 40 and 38.5% in those with three relatives diagnosed at age 40 [34].

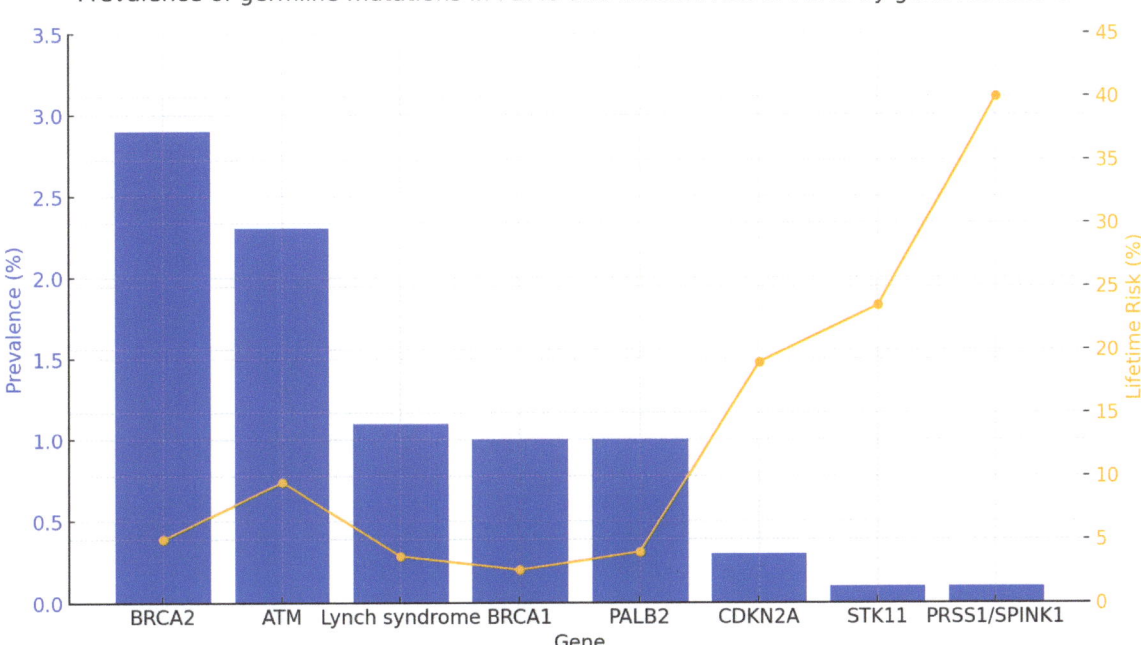

Figure 1. Prevalence and lifetime risk of pancreatic cancer by gene [4,28–31]. The figure summarizes the prevalence (%) of germline mutations in patients diagnosed with PDAC and the lifetime risk (%) of developing PDAC in individuals carrying germline mutations in specific predisposing genes. Data were collected from various studies referenced in the figure. When multiple data points were reported, the median of the published ranges was used.

2.1.2. Modifiable Risk Factors

Tobacco use doubles the risk of PDAC compared to nonusers in the general population [6]. Smoking is associated with increased inflammatory responses in the pancreas, driven by carcinogenic compounds such as N-nitrosamines and aromatic hydrocarbons. These carcinogens can mutate both proto-oncogenes and tumor suppressor genes [7].

Excessive alcohol intake ($\geq$3 drinks/day) modestly increases PDAC risk, with RRs ranging from 1.16 to 1.19, driven by alcohol-induced inflammation and chronic pancreatitis [6]. Obesity also elevates PDAC risk, with an RR of 1.72 for individuals with a body mass index (BMI) $\geq$ 30 kg/m^2 compared to those with a BMI < 23 kg/m^2 [6]. Other dietary factors, such as high intake of red or processed meats, further contribute to PDAC risk, whereas regular physical activity and a diet rich in fruits and vegetables are protective [4].

PDAC risk factors significantly alter the baseline risk in individuals with hereditary predispositions. For example, in FPC kindreds, smoking increases the relative risk to 19.2 compared to 6.25 in non-smokers [33]. Similarly, individuals with *CDKN2A* mutations experience increased sensitivity to carcinogens with tobacco exposure [4]. These interactions highlight the amplified impact of modifiable risks on an already high genetic predisposition.

2.2. Advances in Genetic Testing

2.2.1. Universal Germline Testing

- Recommendations by the National Comprehensive Cancer Network

The NCCN first recommended universal GT for all patients diagnosed with PDAC in 2019 [35]. This groundbreaking recommendation was based on the considerable rate of predisposing PVs in patients with PDAC and the accumulating evidence indicating that typical clinical factors (such as young onset and family history of cancer) are not effective predictors for identifying patients with a PV [36]. For example, a prospective study revealed that 41.8% of patients with PV variants did not meet the classical criteria for GT and were potentially misdiagnosed using these criteria [36].

The NCCN guidelines indicate that germline PVs should be analyzed using a multigene panel that includes *BRCA 1*, *BRCA2*, *CDKN2A*, MMR genes associated with LS (*MSH2*, *MLH1*, *MSH6*, and *EPCAM*), *ATM*, *PALB2*, *STK11*, and *TP53*. *PRSS1* and *SPINK1* are associated with hereditary pancreatitis as well as PDAC and should be included in panels based on clinical features [37].

- Universal Germline Testing: implementation and outcomes of universal testing

Traditionally, clinicians referred selected patients to genetic counseling, where genetic counselors ordered a GT if a hereditary cancer was suspected [38,39]. Based on the recommendations of universal testing, this traditional approach must overcome several challenges, including delays in the first consultation, the increased demand for testing, and the need for a faster turnaround time. These factors are important because these tests have therapeutic implications and due to the poor prognosis of this malignancy [38,40].

Despite recent guideline updates, GT remains significantly underutilized. A study found that only 36% of the patients had a documented discussion about GT, and 78% of those proceeded with the testing [1].

There are different strategies to overcome these challenges. The most commonly used approach for obtaining consent for GT by the treating clinician involves the use of a video educational tool or verbal education. When a PV is identified, the patient or the family is referred to a genetic counselor [40].

The incorporation of videos as an educational tool for patients with PDAC is a key strategy to facilitate pretest education before ordering GT at the point of care. These videos are designed to provide pretest education, covering the role of DNA in genetics, the potential risks and benefits of GT, and its implications for surveillance and treatment. This approach aims to prepare patients before their oncology consultations, enhancing their understanding and engagement in the GT process [41].

The implementation of this video-based education, combined with electronic health record tools and behavioral nudges, led to a high GT acceptance and completion rate, with over 85–100% of eligible patients undergoing testing [41–44]. This strategy also helped to mitigate disparities in testing uptake among different demographic groups [41,42,44]. Genetic counselors review the results of GT and provide post-test genetic counseling to patients with a significant family history despite negative results, those with PVs, and those with variants of uncertain significance (VUS) who seek clarification [43]. This model avoids overwhelming the genetic counseling services [42].

However, this pathway must overcome challenges to ensure consistency and quality across different cancer types and settings [40,42,44–46].

2.2.2. Next-Generation Sequence Panels

NGS technology has revolutionized the genetic evaluation of patients with hereditary PDAC. Historically, GT for these patients followed a stepwise or "cascade" approach, where individual genes were analyzed based on personal and family cancer history. This method, although effective, was time-consuming and limited in scope, as it allowed for the analysis of only one gene at a time [45–47]. Studies have demonstrated that multigene panel testing not only saves time but is also more cost-effective compared to the older, gene-by-gene approach [33,47–49].

As previously mentioned, the NCCN guidelines currently recommend the use of a multigene panel that includes at least 11 key genes for GT in patients with PDAC [37].

While the standard 11-gene panel has been widely accepted, several studies have investigated the value of expanding the panel. For instance, Gardiner et al. found that using a more comprehensive multigene panel, which included genes like *CHEK2*, *RAD51C*, and *BRIP1*, identified PVs in an additional 11.1% of PDAC patients [50]. Similarly, in a large cohort study by Hu et al., multigene panel testing revealed that 20.73% of patients with PDAC harbored germline PVs in genes such as *ATM*, *BRCA2*, *CHEK2*, *PALB2*, and *CDKN2A*. This study demonstrated the importance of considering a broader gene panel, especially in patients with a family history of cancers such as breast, ovarian, or colorectal cancer, where mutations in these genes are more prevalent [46]. Using broader panels that analyze 133 genes, the rate of PV detection was 33% [47].

However, one major concern with expanded gene panels is the increased detection of VUS [51,52]. Although identified during testing, these variants lack sufficient evidence to determine their impact on cancer risk. As a result, VUS findings can complicate clinical decision-making and increase anxiety for patients, as their implications for cancer susceptibility remain unclear [53].

2.3. Early Detection Strategies

2.3.1. Screening for Hereditary PC: Methods and Evidence

Cascade testing of relatives of germline PV carriers identifies individuals at increased risk of developing PDAC, facilitating their enrollment in targeted screening programs and eligibility for risk-reducing procedures, such as salpingo-oophorectomy and mastectomy [54,55].

An HRI is defined as someone with either a lifetime risk of developing PDAC greater than 5% or a fivefold increased relative risk compared to the general population [56,57]. HRIs are classified as those who meet the criteria for FPC or as carriers of a genetic variant linked to a hereditary cancer syndrome, and the two groups have varying PDAC risks. PVs associated with the highest risk of PDAC include STK11/LKB1, CDKN2A, and PRSS1/SPINK1 [57,58]. Additionally, carriers of PVs in BRCA1/2, ATM, PALB2, CDKN2A, MLH1, and APC also present an elevated risk for PDAC, although to varying degrees. Studies emphasize the need for vigilant surveillance in these populations to improve early detection and intervention [59].

The multicenter Cancer of Pancreas Screening-5 (CAPS5) enrolled 1461 HRIs to evaluate the stage at diagnosis and outcome of individuals diagnosed with PDAC and high-grade dysplasia. These individuals underwent annual endoscopic ultrasound (EUS) and/or magnetic resonance imaging (MRI). The detection rate results revealed that one individual was diagnosed with PDAC per year for every 194 screened [60]. Of note, survival outcomes for resectable PDAC were exceptional [60–62], with a 3-year survival rate of 85% reported in a screening study involving 366 HRIs [60]. Although the impact of screening on mortality has not yet been studied in clinical trials, these data suggest a potential benefit.

This approach allows the early detection of PDAC, potentially improving prognosis. Given the complexity of PDAC and premalignant lesion management, a multidisciplinary approach is essential, integrating clinical care, genetic counseling, radiology, endoscopy, surgery, and other key specialties to optimize patient outcomes.

The NCCN recommends PC screening for individuals who meet the criteria for FPC or carriers of high-risk germline PVs. The criteria for initiating screening include the following [37]:

- Individuals with two or more first-degree relatives with PC;
- Individuals with a PV in STK11 or CDKN2A, for whom screening should begin at age 35–40 years;
- For carriers of BRCA1/2, ATM, PALB2, MLH1/MSH2/MSH6, EPCAM, or TP3 mutations, screening is not recommended unless they have at least one first- or second-degree relative diagnosed with PDAC. Screening is recommended starting at age 50 or 10 years prior to the youngest age of diagnosis of PDAC in the family.

Currently, no standard screening protocols exist for HRIs, but guidelines recommend an annual EUS and MRI [37,56,57]. A systematic review of 13 studies revealed no serious physical or psychosocial harms associated with PC screening [62]. Despite advances in imaging techniques like MRI or EUS, neither modality is 100% sensitive or specific for PDAC screening [63].

Recently, early screening strategies for HRIs have expanded beyond FPC or carriers of germline mutations. They now also include other high-risk groups, such as individuals with a history of pancreatitis, those with cystic pancreatic lesions (e.g., intraductal papillary mucinous neoplasm or mucinous cystic neoplasm), and adults with new-onset diabetes [64], although this is beyond the scope of this review.

2.3.2. Biomarker Research: Liquid Biopsy

Liquid biopsy, a minimally invasive approach for analyzing circulating tumor biomarkers in body fluids like blood, has emerged as a promising tool for early cancer detection [65,66]. Currently, CA19-9 is a commonly used biomarker for PDAC. However, it is important to note that not all patients show elevated levels of CA19-9, especially those with the Lewis-negative phenotype [67,68]. Additionally, CA19-9 does not have enough sensitivity and specificity to detect early-stage PDAC reliably [65]. Its levels can also be elevated in other conditions, such as pancreatitis and other gastrointestinal malignancies, making its diagnostic accuracy more challenging [68].

Liquid biopsy analyzes circulating tumor cells, circulating tumor DNA (ctDNA), circulating free DNA (cfDNA), miRNAs, proteins, and extracellular vesicles (EVs).

ctDNA is a type of cfDNA released into the bloodstream by tumor cells as a result of apoptosis, necrosis, or active transport by tumor cells [69]. Its main limitation for early detection is its low sensitivity in identifying PDAC during early-stage disease due to the minimal amount of ctDNA present in circulation [69]. Proteins play a key role in tumor progression and have been explored as potential biomarkers for PDAC. However, most single proteins, like TIMP-1, show lower sensitivity and specificity compared to CA19-9 [70].

miRNAs are small non-coding RNAs that are typically 18–25 nucleotides long and play crucial roles in gene regulation at the post-transcriptional level [67,71,72]. Their function is mediated through binding to the 3' untranslated region of target messenger RNAs, resulting in translational repression or mRNA degradation [71]. They are implicated in different cellular processes, like cancer development and progression [73]. Circulating miRNAs are altered in PDAC patients compared to controls, making them promising diagnostic tools [71,73].

EVs are lipid-bound particles secreted by various cell types, including neurons, epithelial cells, fibroblasts, and cancer cells [74]. EVs encapsulate many molecules, including lipids, nucleic acids (e.g., miRNAs), metabolites, and proteins [65]. EV-derived biomarkers, including RNAs such as miR-21 and proteins like GPC1, demonstrate high diagnostic potential for PDAC, especially in early stages, with sensitivity and specificity reaching 90% (95% CI: 87–93%) and 94% (95% CI: 92–95%), respectively [75].

Panels combining multiple biomarkers outperform single-biomarker assays in sensitivity and specificity, and the different panels have been reviewed elsewhere [65].

One promising approach is the IMMray PanCan-d test, which combines a signature of eight biomarkers with CA19-9 to improve the detection of PDAC in blood samples. In a study involving HRIs, this biomarker panel demonstrated a sensitivity of 85% and a specificity of 98% for detecting PDAC at early stages (I and II) [52]. When patients with normal CA19-9 levels were excluded, the test's sensitivity and specificity increased to 89% and 99%, respectively, underscoring its potential to outperform CA19-9 alone in early-stage detection [52].

Similarly, the CancerSEEK blood test has emerged as another promising tool for the early detection of various cancers, including PDAC. This test evaluates cfDNA for 16 mutations and combines these findings with the levels of eight circulating proteins. In a cohort of patients with PDAC, CancerSEEK demonstrated a sensitivity of 72% and a specificity of 99% [66]. The sensitivity was lower for patients in stage I and the study lacked the statistical power to provide a detailed sensitivity analysis across different tumor stages [66].

A study led by Nakamura validated a transcriptomic signature based on 13 miRNAs for the detection of PDAC. In the validation cohort, this miRNA signature achieved an AUC of 0.93 for detecting PDAC in early stages (I and II), significantly improving sensitivity and specificity compared to CA19-9 [76]. The use of miRNAs in blood and other bodily fluids represents a non-invasive and highly promising approach for the early detection of PDAC.

The use of liquid biopsy biomarkers for the early detection of PDAC faces several limitations that must be addressed to ensure their clinical applicability. One major challenge is the variability in biomarker expression among patients and tumor subtypes, which affects the consistency and reliability of results across studies [64]. Biomarkers like ctDNA also have a short half-life of 16–114 min, requiring rapid sample processing to prevent degradation and ensure reliable analysis [65,74]. Additionally, clonal hematopoiesis of indeterminate potential or germline mutations in cfDNA might cause false-positive results [65]. Many studies lack validation in independent cohorts, raising concerns about the generalizability of findings [73]. Finally, the high cost and technical complexity of advanced detection techniques and multimarker panels limit their adoption in routine clinical practice [75].

2.3.3. Novel Imaging Techniques: Hyperpolarized 13C Pyruvate-MRS

Studies have evaluated the safety, tolerability, and utility of hyperpolarized 13C pyruvate injection as a diagnostic agent for PDAC and other types of cancers [77,78]. This compound is used in combination with MRS imaging techniques to visualize the metabolism of pyruvate and its metabolites in different tissues, allowing differentiation between areas with normal and abnormal metabolism, particularly in malignant tissues [79,80].

Hyperpolarized 13C-MRS is being investigated for its potential use in diagnosing PDAC and assessing therapeutic responses to chemotherapy. An ongoing phase I study is analyzing the efficacy of hyperpolarized 13C-pyruvate MRS imaging in distinguishing between benign and malignant pancreatic cysts [81]. By analyzing metabolic activity prior to surgical resection, the study aims to correlate these imaging findings with pathological outcomes to improve the detection of invasive carcinoma [81].

2.4. Personalized Treatment Strategies

2.4.1. Prevalence of Mutations in Homologous Recombination Genes

Germline mutations in the BRCA1, BRCA2, and PALB2 genes are associated with HRD, which follows DNA damage and increases vulnerability to agents that cause such damage, including platinum-based agents [82]. In the next section, we will discuss studies involving patients with HRD. Therefore, we will first review the prevalence and characteristics of this subgroup of patients.

The prevalence of mutations in HR genes is approximately 15.4% (95% CI, 13–18) as assessed using NGS [83]. However, when evaluated using whole genome sequencing or whole exome sequencing, the prevalence increases to 24–44% [84–86]. HR-related alterations are more frequently found in the germline than in somatic cells [87–89]. For example, one study reported that 15% of HR mutations were identified through germline testing, compared to 4% using somatic analysis [87].

Core HR genes, including BRCA1/2 and PALB2, are the most frequently mutated (around 15%) and the most extensively studied [88]. Non-core genes also play a role in HR, although they are less studied. In addition, there are ongoing debates regarding the therapeutic implications of many of these mutations [89–91]. The prevalence of non-core mutations ranges between 4% and 7%, depending on the specific genes included in the study. Some of these non-core genes include ARID1A, ATM, RAD51, CHEK2, and the Fanconi anemia genes [92–94].

Functional inactivation of both copies of an HR gene (biallelic inactivation) may play a crucial role in determining the treatment response [95]. Studies indicate that 89% of germline BRCA mutations in PDAC are associated with biallelic inactivation, compared to approximately 60% for somatic mutations [87]. Biallelic inactivation results in a more profound defect in DNA repair mechanisms, leading to increased sensitivity to platinum-based therapies and poly ADP-ribose polymerase (PARP) inhibitors [92].

2.4.2. Importance of Personalized Approaches

The treatment of patients with susceptibility gene mutations for hereditary pancreatic cancer is primarily based on the use of platinum-based agents, PARP inhibitors, and immune checkpoint inhibitors (ICI). Below, each of these treatments is described.

- Platinum-Based Agents

In breast and ovarian cancers, the sensitivity of patients with germline HRR deficiency to platinum-based agents has been demonstrated [96]. In a retrospective study of 71 patients with PDAC associated with BRCA1/2, it was observed that those with unresectable pancreatic cancer treated with platinum-based agents had significantly longer overall survival (OS) compared to those who received non-platinum agents (22 vs. 9 months, p = 0.039) [14]. Additionally, a meta-analysis of six studies comparing platinum-based agents with non-platinum agents in patients with germline BRCA mutations and unresectable pancreatic cancer showed that patients treated with platinum had significantly longer OS (23.7 vs. 12.2 months, mean difference of 10.2 months; 95% CI 5.07–15.37; p < 0.001) [97].

Another study of 262 patients who underwent both germline and somatic analyses using the MSK-IMPACT platform revealed that those with HRD experienced significantly better progression-free survival (PFS) following first-line treatment with platinum-based agents compared to those treated with non-platinum agents (12.6 vs. 4.4 months) [87].

- PARP inhibitors

PARP inhibitors have been investigated in cancers with germline BRCA mutations as second-line or later treatments. These agents inhibit PARP's role in base excision repair, which leads to double-strand breaks in DNA that, due to BRCA1/2 deficiency, cannot be repaired, resulting in cell death [93,94].

In the phase III POLO trial, 154 patients with metastatic PDAC and germline BRCA1/2 mutations who responded to platinum therapy were randomly assigned to receive olaparib or placebo as maintenance therapy. PFS was significantly longer in the olaparib group (7.4 vs. 3.8 months, $p = 0.004$), as was the objective response rate (ORR) (23% vs. 12%) [98]. A phase II study evaluated maintenance rucaparib in patients with PDAC responsive to platinum and a germline or somatic PV in BRCA1, BRCA2, or PALB2. The results were promising, with an ORR of 37% in patients with these mutations [99].

PARP inhibitors were also evaluated as monotherapy. Olaparib and rucaparib were tested in phase II trials involving approximately 20 patients with germline BRCA1/2 mutations and PDAC. The ORRs were 21.1% and 21.7%, respectively [100,101]. Veliparib monotherapy showed disappointing results, with a 0% ORR and median PFS and OS of 1.7 and 3.1 months, respectively. Veliparib's PARP-trapping activity is lower than that of olaparib and rucaparib [102]. Talazoparib, a next-generation selective PARP inhibitor with the strongest PARP-trapping activity, was also evaluated in a phase I study [103].

PARP inhibitors have also been studied in combination with chemotherapy. Although veliparib has the lowest PARP-trapping activity among PARP inhibitors, it was evaluated in first-line treatment in combination with chemotherapy. In a phase II trial, the addition of veliparib to gemcitabine plus cisplatin did not improve the outcomes. However, the impressive mOS of 15.5–16.4 months supports the use of platinum therapy as a standard approach in this subgroup [104].

Tumor mutational burden and inflammatory activity are associated with DNA damage response (DDR) deficiency. Following the promising results in breast and ovarian cancer, PARP inhibitors are being investigated in combination with ICI for PDAC with germline BRCA1/2 mutations [105]. However, the efficacy of PARP inhibitor treatments in patients with BRCAness (ATM, BAP1, BARD1, BLM, BRIP1, CHEK2, FAM175A, FANCA, FANCC, NBN, PALB2, RAD50, RAD51, RAD51C, and RTEL1), or in HRD PDAC patients, remains unclear [106]. Further studies are needed in this population.

- Immune Checkpoint Inhibitors

In the field of immunotherapy, pembrolizumab has been approved to treat solid tumors with high MSI-H or MMR deficiency [107]. However, response rates to ICI in PDAC are modest and inferior to those observed in other gastrointestinal tumors with MSI-H [108,109].

In a series of 12 patients with refractory PDAC or cholangiocarcinoma with germline HRD treated with a combination of ipilimumab and nivolumab, a 42% ORR was observed, suggesting the potential of HRD as a biomarker of ICI response in PDAC patients [110].

Additionally, the use of niraparib and ipilimumab for maintenance treatment after a response to first-line platinum therapy has demonstrated potential efficacy. Among the seven patients with BRCA or PALB2 variants, the mPFS was 10.4 months (95% CI, 1.5–19.2), and the mOS was 38 months (95% CI not estimable) [111].

3. Discussion

The benefits of universal GT in PDAC have been previously demonstrated. When implementing point-of-care GT, various challenges emerge. One of these challenges is ensuring that clinicians are adequately trained to perform high-quality pre-test counseling. Adequate training ensures that patients are fully informed about the implications of GT, potential outcomes, and the process itself. Additionally, the interpretation and management of VUS represent another major challenge. It is crucial that GT results are reviewed by genetic services to provide accurate interpretations and follow-up recommendations.

Furthermore, although oncologists are capable of delivering negative results, thereby alleviating the burden on genetic counseling services, there remains debate about who should provide post-test counseling for VUS. Some argue that clinicians can handle these consultations, while others believe that geneticists should manage these discussions due to their complexity. Continued research into VUS and their classification is essential, as this will advance our understanding and ultimately improve patient care.

The question of which genes should be included in GT remains a controversial topic. It is well established that increasing the number of genes analyzed enhances the detection rate. However, there is ongoing uncertainty regarding the therapeutic implications of these alterations and the risk of PDAC development in families carrying low-to-moderate penetrance genes. Further research is needed to elucidate how these findings should influence clinical decision-making.

Additionally, somatic mutation testing in patients with PDAC is also recommended based on current guidelines. Contrary to what might be assumed, both germline and somatic testing have proven to be complementary, providing essential and often distinct information critical for the appropriate management of these patients [112].

Although PDAC screening has shown potential in improving early detection rates and outcomes, several controversies remain. One of the major controversies is determining who should undergo screening. Current evidence suggests that individuals with familial aggregation, even in the absence of a known pathogenic mutation, should be included in screening programs. Carriers of *CDKN2A* mutations often present with more aggressive tumors, and their resectability rates remain lower despite undergoing annual screening. This has raised the question of whether the frequency of screening should be increased to biannual intervals for this subgroup [113–115]. Additionally, there is ongoing debate about whether individuals with moderate risk for PDAC, such as *BRCA2* or *ATM* mutation carriers without a family history of the disease, should be considered candidates for screening.

The management of indeterminate findings, such as subcentimeter lesions, pancreatic duct dilatation, or parenchymal atrophy, remains unclear. These findings can lead to unnecessary surgical resections, adding complexity to the decision-making process. Therefore, screening programs should ideally be conducted within the framework of clinical trials with multidisciplinary collaboration or in specialized centers.

The future of PDAC screening lies in refining risk stratification models by integrating genetic, clinical, and environmental factors to better identify HRIs. Advances in biomarkers, such as ctDNA, miRNA, or EVs, along with improvements in imaging technologies, hold promise for earlier detection. Personalized surveillance protocols based on individual risk factors and biomarker profiles may improve screening accuracy, balancing early detection with the risk of overdiagnosis, ultimately leading to more effective and targeted screening strategies.

Patients with HRD who receive platinum-based chemotherapy exhibit significantly improved outcomes. However, up to 25% of patients with HRD do not receive such treatment [90]. This is likely due to the deterioration of the patient's condition by the time HRD status is identified [90]. This underscores the critical need for early germline and somatic testing, ensuring that HRD-positive patients are identified and treated before clinical progression limits therapeutic options. Interestingly, clinical benefit appears to be comparable in patients with either germline or somatic mutations [82].

There are numerous genes involved in the DDR pathway, and several studies suggest that platinum therapy may benefit patients with mutations in genes such as *ATM* and *ATR*, those within the MRN complex (e.g., *RAD50*), and Fanconi anemia core genes. However, further investigation is required. Additionally, evidence suggests that patients with biallelic loss exhibit greater genomic instability and are more likely to benefit from platinum-based therapy compared to those with monoallelic loss [91]. This genomic instability may also influence responses to PARP inhibitors and immunotherapy. Efforts to standardize the definition of HRD in PDAC include studying the utility of genomic scarring as a surrogate marker, which could be employed in clinical trials to better stratify patients.

Maintenance therapy with olaparib in patients with germline *BRCA1/2* mutations has demonstrated improved PFS in platinum-sensitive patients [98]. However, emerging strategies aim to enhance these outcomes. For instance, the phase II POLAR trial reported a promising 35% ORR for the combination of olaparib with pembrolizumab in patients with either germline or somatic mutations in *BRCA1/2* and *PALB2* [116]. Although the results of immunotherapy in PDAC have generally been disappointing, recent data on the use of ipilimumab–nivolumab in HRD mutant PDAC and the combination of niraparib with ipilimumab in platinum-responsive patients show promise for identifying subgroups that may benefit from these treatments. Lastly, there is growing interest in novel therapeutic strategies targeting DDR-related pathways, such as ATM, ATR, and WEE1 inhibitors, which could further expand treatment options for HRD-positive patients.

4. Conclusions

The implementation of GT in PDAC is of vital importance. However, the timely and effective application of this approach requires the modification of genetic counseling services. PDAC screening has shown promising results, particularly regarding its potential for early diagnosis. Nevertheless, further research is needed to improve early detection methods. The treatment of patients with HRD mutations opens a window of opportunity to improve the prognosis of PDAC patients.

Author Contributions: C.B.A., S.C.R. and M.Á.A. performed the literature search, analysis, interpretation of data, and drafted the original manuscript; C.B.A. wrote the final manuscript; E.P.M. and R.P.C., reviewed and edited the manuscript; R.P.C. conceptualized, designed, and supervised the study and made critical revisions. C.B.A., P.G.P., S.C.R., M.Á.A., M.I.T.R., M.D.M.G., S.I.Á., E.P.M. and R.P.C. prepared the final draft and approved the final version of the manuscript. All authors have read and agreed to the published version of the manuscript.

Funding: This research received no external funding.

Conflicts of Interest: The following represents disclosure information provided by authors of this manuscript. Relationships may not relate to the subject matter of this manuscript. C.B.A.: Speakers' Bureau Participation: Roche, Servier, AstraZeneca Spain. Travel, Accommodations, and Expenses: Lilly, BMS GmbH & Co. KG, Roche/Genentech, Servier, AstraZeneca Spain. P.G.P.: Speakers' Bureau Participation: Roche, BMS GmbH & Co., AstraZeneca Spain. Travel, Accommodations, and Expenses: Lilly, BMS GmbH & Co. KG, Roche/Genentech, SERVIER, AstraZeneca Spain, MSD. S.C.R.: Speaking or advisory role: AztraZeneca. Attending scientific meetings: Lilly, Servier, BMS, Merck, LEO-Pharma, ROVI. M.Á.A.: Speakers' Bureau Participation: Sanofi, Roche, BMS, Novartis, Amgen, Servier, Merck. Travel, Accommodations, and Expenses: Celgene, Roche, Merck, Amgen, Servier, AstraZeneca. I.T.R.: Consulting or Advisory Roles: AstraZeneca Spain. Speakers' Bureau Participation: BMS GmbH & Co. KG, SERVIER, AstraZeneca Spain, GlaxoSmithKline. Travel, Accommodations, and Expenses: AstraZeneca Spain. R.P.C.: Consulting or Advisory Roles: Roche, Bristol-Myers Squibb/Celgene, Eisai Europe, Astellas Pharma, AstraZeneca Spain, SERVIER, Ipsen. Speakers' Bureau Participation: BMS GmbH & Co. KG, SERVIER, AstraZeneca Spain, Astellas Pharma. Travel, Accommodations, and Expenses: Lilly, BMS GmbH & Co. KG, Roche/Genentech. D.M.G., S.I.A., and E.P.M. have no relevant affiliations or financial involvement with any organization or entity with a financial interest in or financial conflict with the subject matter or materials discussed in the manuscript.

References

1. Klatte, D.C.; Starr, J.S.; Clift, K.E.; Hardway, H.D.; van Hooft, J.E.; van Leerdam, M.E.; Potjer, T.P.; Presutti, R.J.; Riegert-Johnson, D.L.; Wallace, M.B.; et al. Utilization and Outcomes of Multigene Panel Testing in Patients with Pancreatic Ductal Adenocarcinoma. *JCO Oncol. Pract.* **2024**, *20*, 1081–1090. [CrossRef] [PubMed]
2. Singh, H.; Nipp, R.D. Bridging the Divide: From Universal Germline Testing Guidance to Real-World Implementation in Pancreatic Cancer Care. *JCO Oncol. Pract.* **2024**, *20*, 1012–1015. [CrossRef] [PubMed]
3. Rosso, C.; Marciano, N.D.; Nathan, D.; Chen, W.P.; McLaren, C.E.; Osann, K.E.; Flodman, P.L.; Cho, M.T.; Lee, F.C.; Dayyani, F.; et al. Hereditary Can-583 cer Clinics Improve Adherence to NCCN Germline Testing Guidelines for Pancreatic Cancer. *J. Natl. Compr. Cancer Netw.* **2024**, *584*, 299–305. [CrossRef]
4. Klatte, D.C.F.; Wallace, M.B.; Löhr, M.; Bruno, M.J.; van Leerdam, M.E. Hereditary Pancreatic Cancer. *Best Pract. Res. Clin. Gastroenterol.* **2022**, *58–59*, 101783. [CrossRef] [PubMed]
5. Morani, A.C.; Hanafy, A.K.; Ramani, N.S.; Katabathina, V.S.; Yedururi, S.; Dasyam, A.K.; Prasad, S.R. Hereditary and Sporadic Pancreatic Ductal Adenocarcinoma: Current Update on Genetics and Imaging. *Radiol. Imaging Cancer* **2020**, *2*, e190020. [CrossRef] [PubMed]
6. Diaz, K.E.; Lucas, A.L. Familial Pancreatic Ductal Adenocarcinoma. *Am. J. Pathol.* **2019**, *189*, 36–43. [CrossRef] [PubMed]
7. Grigorescu, R.R.; Husar-Sburlan, I.A.; Gheorghe, C. Pancreatic Cancer: A Review of Risk Factors. *Life* **2024**, *14*, 980. [CrossRef]
8. Golan, T.; Kindler, H.L.; Park, J.O.; Reni, M.; Macarulla, T.; Hammel, P.; Van Cutsem, E.; Arnold, D.; Hochhauser, D.; McGuinness, D.; et al. Geographic and Ethnic Heterogeneity of Germline BRCA1 or BRCA2 Mutation Prevalence Among Patients with Metastatic Pancreatic Cancer Screened for Entry Into the POLO Trial. *J. Clin. Oncol.* **2020**, *38*, 1442–1454. [CrossRef] [PubMed]
9. Bannon, S.A.; Montiel, M.F.; Goldstein, J.B.; Dong, W.; Mork, M.E.; Borras, E.; Hasanov, M.; Varadhachary, G.R.; Maitra, A.; Katz, M.H.; et al. High Prevalence of Hereditary Cancer Syndromes and Outcomes in Adults with Early-Onset Pancreatic Cancer. *Cancer Prev. Res.* **2018**, *11*, 679–686. [CrossRef]
10. Abe, K.; Kitago, M.; Kitagawa, Y.; Hirasawa, A. Hereditary Pancreatic Cancer. *Int. J. Clin. Oncol.* **2021**, *26*, 1784–1792. [CrossRef] [PubMed]
11. Gorodetska, I.; Kozeretska, I.; Dubrovska, A. BRCA Genes: The Role in Genome Stability, Cancer Stemness and Therapy Resistance. *J. Cancer* **2019**, *10*, 2109–2127. [CrossRef] [PubMed]
12. Wong, W.; Raufi, A.G.; Safyan, R.A.; Bates, S.E.; Manji, G.A. BRCA Mutations in Pancreas Cancer: Spectrum, Current Management, Challenges and Future Prospects. *Cancer Manag. Res.* **2020**, *12*, 2731–2742. [CrossRef]
13. Lai, E.; Ziranu, P.; Spanu, D.; Dubois, M.; Pretta, A.; Tolu, S.; Camera, S.; Liscia, N.; Mariani, S.; Persano, M.; et al. BRCA-Mutant Pancreatic Ductal Adenocarcinoma. *Br. J. Cancer* **2021**, *125*, 1321–1332. [CrossRef]
14. Golan, T.; Kanji, Z.S.; Epelbaum, R.; Devaud, N.; Dagan, E.; Holter, S.; Aderka, D.; Paluch-Shimon, S.; Kaufman, B.; Gershoni-Baruch, R.; et al. Overall Survival and Clinical Characteristics of Pancreatic Cancer in BRCA Mutation Carriers. *Br. J. Cancer* **2014**, *111*, 1132–1138. [CrossRef]
15. Rosen, M.N.; Goodwin, R.A.; Vickers, M.M. BRCA Mutated Pancreatic Cancer: A Change Is Coming. *World J. Gastroenterol.* **2021**, *27*, 1943–1958. [CrossRef]
16. Keane, F.; O'Connor, C.A.; Park, W.; Seufferlein, T.; O'Reilly, E.M. Pancreatic Cancer: BRCA Targeted Therapy and Beyond. *Cancers* **2023**, *15*, 2955. [CrossRef] [PubMed]
17. Bujanda, L.; Herreros-Villanueva, M. Pancreatic Cancer in Lynch Syndrome Patients. *J. Cancer* **2017**, *8*, 3667–3674. [CrossRef]
18. Seppälä, T.T.; Burkhart, R.A.; Katona, B.W. Hereditary Colorectal, Gastric, and Pancreatic Cancer: Comprehensive Review. *BJS Open* **2023**, *7*, zrad023. [CrossRef] [PubMed]
19. Takamizawa, S.; Morizane, C.; Tanabe, N.; Maruki, Y.; Kondo, S.; Hijioka, S.; Ueno, H.; Sugano, K.; Hiraoka, N.; Okusaka, T. Clinical Characteristics of Pancreatic and Biliary Tract Cancers Associated with Lynch Syndrome. *J. Hepato-Biliary-Pancreat. Sci.* **2022**, *29*, 377–384. [CrossRef]
20. Zalevskaja, K.; Mecklin, J.-P.; Seppälä, T.T. Clinical Characteristics of Pancreatic and Biliary Tract Cancers in Lynch Syndrome: A Retrospective Analysis from the Finnish National Lynch Syndrome Research Registry. *Front. Oncol.* **2023**, *13*, 1123901. [CrossRef] [PubMed]
21. Ghidini, M.; Lampis, A.; Mirchev, M.B.; Okuducu, A.F.; Ratti, M.; Valeri, N.; Hahne, J.C. Immune-Based Therapies and the Role of Microsatellite Instability in Pancreatic Cancer. *Genes* **2021**, *12*, 33. [CrossRef] [PubMed]
22. Pantaleo, A.; Forte, G.; Fasano, C.; Lepore Signorile, M.; Sanese, P.; De Marco, K.; Di Nicola, E.; Latrofa, M.; Grossi, V.; Disciglio, V.; et al. Understanding the Genetic Landscape of Pancreatic Ductal Adenocarcinoma to Support Personalized Medicine: A Systematic Review. *Cancers* **2024**, *16*, 56. [CrossRef] [PubMed]
23. The Cancer Genome Atlas Research Network. Integrated Genomic Characterization of Pancreatic Ductal Adenocarcinoma. *Cancer Cell* **2017**, *32*, 185–203.e13. [CrossRef] [PubMed]
24. Zhan, W.; Shelton, C.A.; Greer, P.J.; Brand, R.E.; Whitcomb, D.C. Germline Variants and Risk for Pancreatic Cancer: A Systematic Review and Emerging Concepts. *Pancreas* **2018**, *47*, 924–936. [CrossRef] [PubMed]

25. Dinarvand, P.; Davaro, E.P.; Doan, J.V.; Ising, M.E.; Evans, N.R.; Phillips, N.J.; Lai, J.; Guzman, M.A. Familial Adenomatous Polyposis Syndrome: An Update and Review of Extraintestinal Manifestations. *Arch. Pathol. Lab. Med.* **2019**, *143*, 1382–1398. [CrossRef]
26. Aedma, S.K.; Kasi, A. Li-Fraumeni Syndrome. In *StatPearls*; StatPearls Publishing: Treasure Island, FL, USA, 2024.
27. Shindo, K.; Yu, J.; Suenaga, M.; Fesharakizadeh, S.; Cho, C.; Macgregor-Das, A.; Siddiqui, A.; Witmer, P.D.; Tamura, K.; Song, T.J.; et al. Deleterious Germline Mutations in Patients with Apparently Sporadic Pancreatic Adenocarcinoma. *J. Clin. Oncol.* **2017**, *35*, 3382–3390. [CrossRef] [PubMed]
28. Hsu, F.-C.; Roberts, N.J.; Childs, E.; Porter, N.; Rabe, K.G.; Borgida, A.; Ukaegbu, C.; Goggins, M.G.; Hruban, R.H.; Zogopoulos, G.; et al. Risk of Pancreatic Cancer Among Individuals with Pathogenic Variants in the ATM Gene. *JAMA Oncol.* **2021**, *7*, 1664–1668. [CrossRef] [PubMed]
29. Bennett, C.; Suguitan, M.; Abad, J.; Chawla, A. Identification of High-Risk Germline Variants for the Development of Pancreatic Cancer: Common Characteristics and Potential Guidance to Screening Guidelines. *Pancreatology* **2022**, *22*, 719–729. [CrossRef] [PubMed]
30. Rosendahl, J.; Landt, O.; Bernadova, J.; Kovacs, P.; Teich, N.; Bödeker, H.; Keim, V.; Ruffert, C.; Mössner, J.; Kage, A.; et al. *CFTR*, *SPINK1*, *CTRC* and *PRSS1* Variants in Chronic Pancreatitis: Is the Role of Mutated *CFTR* Overestimated? *Gut* **2013**, *62*, 582–592. [CrossRef]
31. Rodrigues, L.M.; Maistro, S.; Marques Rocha, V.; Lopez, R.V.M.; Koike Folgueira, M.A.A. Prevalence of Germline Mutations in Pancreatic Carcinoma Patients (PCP) Unselected for Family History (FH). *J. Clin. Oncol.* **2021**, *39* (Suppl. S15), e16263. [CrossRef]
32. Matsubayashi, H.; Takaori, K.; Morizane, C.; Maguchi, H.; Mizuma, M.; Takahashi, H.; Wada, K.; Hosoi, H.; Yachida, S.; Suzuki, M.; et al. Familial Pancreatic Cancer: Concept, Management and Issues. *World J. Gastroenterol.* **2017**, *23*, 935–948. [CrossRef] [PubMed]
33. Klein, A.P.; Brune, K.A.; Petersen, G.M.; Goggins, M.; Tersmette, A.C.; Offerhaus, G.J.A.; Griffin, C.; Cameron, J.L.; Yeo, C.J.; Kern, S.; et al. Prospective Risk of Pancreatic Cancer in Familial Pancreatic Cancer Kindreds. *Cancer Res.* **2004**, *64*, 2634–2638. [CrossRef]
34. Brune, K.A.; Lau, B.; Palmisano, E.; Canto, M.; Goggins, M.G.; Hruban, R.H.; Klein, A.P. Importance of Age of Onset in Pancreatic Cancer Kindreds. *J. Natl. Cancer Inst.* **2010**, *102*, 119–126. [CrossRef] [PubMed]
35. Daly, M.B.; Pal, T.; Berry, M.P.; Buys, S.S.; Dickson, P.; Domchek, S.M.; Elkhanany, A.; Friedman, S.; Goggins, M.; Hutton, M.L.; et al. Genetic/Familial High-Risk Assessment: Breast, Ovarian, and Pancreatic, Version 2.2021, NCCN Clinical Practice Guidelines in Oncology. *J. Natl. Compr. Cancer Netw.* **2021**, *19*, 77–102. [CrossRef] [PubMed]
36. Lowery, M.A.; Wong, W.; Jordan, E.J.; Lee, J.W.; Kemel, Y.; Vijai, J.; Mandelker, D.; Zehir, A.; Capanu, M.; Salo-Mullen, E.; et al. Prospective Evaluation of Germline Alterations in Patients with Exocrine Pancreatic Neoplasms. *J. Natl. Cancer Inst.* **2018**, *110*, 1067–1074. [CrossRef] [PubMed]
37. Daly, M.B.; Pal, T.; Maxwell, K.N.; Churpek, J.; Kohlmann, W.; AlHilli, Z.; Arun, B.; Buys, S.S.; Cheng, H.; Domchek, S.M.; et al. NCCN Guidelines® Insights: Genetic/Familial High-Risk Assessment: Breast, Ovarian, and Pancreatic, Version 2.2024. *J. Natl. Compr. Cancer Netw.* **2023**, *21*, 1000–1010. [CrossRef] [PubMed]
38. Rainone, M.; Singh, I.; Salo-Mullen, E.E.; Stadler, Z.K.; O'Reilly, E.M. An Emerging Paradigm for Germline Testing in Pancreatic Ductal Adenocarcinoma and Immediate Implications for Clinical Practice: A Review. *JAMA Oncol.* **2020**, *6*, 764–771. [CrossRef]
39. Golan, T.; Casolino, R.; Biankin, A.V.; Hammel, P.; Whitaker, K.D.; Hall, M.J.; Riegert-Johnson, D.L. Germline BRCA Testing in Pancreatic Cancer: Improving Awareness, Timing, Turnaround, and Uptake. *Ther. Adv. Med. Oncol.* **2023**, *15*, 17588359231189127. [CrossRef] [PubMed]
40. Scheinberg, T.; Young, A.; Woo, H.; Goodwin, A.; Mahon, K.L.; Horvath, L.G. Mainstream Consent Programs for Genetic Counseling in Cancer Patients: A Systematic Review. *Asia Pac. J. Clin. Oncol.* **2021**, *17*, 163–177. [CrossRef] [PubMed]
41. Kasliwal, S.; Baydogan, S.; Harrison, D.; Mork, M.; Maitra, A.; Mcallister, F. Implementation of a Video-Based Remote Germline Testing for Individuals with Pancreatic Ductal Adenocarcinoma. *Gastroenterology* **2022**, *163*, 316–318.e1. [CrossRef] [PubMed]
42. Lau-Min, K.S.; Symecko, H.; Spielman, K.; Mann, D.; Hood, R.; Rathore, S.; Wolfe, C.; Gabriel, P.E.; Rendle, K.A.; Nathanson, K.L.; et al. Integration of Germline Genetic Testing Into Routine Clinical Practice for Patients with Pancreatic Adenocarcinoma. *JCO Oncol. Pract.* **2024**, OP2400356. [CrossRef] [PubMed]
43. Ramsey, M.L.; Tomlinson, J.; Pearlman, R.; Abushahin, L.; Aeilts, A.; Chen, H.-Z.; Chen, Y.; Compton, A.; Elkhatib, R.; Geiger, L.; et al. Mainstreaming Germline Genetic Testing for Patients with Pancreatic Cancer Increases Uptake. *Fam. Cancer* **2023**, *22*, 91–97. [CrossRef] [PubMed]
44. Hamilton, J.G.; Symecko, H.; Spielman, K.; Breen, K.; Mueller, R.; Catchings, A.; Trottier, M.; Salo-Mullen, E.E.; Shah, I.; Arutyunova, A.; et al. Uptake and Acceptability of a Mainstreaming Model of Hereditary Cancer Multigene Panel Testing among Patients with Ovarian, Pancreatic, and Prostate Cancer. *Genet. Med.* **2021**, *23*, 2105–2113. [CrossRef]
45. Mizukami, K.; Iwasaki, Y.; Kawakami, E.; Hirata, M.; Kamatani, Y.; Matsuda, K.; Endo, M.; Sugano, K.; Yoshida, T.; Murakami, Y.; et al. Genetic Characterization of Pancreatic Cancer Patients and Prediction of Carrier Status of Germline Pathogenic Variants in Cancer-Predisposing Genes. *EBioMedicine* **2020**, *60*, 103033. [CrossRef] [PubMed]

46. Hu, C.; LaDuca, H.; Shimelis, H.; Polley, E.C.; Lilyquist, J.; Hart, S.N.; Na, J.; Thomas, A.; Lee, K.Y.; Davis, B.T.; et al. Multigene Hereditary Cancer Panels Reveal High-Risk Pancreatic Cancer Susceptibility Genes. *JCO Precis. Oncol.* **2018**, *2*, PO.17.00291. [CrossRef] [PubMed]
47. Walker, E.J.; Goldberg, D.; Gordon, K.M.; Pedley, C.; Carnevale, J.; Cinar, P.; Collisson, E.A.; Tempero, M.A.; Ko, A.H.; Blanco, A.M.; et al. Implementation of an Embedded In-Clinic Genetic Testing Station to Optimize Germline Testing for Patients with Pancreatic Adenocarcinoma. *The Oncologist* **2021**, *26*, e1982–e1991. [CrossRef]
48. Hu, C.; Hart, S.N.; Polley, E.C.; Gnanaolivu, R.; Shimelis, H.; Lee, K.Y.; Lilyquist, J.; Na, J.; Moore, R.; Antwi, S.O.; et al. Association Between Inherited Germline Mutations in Cancer Predisposition Genes and Risk of Pancreatic Cancer. *JAMA* **2018**, *319*, 2401–2409. [CrossRef] [PubMed]
49. Chittenden, A.; Haraldsdottir, S.; Ukaegbu, C.; Underhill-Blazey, M.; Gaonkar, S.; Uno, H.; Brais, L.K.; Perez, K.; Wolpin, B.M.; Syngal, S.; et al. Implementing Systematic Genetic Counseling and Multigene Germline Testing for Individuals with Pancreatic Cancer. *JCO Oncol. Pract.* **2021**, *17*, e236–e247. [CrossRef]
50. Gardiner, A.; Kidd, J.; Elias, M.C.; Young, K.; Mabey, B.; Taherian, N.; Cummings, S.; Malafa, M.; Rosenthal, E.; Permuth, J.B. Pancreatic Ductal Carcinoma Risk Associated with Hereditary Cancer-Risk Genes. *J. Natl. Cancer Inst.* **2022**, *114*, 996–1002. [CrossRef]
51. Grant, R.C.; Selander, I.; Connor, A.A.; Selvarajah, S.; Borgida, A.; Briollais, L.; Petersen, G.M.; Lerner-Ellis, J.; Holter, S.; Gallinger, S. Prevalence of Germline Mutations in Cancer Predisposition Genes in Patients with Pancreatic Cancer. *Gastroenterology* **2015**, *148*, 556–564. [CrossRef]
52. Brand, R.E.; Persson, J.; Bratlie, S.O.; Chung, D.C.; Katona, B.W.; Carrato, A.; Castillo, M.; Earl, J.; Kokkola, A.; Lucas, A.L.; et al. Detection of Early-Stage Pancreatic Ductal Adenocarcinoma From Blood Samples: Results of a Multiplex Biomarker Signature Validation Study. *Clin. Transl. Gastroenterol.* **2022**, *13*, e00468. [CrossRef] [PubMed]
53. Drogan, C.M.; Kindler, H.L.; Gao, G.; Kupfer, S.S. Outcomes of Universal Point-of-Care Genetic Testing in Diverse Patients with Pancreatic Ductal Adenocarcinoma. *JCO Precis. Oncol.* **2023**, *7*, e2200196. [CrossRef] [PubMed]
54. Bono, M.; Fanale, D.; Incorvaia, L.; Cancelliere, D.; Fiorino, A.; Calò, V.; Dimino, A.; Filorizzo, C.; Corsini, L.R.; Brando, C.; et al. Impact of Deleterious Variants in Other Genes beyond BRCA1/2 Detected in Breast/Ovarian and Pancreatic Cancer Patients by NGS-Based Multi-Gene Panel Testing: Looking over the Hedge. *ESMO Open* **2021**, *6*, 100235. [CrossRef] [PubMed]
55. Goggins, M.; Overbeek, K.A.; Brand, R.; Syngal, S.; Del Chiaro, M.; Bartsch, D.K.; Bassi, C.; Carrato, A.; Farrell, J.; Fishman, E.K.; et al. International Cancer of the Pancreas Screening (CAPS) consortium. Management of Patients with Increased Risk for Familial Pancreatic Cancer: Updated Recommendations from the International Cancer of the Pancreas Screening (CAPS) Consortium. *Gut* **2020**, *69*, 7–17. [CrossRef] [PubMed]
56. Ohmoto, A.; Yachida, S.; Morizane, C. Genomic Features and Clinical Management of Patients with Hereditary Pancreatic Cancer Syndromes and Familial Pancreatic Cancer. *Int. J. Mol. Sci.* **2019**, *20*, 561. [CrossRef]
57. Matsubayashi, H.; Takaori, K.; Morizane, C.; Kiyozumi, Y. Familial Pancreatic Cancer and Surveillance of High-Risk Individuals. *Gut Liver* **2019**, *13*, 498–505. [CrossRef] [PubMed]
58. Brentnall, T.A. Progress in the Earlier Detection of Pancreatic Cancer. *J. Clin. Oncol.* **2016**, *34*, 1973–1974. [CrossRef]
59. Dbouk, M.; Katona, B.W.; Brand, R.E.; Chak, A.; Syngal, S.; Farrell, J.J.; Kastrinos, F.; Stoffel, E.M.; Blackford, A.L.; Rustgi, A.K.; et al. The Multicenter Cancer of Pancreas Screening Study: Impact on Stage and Survival. *J. Clin. Oncol.* **2022**, *40*, 3257–3266. [CrossRef] [PubMed]
60. Canto, M.I.; Almario, J.A.; Schulick, R.D.; Yeo, C.J.; Klein, A.; Blackford, A.; Shin, E.J.; Sanyal, A.; Yenokyan, G.; Lennon, A.M.; et al. Risk of Neoplastic Progression in Individuals at High Risk for Pancreatic Cancer Undergoing Long-Term Surveillance. *Gastroenterology* **2018**, *155*, 740–751.e2. [CrossRef]
61. Overbeek, K.A.; Levink, I.J.M.; Koopmann, B.D.M.; Harinck, F.; Konings, I.C.A.W.; Ausems, M.G.E.M.; Wagner, A.; Fockens, P.; van Eijck, C.H.; Groot Koerkamp, B.; et al. Dutch Familial Pancreatic Cancer Surveillance Study Group. Long-Term Yield of Pancreatic Cancer Surveillance in High-Risk Individuals. *Gut* **2022**, *71*, 1152–1160. [CrossRef]
62. Henrikson, N.B.; Aiello Bowles, E.J.; Blasi, P.R.; Morrison, C.C.; Nguyen, M.; Pillarisetty, V.G.; Lin, J.S. Screening for Pancreatic Cancer: Updated Evidence Report and Systematic Review for the US Preventive Services Task Force. *JAMA* **2019**, *322*, 445–454. [CrossRef] [PubMed]
63. Singhi, A.D.; Koay, E.J.; Chari, S.T.; Maitra, A. Early Detection of Pancreatic Cancer: Opportunities and Challenges. *Gastroenterology* **2019**, *156*, 2024–2040. [CrossRef] [PubMed]
64. Wu, W. Early Detection of Pancreatic Cancer: Are We Ready for Prime Time? *Gastroenterology* **2022**, *163*, 1157–1159. [CrossRef] [PubMed]
65. Reese, K.-L.; Pantel, K.; Smit, D.J. Multibiomarker Panels in Liquid Biopsy for Early Detection of Pancreatic Cancer—A Comprehensive Review. *J. Exp. Clin. Cancer Res.* **2024**, *43*, 250. [CrossRef] [PubMed]

66. Cohen, J.D.; Li, L.; Wang, Y.; Thoburn, C.; Afsari, B.; Danilova, L.; Douville, C.; Javed, A.A.; Wong, F.; Mattox, A.; et al. Detection and Localization of Surgically Resectable Cancers with a Multi-Analyte Blood Test. *Science* **2018**, *359*, 926–930. [CrossRef] [PubMed]
67. Nishiwada, S.; Sho, M.; Banwait, J.K.; Yamamura, K.; Akahori, T.; Nakamura, K.; Baba, H.; Goel, A. A microRNA Signature Identifies Pancreatic Ductal Adenocarcinoma Patients at Risk for Lymph Node Metastases. *Gastroenterology* **2020**, *159*, 562–574. [CrossRef]
68. Treekitkarnmongkol, W.; Dai, J.; Liu, S.; Sankaran, D.; Nguyen, T.; Balasenthil, S.; Hurd, M.W.; Chen, M.; Katayama, H.; Roy-Chowdhuri, S.; et al. Blood-Based microRNA Biomarker Signature of Early-Stage Pancreatic Ductal Adenocarcinoma with Lead-Time Trajectory in Prediagnostic Samples. *Gastro Hep Adv.* **2024**, *3*, 1098–1115. [CrossRef]
69. Jaworski, J.J.; Morgan, R.D.; Sivakumar, S. Circulating Cell-Free Tumour DNA for Early Detection of Pancreatic Cancer. *Cancers* **2020**, *12*, 3704. [CrossRef] [PubMed]
70. Kane, L.E.; Mellotte, G.S.; Mylod, E.; O'Brien, R.M.; O'Connell, F.; Buckley, C.E.; Arlow, J.; Nguyen, K.; Mockler, D.; Meade, A.D.; et al. Diagnostic Accuracy of Blood-Based Biomarkers for Pancreatic Cancer: A Systematic Review and Meta-Analysis. *Cancer Res. Commun.* **2022**, *2*, 1229–1243. [CrossRef] [PubMed]
71. Mok, E.T.Y.; Chitty, J.L.; Cox, T.R. miRNAs in Pancreatic Cancer Progression and Metastasis. *Clin. Exp. Metastasis* **2024**, *41*, 163–186. [CrossRef]
72. Sharma, G.G.; Okada, Y.; Von Hoff, D.; Goel, A. Non-Coding RNA Biomarkers in Pancreatic Ductal Adenocarcinoma. *Semin. Cancer Biol.* **2021**, *75*, 153–168. [CrossRef]
73. Madadjim, R.; An, T.; Cui, J. MicroRNAs in Pancreatic Cancer: Advances in Biomarker Discovery and Therapeutic Implications. *Int. J. Mol. Sci.* **2024**, *25*, 3914. [CrossRef] [PubMed]
74. Li, Y.; Sui, S.; Goel, A. Extracellular Vesicles Associated microRNAs: Their Biology and Clinical Significance as Biomarkers in Gastrointestinal Cancers. *Semin. Cancer Biol.* **2024**, *99*, 5–23. [CrossRef]
75. Jia, E.; Ren, N.; Shi, X.; Zhang, R.; Yu, H.; Yu, F.; Qin, S.; Xue, J. Extracellular Vesicle Biomarkers for Pancreatic Cancer Diagnosis: A Systematic Review and Meta-Analysis. *BMC Cancer* **2022**, *22*, 573. [CrossRef] [PubMed]
76. Nakamura, K.; Zhu, Z.; Roy, S.; Jun, E.; Han, H.; Munoz, R.M.; Nishiwada, S.; Sharma, G.; Cridebring, D.; Zenhausern, F.; et al. An Exosome-Based Transcriptomic Signature for Noninvasive, Early Detection of Patients with Pancreatic Ductal Adenocarcinoma: A Multicenter Cohort Study. *Gastroenterology* **2022**, *163*, 1252–1266.e2. [CrossRef]
77. Albers, M.J.; Bok, R.; Chen, A.P.; Cunningham, C.H.; Zierhut, M.L.; Zhang, V.Y.; Kohler, S.J.; Tropp, J.; Hurd, R.E.; Yen, Y.-F.; et al. Hyperpolarized 13C Lactate, Pyruvate, and Alanine: Noninvasive Biomarkers for Prostate Cancer Detection and Grading. *Cancer Res.* **2008**, *68*, 8607–8615. [CrossRef]
78. Chen, S.; Zhang, L.; Li, S.; Yuan, Y.; Jiang, B.; Jiang, Z.; Zhang, X.; Zhou, X.; Liu, M. Detecting Biomarkers by Dynamic Nuclear Polarization Enhanced Magnetic Resonance. *Natl. Sci. Rev.* **2024**, *11*, nwae228. [CrossRef] [PubMed]
79. Day, S.E.; Kettunen, M.I.; Gallagher, F.A.; Hu, D.-E.; Lerche, M.; Wolber, J.; Golman, K.; Ardenkjaer-Larsen, J.H.; Brindle, K.M. Detecting Tumor Response to Treatment Using Hyperpolarized 13C Magnetic Resonance Imaging and Spectroscopy. *Nat. Med.* **2007**, *13*, 1382–1387. [CrossRef] [PubMed]
80. Dos Santos, K.; Bertho, G.; Baudin, M.; Giraud, N. Glutamine: A Key Player in Human Metabolism as Revealed by Hyperpolarized Magnetic Resonance. *Prog. Nucl. Magn. Reson. Spectrosc.* **2024**, *144–145*, 15–39. [CrossRef]
81. M.D. Anderson Cancer Center. Pilot Study Using Hyperpolarized 13C-Pyruvate Magnetic Resonance Spectroscopic Imaging in Patients with Pancreatic Cysts Undergoing Surgical Resection. Clinical Trial Registration NCT05873699; clinicaltrials.gov; 2024. Available online: https://clinicaltrials.gov/study/NCT05873699 (accessed on 21 December 2024).
82. Lord, C.J.; Ashworth, A. BRCAness Revisited. *Nat. Rev. Cancer* **2016**, *16*, 110–120. [CrossRef]
83. Heeke, A.L.; Pishvaian, M.J.; Lynce, F.; Xiu, J.; Brody, J.R.; Chen, W.-J.; Baker, T.M.; Marshall, J.L.; Isaacs, C. Prevalence of Homologous Recombination-Related Gene Mutations Across Multiple Cancer Types. *JCO Precis. Oncol.* **2018**, *2018*, PO.17.00286. [CrossRef]
84. Casolino, R.; Paiella, S.; Azzolina, D.; Beer, P.A.; Corbo, V.; Lorenzoni, G.; Gregori, D.; Golan, T.; Braconi, C.; Froeling, F.E.M.; et al. Homologous Recombination Deficiency in Pancreatic Cancer: A Systematic Review and Prevalence Meta-Analysis. *J. Clin. Oncol.* **2021**, *39*, 2617–2631. [CrossRef] [PubMed]
85. Wattenberg, M.M.; Asch, D.; Yu, S.; O'Dwyer, P.J.; Domchek, S.M.; Nathanson, K.L.; Rosen, M.A.; Beatty, G.L.; Siegelman, E.S.; Reiss, K.A. Platinum Response Characteristics of Patients with Pancreatic Ductal Adenocarcinoma and a Germline BRCA1, BRCA2 or PALB2 Mutation. *Br. J. Cancer* **2020**, *122*, 333–339. [CrossRef]
86. Pishvaian, M.J.; Blais, E.M.; Brody, J.R.; Rahib, L.; Lyons, E.; De Arbeloa, P.; Hendifar, A.; Mikhail, S.; Chung, V.; Sohal, D.P.S.; et al. Outcomes in Patients with Pancreatic Adenocarcinoma with Genetic Mutations in DNA Damage Response Pathways: Results From the Know Your Tumor Program. *JCO Precis. Oncol.* **2019**, *3*, 1–10. [CrossRef]

87. Park, W.; Chen, J.; Chou, J.F.; Varghese, A.M.; Yu, K.H.; Wong, W.; Capanu, M.; Balachandran, V.; McIntyre, C.A.; El Dika, I.; et al. Genomic Methods Identify Homologous Recombination Deficiency in Pancreas Adenocarcinoma and Optimize Treatment Selection. *Clin. Cancer Res.* **2020**, *26*, 3239–3247. [CrossRef] [PubMed]
88. Waddell, N.; Pajic, M.; Patch, A.-M.; Chang, D.K.; Kassahn, K.S.; Bailey, P.; Johns, A.L.; Miller, D.; Nones, K.; Quek, K.; et al. Whole Genomes Redefine the Mutational Landscape of Pancreatic Cancer. *Nature* **2015**, *518*, 495–501. [CrossRef] [PubMed]
89. Bailey, P.; Chang, D.K.; Nones, K.; Johns, A.L.; Patch, A.-M.; Gingras, M.-C.; Miller, D.K.; Christ, A.N.; Bruxner, T.J.C.; Quinn, M.C.; et al. Genomic Analyses Identify Molecular Subtypes of Pancreatic Cancer. *Nature* **2016**, *531*, 47–52. [CrossRef] [PubMed]
90. Stossel, C.; Raitses-Gurevich, M.; Atias, D.; Beller, T.; Glick Gorman, Y.; Halperin, S.; Peer, E.; Denroche, R.E.; Zhang, A.; Notta, F.; et al. Spectrum of Response to Platinum and PARP Inhibitors in Germline BRCA-Associated Pancreatic Cancer in the Clinical and Preclinical Setting. *Cancer Discov.* **2023**, *13*, 1826–1843. [CrossRef] [PubMed]
91. Momtaz, P.; O'Connor, C.A.; Chou, J.F.; Capanu, M.; Park, W.; Bandlamudi, C.; Berger, M.F.; Kelsen, D.P.; Suehnholz, S.P.; Chakravarty, D.; et al. Pancreas Cancer and BRCA: A Critical Subset of Patients with Improving Therapeutic Outcomes. *Cancer* **2021**, *127*, 4393–4402. [CrossRef] [PubMed]
92. Tan, H.; Hosein, P.J. Detection and Therapeutic Implications of Homologous Recombination Repair Deficiency in Pancreatic Cancer: A Narrative Review. *J. Gastrointest. Oncol.* **2023**, *14*, 2249–2259. [CrossRef] [PubMed]
93. Perkhofer, L.; Gout, J.; Roger, E.; Kude de Almeida, F.; Baptista Simões, C.; Wiesmüller, L.; Seufferlein, T.; Kleger, A. DNA Damage Repair as a Target in Pancreatic Cancer: State-of-the-Art and Future Perspectives. *Gut* **2021**, *70*, 606–617. [CrossRef] [PubMed]
94. Curtin, N.J. DNA Repair Dysregulation from Cancer Driver to Therapeutic Target. *Nat. Rev. Cancer* **2012**, *12*, 801–817. [CrossRef] [PubMed]
95. Cleary, J.M.; Wolpin, B.M.; Dougan, S.K.; Raghavan, S.; Singh, H.; Huffman, B.; Sethi, N.S.; Nowak, J.A.; Shapiro, G.I.; Aguirre, A.J.; et al. Opportunities for Utilization of DNA Repair Inhibitors in Homologous Recombination Repair-Deficient and Proficient Pancreatic Adenocarcinoma. *Clin. Cancer Res.* **2021**, *27*, 6622–6637. [CrossRef] [PubMed]
96. Chartron, E.; Theillet, C.; Guiu, S.; Jacot, W. Targeting Homologous Repair Deficiency in Breast and Ovarian Cancers: Biological Pathways, Preclinical and Clinical Data. *Crit. Rev. Oncol. Hematol.* **2019**, *133*, 58–73. [CrossRef]
97. Rebelatto, T.F.; Falavigna, M.; Pozarri, M.; Spada, F.; Cella, C.A.; Laffi, A.; Pellicori, S.; Fazio, N. Should platinum-based chemotherapy be preferred for germline BReast CAncer genes (BRCA) 1 and 2-mutated pancreatic ductal adenocarcinoma (PDAC) patients? A systematic review and meta-analysis. *Cancer Treat. Rev.* **2019**, *80*, 101895. [CrossRef]
98. Golan, T.; Hammel, P.; Reni, M.; Van Cutsem, E.; Macarulla, T.; Hall, M.J.; Park, J.-O.; Hochhauser, D.; Arnold, D.; Oh, D.-Y.; et al. Maintenance Olaparib for Germline BRCA-Mutated Metastatic Pancreatic Cancer. *N. Engl. J. Med.* **2019**, *381*, 317–327. [CrossRef] [PubMed]
99. Reiss, K.A.; Mick, R.; O'Hara, M.H.; Teitelbaum, U.; Karasic, T.B.; Schneider, C.; Cowden, S.; Southwell, T.; Romeo, J.; Izgur, N.; et al. Phase II Study of Maintenance Rucaparib in Patients with Platinum-Sensitive Advanced Pancreatic Cancer and a Pathogenic Germline or Somatic Variant in BRCA1, BRCA2, or PALB2. *J. Clin. Oncol.* **2021**, *39*, 2497–2505. [CrossRef] [PubMed]
100. Kaufman, B.; Shapira-Frommer, R.; Schmutzler, R.K.; Audeh, M.W.; Friedlander, M.; Balmaña, J.; Mitchell, G.; Fried, G.; Stemmer, S.M.; Hubert, A.; et al. Olaparib Monotherapy in Patients with Advanced Cancer and a Germline BRCA1/2 Mutation. *J. Clin. Oncol.* **2015**, *33*, 244–250. [CrossRef] [PubMed]
101. Shroff, R.T.; Hendifar, A.; McWilliams, R.R.; Geva, R.; Epelbaum, R.; Rolfe, L.; Goble, S.; Lin, K.K.; Biankin, A.V.; Giordano, H.; et al. Rucaparib Monotherapy in Patients with Pancreatic Cancer and a Known Deleterious BRCA Mutation. *JCO Precis. Oncol.* **2018**, *2018*, PO.17.00316. [CrossRef]
102. Lowery, M.A.; Kelsen, D.P.; Capanu, M.; Smith, S.C.; Lee, J.W.; Stadler, Z.K.; Moore, M.J.; Kindler, H.L.; Golan, T.; Segal, A.; et al. Phase II Trial of Veliparib in Patients with Previously Treated BRCA-Mutated Pancreas Ductal Adenocarcinoma. *Eur. J. Cancer* **2018**, *89*, 19–26. [CrossRef] [PubMed]
103. de Bono, J.; Ramanathan, R.K.; Mina, L.; Chugh, R.; Glaspy, J.; Rafii, S.; Kaye, S.; Sachdev, J.; Heymach, J.; Smith, D.C.; et al. A Phase I, Dose-Escalation, Two-Part Trial of the PARP Inhibitor Talazoparib in Patients with Advanced Germline BRCA1/2 Mutations and Selected Sporadic Cancers. *Cancer Discov.* **2017**, *7*, 620–629. [CrossRef]
104. O'Reilly, E.M.; Lee, J.W.; Zalupski, M.; Capanu, M.; Park, J.; Golan, T.; Tahover, E.; Lowery, M.A.; Chou, J.F.; Sahai, V.; et al. Randomized, Multicenter, Phase II Trial of Gemcitabine and Cisplatin with or without Veliparib in Patients with Pancreas Adenocarcinoma and a Germline BRCA/PALB2 Mutation. *J. Clin. Oncol.* **2020**, *38*, 1378–1388. [CrossRef]
105. Domchek, S.M.; Postel-Vinay, S.; Im, S.-A.; Park, Y.H.; Delord, J.-P.; Italiano, A.; Alexandre, J.; You, B.; Bastian, S.; Krebs, M.G.; et al. Olaparib and Durvalumab in Patients with Germline BRCA-Mutated Metastatic Breast Cancer (MEDIOLA): An Open-Label, Multicentre, Phase 1/2, Basket Study. *Lancet Oncol.* **2020**, *21*, 1155–1164. [CrossRef] [PubMed]
106. Javle, M.; Shacham-Shmueli, E.; Xiao, L.; Varadhachary, G.; Halpern, N.; Fogelman, D.; Boursi, B.; Uruba, S.; Margalit, O.; Wolff, R.A.; et al. Olaparib Monotherapy for Previously Treated Pancreatic Cancer with DNA Damage Repair Genetic Alterations Other Than Germline BRCA Variants: Findings From 2 Phase 2 Nonrandomized Clinical Trials. *JAMA Oncol.* **2021**, *7*, 693–699. [CrossRef] [PubMed]

107. Diaz, L.A.; Le, D.T. PD-1 Blockade in Tumors with Mismatch-Repair Deficiency. *N. Engl. J. Med.* **2015**, *373*, 1979. [CrossRef] [PubMed]
108. Marabelle, A.; Le, D.T.; Ascierto, P.A.; Di Giacomo, A.M.; De Jesus-Acosta, A.; Delord, J.-P.; Geva, R.; Gottfried, M.; Penel, N.; Hansen, A.R.; et al. Efficacy of Pembrolizumab in Patients with Noncolorectal High Microsatellite Instability/Mismatch Repair-Deficient Cancer: Results From the Phase II KEYNOTE-158 Study. *J. Clin. Oncol.* **2020**, *38*, 1–10. [CrossRef] [PubMed]
109. André, T.; Shiu, K.-K.; Kim, T.W.; Jensen, B.V.; Jensen, L.H.; Punt, C.; Smith, D.; Garcia-Carbonero, R.; Benavides, M.; Gibbs, P.; et al. KEYNOTE-177 Investigators. Pembrolizumab in Microsatellite-Instability-High Advanced Colorectal Cancer. *N. Engl. J. Med.* **2020**, *383*, 2207–2218. [CrossRef]
110. Terrero, G.; Datta, J.; Dennison, J.; Sussman, D.A.; Lohse, I.; Merchant, N.B.; Hosein, P.J. Ipilimumab/Nivolumab Therapy in Patients with Metastatic Pancreatic or Biliary Cancer with Homologous Recombination Deficiency Pathogenic Germline Variants. *JAMA Oncol.* **2022**, *8*, 938–940. [CrossRef] [PubMed]
111. Reiss, K.A.; Mick, R.; Teitelbaum, U.; O'Hara, M.; Schneider, C.; Massa, R.; Karasic, T.; Tondon, R.; Onyiah, C.; Gosselin, M.K.; et al. Niraparib plus Nivolumab or Niraparib plus Ipilimumab in Patients with Platinum-Sensitive Advanced Pancreatic Cancer: A Randomised, Phase 1b/2 Trial. *Lancet Oncol.* **2022**, *23*, 1009–1020. [CrossRef]
112. Lincoln, S.E.; Nussbaum, R.L.; Kurian, A.W.; Nielsen, S.M.; Das, K.; Michalski, S.; Yang, S.; Ngo, N.; Blanco, A.; Esplin, E.D. Yield and Utility of Germline Testing Following Tumor Sequencing in Patients with Cancer. *JAMA Netw. Open* **2020**, *3*, e2019452. [CrossRef] [PubMed]
113. Stoffel, E.M.; Brand, R.E.; Goggins, M. Pancreatic Cancer: Changing Epidemiology and New Approaches to Risk Assessment, Early Detection, and Prevention. *Gastroenterology* **2023**, *164*, 752–765. [CrossRef] [PubMed]
114. Mazer, B.L.; Lee, J.W.; Roberts, N.J.; Chu, L.C.; Lennon, A.M.; Klein, A.P.; Eshleman, J.R.; Fishman, E.K.; Canto, M.I.; Goggins, M.G.; et al. Screening for Pancreatic Cancer Has the Potential to Save Lives, but Is It Practical? *Expert Rev. Gastroenterol. Hepatol.* **2023**, *17*, 555–574. [CrossRef] [PubMed]
115. Everett, J.N.; Burgos, G.; Chun, J.; Baptiste, A.; Khanna, L.G.; Oberstein, P.E.; Simeone, D.M. Cancer Surveillance Awareness and Practice among Families at Increased Risk for Pancreatic Adenocarcinoma. *Cancer* **2021**, *127*, 2271–2278. [CrossRef] [PubMed]
116. Park, W.; O'Connor, C.; Chou, J.F.; Schwartz, C.; Varghese, A.M.; Larsen, M.; Balogun, F.; Brenner, R.; Yu, K.H.; Diguglielmo, E.; et al. Phase 2 Trial of Pembrolizumab and Olaparib (POLAR) Maintenance for Patients (Pts) with Metastatic Pancreatic Cancer (mPDAC): Two Cohorts B Non-Core Homologous Recombination Deficiency (HRD) and C Exceptional Response to Platinum-Therapy. *J. Clin. Oncol.* **2023**, *41* (Suppl. S16), 4140. [CrossRef]

Disclaimer/Publisher's Note: The statements, opinions and data contained in all publications are solely those of the individual author(s) and contributor(s) and not of MDPI and/or the editor(s). MDPI and/or the editor(s) disclaim responsibility for any injury to people or property resulting from any ideas, methods, instructions or products referred to in the content.

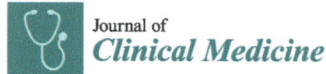 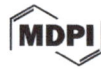

Review

An Approach to and Treatment of Indeterminate Biliary Strictures: A Comprehensive Review of the Literature

Giovanna Impellizzeri [1], Maria Vittoria Grassini [2], Giulio Donato [1], Claudio Giovanni De Angelis [1] and Nico Pagano [1,*]

[1] Gastroenterology Unit, Department of Oncological and Specialty Medicine, Azienda Ospedaliero-Universitaria Maggiore della Carità, 28100 Novara, Italy; g.impellizzeri@maggioreosp.novara.it (G.I.); eusdeang@hotmail.com (C.G.D.A.)
[2] Section of Gastroenterology & Hepatology, Department of Health Promotion Sciences Maternal and Infant Care, Internal Medicine and Medical Specialties, PROMISE, University of Palermo, 90127 Palermo, Italy; mvittoriagrassini@gmail.com
* Correspondence: nicopagano@gmail.com

Abstract: This review aims to focus on what we know about the management of biliary strictures of unknown etiology, especially exploring our diagnostic armamentarium in the setting of indeterminate biliary strictures. Presently, this is a current issue that has a relevant impact both on patient prognosis, often delaying diagnosis, and on overall costs associated with repeating diagnostic procedures, sometimes performed with very expensive devices. We also focus on current biliary drainage approaches, providing an overview of therapeutic options, endoscopic or not.

Keywords: strictures; ERCP; EUS; cholangioscopy; cholangiocarcinoma

1. Introduction

Indeterminate biliary strictures still represent a diagnostic and therapeutic challenge mainly because of the lack of a clear, shared definition. This original subject often generates ambiguity in the interpretation of literature studies and hampers a universal approach. Currently, there is not a clear agreement in indeterminate biliary stricture management, even from two of the major gastroenterological societies' guidelines. The European Society of Gastrointestinal Endoscopy *(ESGE)* guidelines [1] actually still focus on a single technique to obtain a diagnosis, depending on stricture position, whereas the latest American Society for Gastrointestinal Endoscopy *(ASGE)* ones [2] more so stress the concept that, if we have a stricture of uncertain etiology, all the available tools have to be used as soon as possible to procure a diagnosis. Today, one of the most common definitions of indeterminate stricture is a stenosis in which a diagnosis of nature is still lacking after the results of laboratory tests, cross-sectional imaging (such as ultrasonography, computed tomography (CT), magnetic resonance imaging with cholangiopancreatography (MRI/MRCP)) and endoscopic procedures, such as retrograde cholangiopancreatography (ERCP) or endoscopic ultrasonography (EUS) with standard diagnostic tools (cytology, biopsies or FNB/FNA).

Most indeterminate biliary strictures are malignant, due to cholangiocarcinoma (CCA) or pancreatic adenocarcinoma, but they also could be benign ones (iatrogenic injury, inflammatory or infectious causes, etc.) (Table 1). A quick diagnosis can lead to a better prognosis and less morbidity/mortality in both cases, one side providing an earlier curative or palliative treatment and the other avoiding useless overtreatment.

Table 1. Main causes of malignant and benign biliary strictures.

Malignant	Benign
Pancreatic cancer	*Inflammatory:* chronic pancreatitis, PSC, IgG4-related cholangitis/pancreatitis
Cholangiocarcinoma	*Iatrogenic:* cholecystectomy, liver transplant, chemotherapy, radiation
Gallbladder malignancy	*Vascular:* ischemic biliary injury, portal hypertensive biliopathy, vasculitis
Hepatocellular carcinoma	*Infectious:* recurrent pyogenic cholangitis, HIV cholangiopathy, parasitic infections
Ampullary cancer	*Traumatic*
Lymphoma	Mirizzi syndrome
Metastasis	*Other:* sarcoidosis, eosinophilic cholangitis, mastocytosis

In this setting, obtaining a histological diagnosis is the key to assessing appropriate, subsequent, and patient-tailored management.

This review will focus on the many possible causes of indeterminate biliary strictures. We performed a comprehensive literature review researching the most relevant studies about this topic on the PubMed and Scopus databases using the keywords "biliary strictures", "cholangiocarcinoma", "ERCP-guided drainage", "EUS-guided drainage", and "cholangioscopy". Starting from the different diagnostic tools, we also focus on the best therapeutic approaches to manage them.

2. Indeterminate Biliary Stricture Characteristics

Biliary stricture signs and symptoms are heterogeneous. Sometimes, diagnosis is accidental in patients undergoing cross-sectional imaging for other reasons. Other times, there are signs such as jaundice and fever or symptoms like abdominal pain or nausea. Clearly, a patient's personal history plays a key role. If we have asymptomatic jaundice or weight loss, we can suspect malignancy. Conversely, if we have a history of chronic pancreatitis or of previous hepatobiliary surgery, we can suspect a benign stricture. Biliary strictures can be classified according to their location (proximal or distal to the hepatic hilum), to their growth pattern (extrinsic or intrinsic, as to say from an external compression or an intraductal growth), and to their etiology (benign or malignant). In most cases, biliary strictures are malignant: in a retrospective analysis of 342 patients with obstructive jaundice and a biliary stricture who underwent EUS/EUS + FNA, 72.5% of cases were diagnosed as malignant ones [3]. Another retrospective study evaluating EUS + FNA specifically in proximal biliary strictures identified the same proportions between benign and malignant lesions: in 71% of patients, there were findings showing adenocarcinoma [4]. Among malignant causes, we can have cholangiocarcinoma (CCA), pancreatic adenocarcinoma, hepatocellular carcinoma (HCC), gallbladder cancer, lymphomas, and metastasis.

Among the benign causes, we can have previous hepatobiliary surgery (such as cholecystectomy or liver transplant), chronic pancreatitis, chronic diseases such as primary sclerosing cholangitis (PSC) or autoimmune cholangiopathies, and infectious or ischemic causes. Despite that, today, indeterminate lesions still account for up to 20% of cases [5] after the use of first-line diagnostic tools, and so we often need further investigations.

3. Main Diagnostic Tools

If a biliary stricture is suspected or recognized through ultrasonography, CT, or MRI/MRCP, we need a histological sampling to define its nature. Many tests are available to reach a diagnosis, considering that none of them is always conclusive and often the final diagnosis is made by a combination of them.

3.1. ERCP

ERCP has both a diagnostic and therapeutic role in this setting. During ERCP, after a successful cannulation, we perform a cholangiography that shows us the site and suggests to us a stricture nature: an abrupt narrowing is mostly typical of malignancy (Figures 1 and 2) as compared to a smooth or a progressive one. ERCP is still the first-line approach technique to obtain cytological and histological samples in biliary strictures, but it is also essential in the subsequent therapeutic approach because of its palliative role. Traditionally, brush cytology, inexpensive and routinely performed, has high specificity but low sensitivity in detecting malignant biliary strictures. Intraductal biopsies, which require sphincterotomy, do not have a clear advantage over the brushing technique. A 2015 meta-analysis comparing the effectiveness of brush cytology and intraductal biopsies in biliary strictures showed that the pooled sensitivity of the brushing technique and intraductal biopsies were, respectively, 45% and 48.1%. Combining both modalities, the sensitivity modestly increased (59.4%) [6]. Brushing also allows us to obtain material for FISH (fluorescence in situ hybridization). FISH is a cytogenic technique that permits abnormality identification in a specific DNA sequence, and it was demonstrated that adding it to standard cytology analysis improves diagnostic chances. A single-center retrospective study showed that the dual-modality sampling (transductal biopsies + brushing cytology or brushing cytology + FISH) or the trimodality one (transductal biopsies + brushing cytology + FISH) performed better than brushing cytology alone in detecting malignancy, respectively, by 58.7% and 40.4% in the dual-modality samplings and by 68.3% in the trimodality one versus by 17.3% in brushing cytology alone [7]. Furthermore, another retrospective study including 168 patients with suspicious malignant biliary strictures who underwent double-tissue sampling (DTS) or triple-tissue sampling (TTS) via ERCP, showed a diagnostic sensitivity for cancer significantly higher in the TTS group than the DTS group (85.0% vs. 64.9%, respectively). Remarkably, regarding cancer type (cholangiocarcinoma vs. non-cholangiocarcinoma), the diagnostic sensitivity was higher for cholangiocarcinoma in the TTS group than in the DTS group (100% vs. 69.4%, respectively; $p < 0.001$) but not for the non-cholangiocarcinoma patients (57.1% vs. 57.1%, respectively). Thus, triple-tissue sampling can offer relevant diagnostic accuracy in suspicious biliary strictures, especially due to cholangiocarcinoma [8].

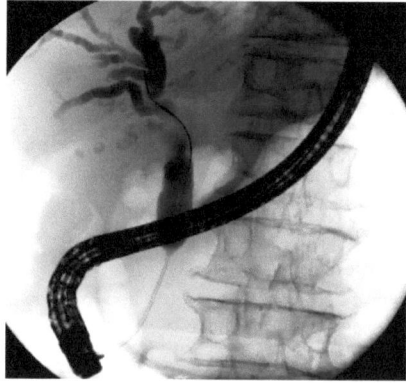

Figure 1. Double biliary stricture in pancreatic cancer with liver perihilar metastasis.

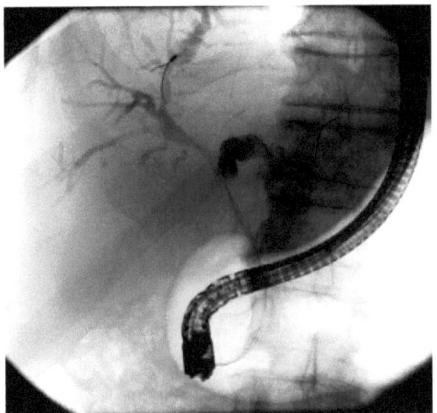

Figure 2. Hilar cholangiocarcinoma stricture.

3.2. EUS

EUS's role in defining biliopancreatic neoplasms and bile duct strictures has constantly increased over the last few years. EUS can provide a high-quality real-time image of the biliopancreatic system and allows for the obtention samples for cytology and histology through fine-needle aspiration (FNA) and fine-needle biopsy (FNB, Figure 3). Some studies demonstrated EUS's better sensitivity in detecting distal strictures over proximal ones, which is the reason why ERCP remains the preferred initial approach in patients with proximal strictures. A single-center observational study showed that in a population of patients affected by CCA, EUS detected it in all distal tumors (100%) and in 83% of proximal tumors, with better performance of EUS over CT scans in tumor detection (94% vs. 30%, respectively) [9]. In particular, the yield of EUS with FNA in distal biliary strictures is excellent, with a reported sensitivity of 84% to 91% and specificity of 71% to 100%. The diagnostic yield of EUS with FNA in proximal biliary strictures is more variable. The reported sensitivity and specificity in this setting range from 45% to 89% and 79% to 100%, respectively [10]. Another interesting point is that combining EUS + ERCP further increases diagnostic chances: a multicenter study including 263 patients with suspected malignant biliary obstruction who underwent same-session EUS and ERCP concluded that overall diagnostic sensitivity and accuracy were 73.6% and 76.1% for EUS-FNA, 56.5% and 60.5% for ERCP, and 85.8% and 87.1% for the EUS/ERCP combination [11]. A recent meta-analysis involving 497 patients focused on same-session EUS and ERCP for tissue diagnosis compared to each method alone: the sensitivity, specificity, and accuracy for EUS-FNA alone were, respectively, 76%, 100%, and 94.5%; for ERCP-based tissue sampling, these variables were 58%, 98%, and 78.1%. For the same-session combined techniques, the sensitivity, specificity, and accuracy increased to 86%, 98%, and 96.5%, respectively. Interestingly, the analysis of each method in detecting pancreatic and biliary etiologies showed that EUS-FNA was superior to ERCP-based tissue sampling for pancreatic lesions, whereas for biliary ones, both methods had similar sensitivities [12]. A controversial consideration is the risk of needle tract seeding leading to metastases. Heimbach et al. [13] have demonstrated peritoneal metastases in 83% (5/6) of patients who underwent the FNA of unresectable hilar cholangiocarcinoma. Unfortunately, they did not distinguish between the percutaneous and EUS approaches. A few studies have examined the risk of seeding among distal common bile duct malignant strictures but with conflicting results [14–19]. Overall, based on the evidence to date, EUS with FNA/FNB is not recommended for proximal biliary strictures (in this case, lymphadenopathies can be a good FNA/FNB target to improve diagnostic chances), whereas the risk associated with distal biliary strictures remains unclear [20].

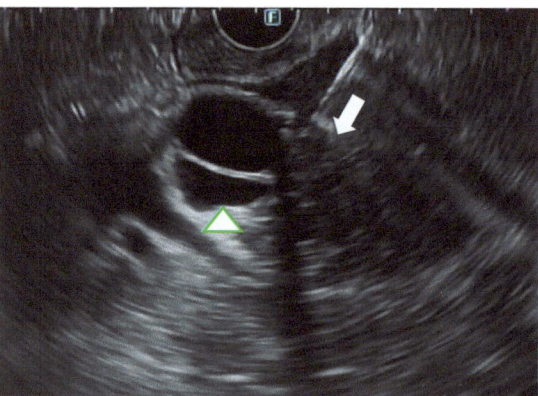

Figure 3. FNB of a suspicious extrahepatic cholangiocarcinoma (white arrow) with cystic duct involvement (arrowhead).

3.3. Intraductal Ultrasound (Miniprobe Endoscopic Ultrasound)

Intraductal ultrasound (IDUS) is performed during ERCP by inserting a small (2.4 mm in diameter), high-frequency (usually 20 MHz) catheter probe over a wire via a monorail design into the bile duct. The transducer rotates at the end of the probe and generates 360° images in a plane perpendicular to the catheter axis (similar to the radial echoendoscope). Malignant strictures tend to disrupt the normal three-layer appearance of the bile duct, have an asymmetric echo-poor mass with irregular margins, and infiltrate the surrounding tissue. Benign strictures often show the preservation of the bile duct wall layers and have a symmetric echo-rich mass with smooth margins [21]. The yield of IDUS in predicting malignant biliary stricture is good, with a sensitivity of 83% to 91% and a specificity of 80% to 93%. IDUS may be the most clinically useful tool when no mass is seen on cross-sectional or EUS imaging, or when EUS with FNA is negative and there is a suspicion of malignancy, thus increasing ERCP with brush sensitivity [10].

3.4. Cholangioscopy

Cholangioscopy is an endoscopic technique that allows direct bile duct lesions visualization with the opportunity to take samples with specific miniature biopsy forceps (Figure 4). During cholangioscopy, the visual impression of the bile ducts constitutes an integral part of the study (Figure 5). Signs of malignancy are, for example, tortuous dilated vessels, infiltrative strictures, polypoid or vegetative lesions, and easily bleeding ones (Figure 6). Benign features are villous or polypoid patterns without vascularity, fibrous or congestive patterns with inflammation signs, or a smooth epithelium [22]. In a recent meta-analysis including 283 procedures, the overall pooled sensitivity and specificity of direct single-operator cholangioscopy in the visual interpretation of biliary malignancies was 94% and 95%, respectively [23]. Direct biopsy collection through cholangioscopy is another advantage of this procedure: a meta-analysis revealed a pooled sensitivity of 71.9% of cholangioscopy-directed biopsies in diagnosing malignancy and a pooled specificity of 99.1% [24]. Despite these advantages, cholangioscopy has some limitations: it is not universally accessible and is an operator-dependent technique, with high costs and associations with serious and frequent adverse events due to bile duct direct access (such as cholangitis, pancreatitis, and bleeding). We summarize below the diagnostic tools available in biliary stricture settings (Scheme 1).

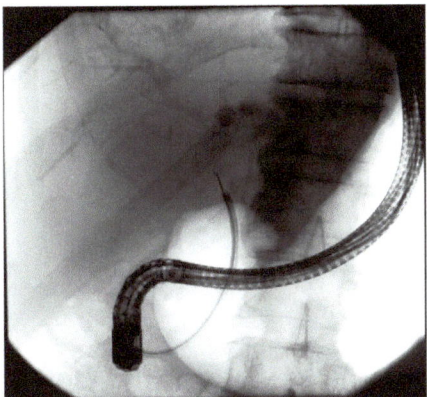

Figure 4. Spyglass device with spybite forceps during cholangioscopy.

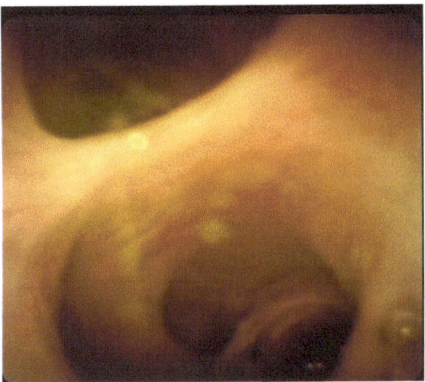

Figure 5. Regular hepatic confluence appearance during cholangioscopy.

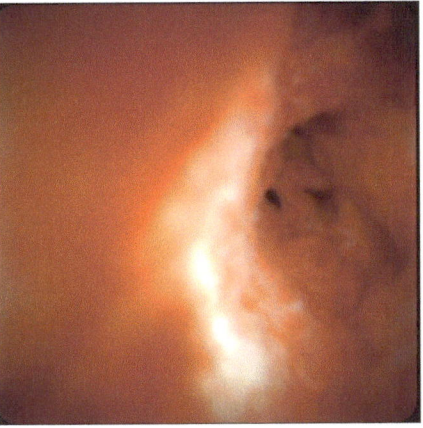

Figure 6. Hilar cholangiocarcinoma stricture appearance during cholangioscopy.

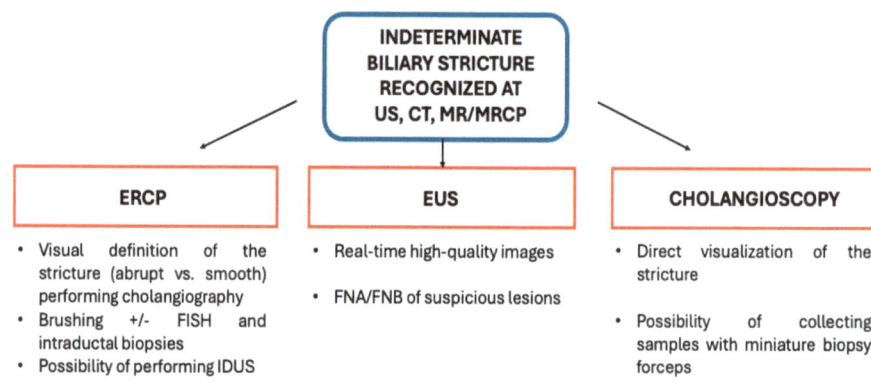

Scheme 1. Schematic diagnostic approaches available to manage indeterminate biliary strictures.

3.5. Confocal Laser Endomicroscopy

Probe-based confocal laser endomicroscopy (CLE) can provide in vivo imaging of biliary lesions during ERCP and additional diagnostic information [25,26]. A contrast agent is typically injected intravenously, and the biliary tissue is imaged with a CLE probe. This technique results in specific patterns that correlate with histology and help differentiate between malignant and normal biliary mucosa [27]. Miami classification is used to differentiate probe-based CLE visual findings as benign or malignant strictures. The presence of thick dark bands (>40 m), thick white bands (>20 m), dark clumps, epithelial strictures, villous glands, and contrast leakage can distinguish the nature of strictures [28]. Paris classification is a newer classification that includes additional features like vascular congestion, dark glandular patterns, interglandular spaces, and a thickened reticular structure [25]. CLE can be a promising tool but currently, its use is limited due to its cost and the lack of interobserver agreement [29].

3.6. Other Diagnostic Approaches

Vascular endothelial growth factor level in bile, fluorescence in situ hybridization for brush cytology, and methionyl-tRNA synthetase 1 staining for brush cytology are reported to be promising in pilot studies, but we need stronger evidence about their clinical value [29–31].

4. Management and Therapeutic Approach

When we suspect a biliary stricture, whatever its etiology, it is crucial to re-establish regular biliary flow into the duodenum. Restoring lower or normal bilirubin levels relieves patient symptoms such as itching due to jaundice and, in oncological patients, allows for the starting of chemotherapies. Indeterminate biliary strictures should be considered malignant unless proven otherwise. In patients with an extrahepatic or hilar indeterminate stricture, with high-serum bilirubin levels or with cholangitis or intractable itching, we need appropriate biliary drainage. Endoscopic treatment, particularly ERCP with stent placement, remains the first-line treatment in this setting. EUS-guided biliary drainage could be a good option in cases of failed ERCP. The percutaneous approach could still be an acceptable alternative in all cases of endoscopic approach failure or ineffectiveness.

4.1. ERCP in Distal Strictures

In extrahepatic strictures amenable to surgical approach, generally, the current guidelines recommend against routine preoperative biliary drainage (PBD), which should be reserved for symptomatic patients (cholangitis, itching, etc.) or for those who will undergo delayed surgery or neoadjuvant chemotherapy. Many meta-analyses and literature reviews have focused on the benefits and adverse events of preoperative biliary drainage: one of them [32] showed that preoperative biliary drainage increases wound and bile infection rates, but without affecting mortality and morbidity. A 2016 meta-analysis comparing mortality and adverse events in patients treated with PBD vs. direct surgery (DS) showed that in patients with malignant biliary jaundice requiring surgery, the PBD group had significantly fewer major adverse effects than the DS group [33]. Conversely, another study evaluating the incidence of overall complications and wound infection in these two groups found that there was a greater increase in overall complications and wound infections in the PBD group than in the DS group [34]. However, when the choice of biliary drainage in a preoperative setting is made, the current guidelines [35,36] recommend a self-expandable metal stent (SEMS) placement over a plastic one. It has been demonstrated by many meta-analyses that placing SEMS over plastic stents reduces the risk of stent dysfunction/cholangitis, requires fewer reinterventions, and ensures better patency periods and longer patient survival [37–39]. Then, when we have to choose between covered or uncovered SEMS, we must consider that the current guidelines [35] recommend against uncovered SEMSs (uSEMSs) in strictures of unconfirmed etiology. uSEMSs indeed have a poor long-term patency in obstructions that eventually turn out to be benign, because even in these ones, there could be tissue hyperplasia and ingrowth or sludge formation: complete stent embedding could lead to recurrent occlusion or cholangitis. Moreover, they are difficult to remove even with a "stent-in-stent" technique, which could be related to adverse events.

4.2. ERCP in Perihilar Strictures

Perihilar obstruction management is more difficult than distal ones and often requires a multidisciplinary approach in a referral center. Even in these kinds of strictures, the role of preoperative drainage in surgical candidates is debated due to increased postoperative morbidities, such as a greater infection rate or more adverse events. For these reasons, also in this setting, PBD is reserved for selected cases (delayed surgery, high serum bilirubin, and itching) and is not a routine suggested technique. When performed in the preoperative setting, the first choice is PBD by means of plastic stents with a side-by-side (SBS) bilateral stenting technique. Conversely, in palliative cases, many meta-analyses have indicated that SEMSs are superior to plastic ones in terms of prolonged overall survival, a lower rate of cholangitis, higher clinical success, and longer stent patency [40–42]. Particularly, the current guidelines [35] suggest uSEMSs in these cases. In uncertain-etiology strictures, multiple plastic stents are the best choice. Under fluoroscopic guidance, we can obtain appropriate liver drainage by a SBS stenting approach. In these cases, especially if the stricture is tight, it is often easier to place two 7 Fr stents initially to gradually dilate the bile duct and then replace them later with 10 Fr stents [43]. It is crucial to remember that the technical goal in hilar drainage has to be evaluated in volumetric sectorial terms and not in bilateral or unilateral terms: the final target is to promote the drainage of as much of the remaining liver as possible.

4.3. EUS-Guided Biliary Drainage (EUS-BD)

In the case of failed ERCP (papillary or duodenal infiltration, for example) an EUS-guided approach could be the solution. EUS could be helpful in obtaining anterograde access to the bile duct when papilla cannulation is not possible through a rendezvous technique, which consists of puncturing a bile duct with an access needle and introducing from there a guidewire through the papilla. In other cases, EUS is used to create a biliary–enteric fistula through a LAMS (lumen-apposing metal stent) that could provide a drainage proximal to the stricture. Examples of biliary–enteric EUS-guided fistulas are choledochoduodenostomy or hepaticogastrostomy, which are selected depending on several factors (such as stricture position or vascular interposition). Many meta-analyses have investigated EUS-BD's role and its technical success. In 2017, Moole et al. [44] compared EUS-BD to the percutaneous transhepatic approach (PTBD), describing a successful biliary drainage with EUS in 90.91% of the pooled patient population with a pooled odds ratio of 3.06 for successful biliary drainage in the EUS-PD versus PTBD groups. Another meta-analysis evaluating the intrahepatic and extrahepatic approaches in EUS-BD showed a weighted pooled rate of 94% for technical success. Notably, in the meta-regression model, distal CBD strictures and transpapillary drainage were associated with higher technical success while the intrahepatic access route was linked to a higher adverse event rate [45]. Finally, another comprehensive literature review about the overall efficacy and safety of EUS-BD reported a pooled technical success rate of 91.5% and a clinical success rate of 87%, respectively [46].

4.4. Percutaneous Transhepatic Biliary Drainage (PTBD)

Percutaneous transhepatic biliary drainage consists of puncturing a bile duct under fluoroscopic or ultrasound guidance and obtaining a cholangiography by injecting contrast. Then, a guidewire is inserted through the needle to gain access to the biliary tree. To establish biliary drainage, we need to insert a catheter over the guidewire across the obstruction, providing an external drainage route transcutaneously. Today, this approach is not the first choice, especially if we have other options and if the stricture's nature is not established. However, it may be a mandatory choice if endoscopic treatment is contraindicated, is not feasible, or has failed. Some recent meta-analyses [47,48], comparing endoscopic biliary drainage and percutaneous transhepatic biliary drainage, showed no difference in terms of technical success. One study, comparing specifically EUS-BD to PTBD, interestingly indicated that EUS-BD was associated with lower reintervention rates and lower odds of adverse events. Even the total treatment costs and the hospital stay were significantly lower in the EUS-BD group than in the PTBD group [49]. Thus, PTBD is reserved exclusively for endoscopic approach failure or non-feasibility.

5. Conclusions and Future Directions

Indeterminate biliary strictures still represent a diagnostic and therapeutic challenge for endoscopists. What we know is that the approach must be a multidisciplinary one, tailored to a single patient, and based on his or her personal history, preferably in a referral center. Often, a single diagnostic technique is not adequate to secure a proper diagnosis. What is determined is, therefore, that the key is to integrate different techniques in order to increase diagnostic chances and that a single-tissue sampling method is not always quite enough. Our future goal is to improve our diagnostic skills to minimize the total number of uncertain-etiology strictures to "determinate the indeterminate".

Funding: This research received no external funding.

Conflicts of Interest: The authors declare no conflicts of interest.

References

1. Pouw, R.E.; Barret, M.; Biermann, K.; Bisschops, R.; Czakó, L.; Gecse, K.B.; de Hertogh, G.; Hucl, T.; Iacucci, M.; van Hooft, J.E.; et al. Endoscopic tissue sampling—Part 1: Upper gastrointestinal and hepatopancreatobiliary tracts. European Society of Gastrointestinal Endoscopy (ESGE) Guideline. *Endoscopy* **2021**, *53*, 1174–1188. [CrossRef]
2. Fujii-Lau, L.L.; Thosani, N.C.; Al-Haddad, M.; Acoba, J.; Wray, C.J.; Zvavanjanja, R.; Dabr, F.; Amateau, S.K.; Buxbaum, J.L.; Qumseya, B.J.; et al. American Society for Gastrointestinal Endoscopy guideline on the role of endoscopy in the diagnosis of malignancy in biliary strictures of undetermined etiology: Summary and recommendations. *Gastrointest Endosc.* **2023**, *98*, 685–693. [CrossRef]

3. Tummala, P.; Munigala, S.; Eloubeidi, M.A.; Agarwal, B. Patients with obstructive jaundice and biliary stricture ± mass lesion on imaging: Prevalence of malignancy and potential role of EUS-FNA. *J. Clin. Gastroenterol.* **2013**, *47*, 532–537. [CrossRef]
4. DeWitt, J.; Misra, V.L.; Leblanc, J.K.; McHenry, L.; Sherman, S. EUS-guided FNA of proximal biliary strictures after negative ERCP brush cytology results. *Gastrointest. Endosc.* **2006**, *64*, 325–333. [CrossRef] [PubMed]
5. Bowlus, C.L.; Olson, K.A.; Gershwin, M.E. Evaluation of indeterminate biliary strictures. *Nat. Rev. Gastroenterol. Hepatol.* **2016**, *13*, 28–37, Erratum in: *Nat. Rev. Gastroenterol. Hepatol.* **2017**, *14*, 749. [CrossRef]
6. Navaneethan, U.; Njei, B.; Lourdusamy, V.; Konjeti, R.; Vargo, J.J.; Parsi, M.A. Comparative effectiveness of biliary brush cytology and intraductal biopsy for detection of malignant biliary strictures: A systematic review and meta-analysis. *Gastrointest. Endosc.* **2015**, *81*, 168–176. [CrossRef]
7. Baroud, S.; Sahakian, A.J.; Sawas, T.; Storm, A.C.; Martin, J.A.; Abu Dayyeh, B.K.; Topazian, M.D.; Levy, M.J.; Roberts, L.R.; Gores, G.J.; et al. Impact of trimodality sampling on detection of malignant biliary strictures compared with patients with primary sclerosing cholangitis. *Gastrointest. Endosc.* **2022**, *95*, 884–892. [CrossRef]
8. Lee, S.J.; Lee, Y.S.; Lee, M.G.; Lee, S.H.; Shin, E.; Hwang, J.H. Triple-tissue sampling during endoscopic retrograde cholangiopancreatography increases the overall diagnostic sensitivity for cholangiocarcinoma. *Gut Liver* **2014**, *8*, 669–673. [CrossRef]
9. Mohamadnejad, M.; DeWitt, J.M.; Sherman, S.; LeBlanc, J.K.; Pitt, H.A.; House, M.G.; Jones, K.J.; Fogel, E.L.; McHenry, L.; Watkins, J.L.; et al. Role of EUS for preoperative evaluation of cholangiocarcinoma: A large single-center experience. *Gastrointest. Endosc.* **2011**, *73*, 71–78. [CrossRef]
10. Conway, J.D.; Mishra, G. The Role of Endoscopic Ultrasound in Biliary Strictures. *Curr. Gastroenterol. Rep.* **2008**, *10*, 157–162. [CrossRef] [PubMed]
11. Jo, J.H.; Cho, C.M.; Jun, J.H.; Chung, M.J.; Kim, T.H.; Seo, D.W.; Kim, J.; Park, D.H.; Research Group for Endoscopic Ultrasonography in KSGE. Same-session endoscopic ultrasound-guided fine needle aspiration and endoscopic retrograde cholangiopancreatography-based tissue sampling in suspected malignant biliary obstruction: A multicenter experience. *J. Gastroenterol. Hepatol.* **2019**, *34*, 799–805. [CrossRef] [PubMed]
12. De Moura, D.T.H.; Ryou, M.; De Moura, E.G.H.; Ribeiro, I.B.; Bernardo, W.M.; Thompson, C.C. Endoscopic Ultrasound-Guided Fine Needle Aspiration and Endoscopic Retrograde Cholangiopancreatography-Based Tissue Sampling in Suspected Malignant Biliary Strictures: A Meta-Analysis of Same-Session Procedures. *Clin. Endosc.* **2020**, *53*, 417–428. [CrossRef]
13. Heimbach, J.K.; Sanchez, W.; Rosen, C.B.; Gores, G.J. Trans-peritoneal fine needle aspiration biopsy of hilar cholangiocarcinoma is associated with disease dissemination. *HPB* **2011**, *13*, 356–360. [CrossRef] [PubMed]
14. Levy, M.J.; Gleeson, F.C.; Campion, M.B.; Caudill, J.L.; E Clain, J.; Halling, K.; Rajan, E.; Topazian, M.D.; Wang, K.K.; Wiersema, M.J.; et al. Prospective cytological assessment of gastrointestinal luminal fluid acquired during EUS: A potential source of false-positive FNA and needle tract seeding. *Am. J. Gastroenterol.* **2010**, *105*, 1311–1318. [CrossRef]
15. Ngamruengphong, S.; Xu, C.; Woodward, T.A.; Raimondo, M.; Stauffer, J.A.; Asbun, H.J.; Wallace, M.B. Risk of gastric or peritoneal recurrence, and long-term outcomes, following pancreatic cancer resection with preoperative endosonographically guided fine needle aspiration. *Endoscopy* **2013**, *45*, 619–626. [CrossRef]
16. Ikezawa, K.; Uehara, H.; Sakai, A.; Fukutake, N.; Imanaka, K.; Ohkawa, K.; Tanakura, R.; Ioka, T.; Tanaka, S.; Ishikawa, O.; et al. Risk of peritoneal carcinomatosis by endoscopic ultrasound-guided fine needle aspiration for pancreatic cancer. *J. Gastroenterol.* **2013**, *48*, 966–972. [CrossRef] [PubMed]
17. El Chafic, A.H.; Dewitt, J.; Leblanc, J.K.; El Hajj, I.I.; Cote, G.; House, M.G.; Sherman, S.; McHenry, L.; Pitt, H.A.; Johnson, C.; et al. Impact of preoperative endoscopic ultrasound-guided fine needle aspiration on postoperative recurrence and survival in cholangiocarcinoma patients. *Endoscopy* **2013**, *45*, 883–889. [CrossRef] [PubMed]
18. Yoon, W.J.; Daglilar, E.S.; Fernández-del Castillo, C.; Mino-Kenudson, M.; Pitman, M.B.; Brugge, W.R. Peritoneal seeding in intraductal papillary mucinous neoplasm of the pancreas patients who underwent endoscopic ultrasound-guided fine-needle aspiration: The PIPE study. *Endoscopy* **2014**, *46*, 382–387. [CrossRef] [PubMed]
19. Tsutsumi, H.; Hara, K.; Mizuno, N.; Hijioka, S.; Imaoka, H.; Tajika, M.; Tanaka, T.; Ishihara, M.; Yoshimura, K.; Shimizu, Y.; et al. Clinical impact of preoperative endoscopic ultrasound-guided fine-needle aspiration for pancreatic ductal adenocarcinoma. *Endosc. Ultrasound* **2016**, *5*, 94–100. [PubMed]
20. Chiang, A.; Theriault, M.; Salim, M.; James, P.D. The incremental benefit of EUS for the identification of malignancy in indeterminate extrahepatic biliary strictures: A systematic review and meta-analysis. *Endosc. Ultrasound* **2019**, *8*, 310–317.
21. Tamada, K.; Ueno, N.; Tomiyama, T.; Oohashi, A.; Wada, S.; Nishizono, T.; Tano, S.; Aizawa, T.; Ido, K.; Kimura, K. Characterization of biliary strictures using intraductal ultrasonography: Comparison with percutaneous cholangioscopic biopsy. *Gastrointest. Endosc.* **1998**, *47*, 341–349. [CrossRef]
22. Robles-Medranda, C.; Valero, M.; Soria-Alcivar, M.; Puga-Tejada, M.; Oleas, R.; Ospina-Arboleda, J.; Alvarado-Escobar, H.; Baquerizo-Burgos, J.; Robles-Jara, C.; Pitanga-Lukashok, H.; et al. Reliability and accuracy of a novel classification system using peroral cholangioscopy for the diagnosis of bile duct lesions. *Endoscopy* **2018**, *50*, 1059–1070. [CrossRef] [PubMed]

23. De Oliveira, P.V.A.G.; de Moura, D.T.H.; Ribeiro, I.B.; Bazarbashi, A.N.; Franzini, T.A.P.; dos Santos, M.E.L.; Bernardo, W.M.; de Moura, E.G.H. Efficacy of digital single-operator cholangioscopy in the visual interpretation of indeterminate biliary strictures: A systematic review and meta-analysis. *Surg. Endosc.* 2020, *34*, 3321–3329. [CrossRef] [PubMed]
24. Badshah, M.B.; Vanar, V.; Kandula, M.; Kalva, N.; Badshah, M.B.; Revenur, V.; Bechtold, M.L.; Forcione, D.G.; Donthireddy, K.; Puli, S.R. Peroral cholangioscopy with cholangioscopy-directed biopsies in the diagnosis of biliary malignancies: A systemic review and meta-analysis. *Eur. J. Gastroenterol. Hepatol.* 2019, *31*, 935–940. [CrossRef] [PubMed]
25. Caillol, F.; Filoche, B.; Gaidhane, M.; Kahaleh, M. Refined probe-based confocal laser endomicroscopy classification for biliary strictures: The Paris Classification. *Dig. Dis. Sci.* 2013, *58*, 1784–1789. [CrossRef]
26. Kahaleh, M.; Giovannini, M.; Jamidar, P.; Gan, S.I.; Cesaro, P.; Caillol, F.; Filoche, B.; Karia, K.; Smith, I.; Gaidhane, M.; et al. Probe-based confocal laser endomicroscopy for indeterminate biliary strictures: Refinement of the image interpretation classification. *Gastroenterol. Res. Pract.* 2015, *2015*, 675210. [CrossRef] [PubMed]
27. Yadlapati, S.; Mulki, R.; Sánchez-Luna, A.S.; Ahmed, A.M.; Baig, K.R.K.K.; Peter, S. Clinical approach to indeterminate biliary strictures: Clinical presentation, diagnosis, and workup. *World J. Gastroenterol.* 2023, *29*, 5198–5210. [CrossRef] [PubMed]
28. Meining, A.; Shah, R.J.; Slivka, A.; Pleskow, D.; Chuttani, R.; Stevens, P.D.; Becker, V.; Chen, Y.K. Classification of probe-based confocal laser endomicroscopy findings in pancreaticobiliary strictures. *Endoscopy* 2012, *44*, 251–257. [CrossRef]
29. Sato, T.; Nakai, Y.; Fujishiro, M. Current endoscopic approaches to biliary strictures. *Curr. Opin. Gastroenterol.* 2022, *38*, 450–460. [CrossRef]
30. Navaneethan, U.; Gutierrez, N.G.; Jegadeesan, R.; Venkatesh, P.G.K.; Poptic, E.; Liu, X.; Sanaka, M.R.; Jang, S.; Vargo, J.J.; Parsi, M.A. Vascular endothelial growth factor levels in bile distinguishes pancreatic cancer from other etiologies of biliary stricture: A pilot study. *Dig. Dis. Sci.* 2013, *58*, 2986–2992. [CrossRef] [PubMed]
31. Liew, Z.H.; Loh, T.J.; Lim, T.K.H.; Lim, T.H.; Khor CJ, L.; Mesenas, S.J.; Kong, C.S.C.; Ong, W.C.; Tan, D.M.Y. Role of fluorescence in situ hybridization in diagnosing cholangiocarcinoma in indeterminate biliary strictures. *J. Gastroenterol. Hepatol.* 2018, *33*, 315–319. [CrossRef]
32. Garcea, G.; Chee, W.; Ong, S.L.; Maddern, G.J. Preoperative biliary drainage for distal obstruction: The case against revisited. *Pancreas* 2010, *39*, 119–126. [CrossRef] [PubMed]
33. Moole, H.; Bechtold, M.; Puli, S.R. Efficacy of preoperative biliary drainage in malignant obstructive jaundice: A meta-analysis and systematic review. *World J. Surg. Oncol.* 2016, *14*, 182. [CrossRef]
34. Scheufele, F.; Schorn, S.; Demir, I.E.; Sargut, M.; Tieftrunk, E.; Calavrezos, L.; Jäger, C.; Friess, H.; Ceyhan, G.O. Preoperative biliary stenting versus operation first in jaundiced patients due to malignant lesions in the pancreatic head: A meta-analysis of current literature. *Surgery* 2017, *161*, 939–950. [CrossRef]
35. Dumonceau, J.M.; Tringali, A.; Papanikolaou, I.S.; Blero, D.; Mangiavillano, B.; Schmidt, A.; Vanbiervliet, G.; Costamagna, G.; Devière, J.; García-Cano, J.; et al. Endoscopic biliary stenting: Indications, choice of stents, and results: European Society of Gastrointestinal Endoscopy (ESGE) Clinical Guideline—Updated October 2017. *Endoscopy* 2018, *50*, 910–930. [CrossRef]
36. Elmunzer, B.J.; Maranki, J.L.; Gómez, V.; Tavakkoli, A.; Sauer, B.G.; Limketkai, B.N.; Brennan, E.A.; Attridge, E.M.; Brigham, T.J.; Wang, A.Y. ACG Clinical Guideline: Diagnosis and Management of Biliary Strictures. *Am. J. Gastroenterol.* 2023, *118*, 405–426. [CrossRef]
37. Moole, H.; Jaeger, A.; Cashman, M.; Volmar, F.H.; Dhillon, S.; Bechtold, M.L.; Puli, S.R. Are self-expandable metal stents superior to plastic stents in palliating malignant distal biliary strictures? A meta-analysis and systematic review. *Med. J. Armed Forces India* 2017, *73*, 42–48. [CrossRef] [PubMed]
38. Zorrón, P.L.; de Moura, E.G.; Bernardo, W.M.; Baracat, F.I.; Mendonça, E.Q.; Kondo, A.; Luz, G.Q.; Júnior, C.K.F.; Artifon, E.L.d.A. Endoscopic stenting for inoperable malignant biliary obstruction: A systematic review and meta-analysis. *World J Gastroenterol.* 2015, *21*, 13374–13385.
39. Almadi, M.A.; Barkun, A.; Martel, M. Plastic vs. Self-Expandable Metal Stents for Palliation in Malignant Biliary Obstruction: A Series of Meta-Analyses. *Am. J. Gastroenterol.* 2017, *112*, 260–273. [CrossRef]
40. Xia, M.X.; Pan, Y.L.; Cai, X.B.; Wu, J.; Gao, D.; Ye, X.; Wang, T.; Hu, B. Comparison of endoscopic bilateral metal stent drainage with plastic stents in the palliation of unresectable hilar biliary malignant strictures: Large multicenter study. *Dig. Endosc.* 2021, *33*, 179–189. [CrossRef]
41. Kim, J.Y.; Lee, S.G.; Kang, D.; Lee, D.K.; Park, J.K.; Lee, K.T.; Lee, J.K.; Lee, K.H. The Comparison of Endoscopic Biliary Drainage in Malignant Hilar Obstruction by Cholangiocarcinoma: Bilateral Metal Stents versus Multiple Plastic Stents. *Gut Liver* 2021, *15*, 922–929. [CrossRef] [PubMed]
42. Kerdsirichairat, T.; Arain, M.A.; Attam, R.; Glessing, B.; Bakman, Y.; Amateau, S.K.; Freeman, M.L. Endoscopic Drainage of >50% of Liver in Malignant Hilar Biliary Obstruction Using Metallic or Fenestrated Plastic Stents. *Clin. Transl. Gastroenterol.* 2017, *8*, e115. [CrossRef] [PubMed]

43. Mangiavillano, B.; Pagano, N.; Baron, T.H.; Arena, M.; Iabichino, G.; Consolo, P.; Opocher, E.; Luigiano, C. Biliary and pancreatic stenting: Devices and insertion techniques in therapeutic endoscopic retrograde cholangiopancreatography and endoscopic ultrasonography. *World J. Gastrointest. Endosc.* **2016**, *8*, 143–156. [CrossRef] [PubMed]
44. Moole, H.; Bechtold, M.L.; Forcione, D.; Puli, S.R. A meta-analysis and systematic review: Success of endoscopic ultrasound guided biliary stenting in patients with inoperable malignant biliary strictures and a failed ERCP. *Medicine* **2017**, *96*, e5154. [CrossRef] [PubMed]
45. Khan, M.A.; Akbar, A.; Baron, T.H.; Khan, S.; Kocak, M.; Alastal, Y.; Hammad, T.; Lee, W.M.; Sofi, A.; Artifon, E.L.A.; et al. Endoscopic Ultrasound-Guided Biliary Drainage: A Systematic Review and Meta-Analysis. *Dig. Dis. Sci.* **2016**, *61*, 684–703. [CrossRef]
46. Dhindsa, B.S.; Mashiana, H.S.; Dhaliwal, A.; Dhaliwal, A.; Mohan, B.; Jayaraj, M.; Sayles, H.; Singh, S.; Ohning, G.; Bhat, I. EUS-guided biliary drainage: A systematic review and meta-analysis. *Endosc. Ultrasound* **2020**, *9*, 101–109.
47. Liu, J.G.; Wu, J.; Wang, J.; Shu, G.-M.; Wang, Y.-J.; Lou, C.; Zhang, J.; Du, Z. Endoscopic Biliary Drainage Versus Percutaneous Transhepatic Biliary Drainage in Patients with Resectable Hilar Cholangiocarcinoma: A Systematic Review and Meta-Analysis. *J. Laparoendosc. Adv. Surg. Tech. A* **2018**, *28*, 1053–1060. [CrossRef]
48. Moll, C.F.; de Moura, D.T.H.; Ribeiro, I.B.; Proença, I.M.; Monte ES, D.; Sánchez-Luna, S.A.; Merchán, M.F.S.; Intriago, J.M.V.; Bernardo, W.M.; de Moura, E.G.H.; et al. Endoscopic Biliary Darinage (EBD) versus Percutaneous Transhepatic Biliary Drainage (PTBD) for biliary drainage in patients with Perihilar Cholangiocarcinoma (PCCA): A systematic review and meta-analysis. *Clinics* **2023**, *78*, 100163. [CrossRef]
49. Giri, S.; Seth, V.; Afzalpurkar, S.; Angadi, S.M.; Jearth, V.M.; Sundaram, S.M. Endoscopic Ultrasound-guided Versus Percutaneous Transhepatic Biliary Drainage After Failed ERCP: A Systematic Review and Meta-analysis. *Surg. Laparosc. Endosc. Percutan Tech.* **2023**, *33*, 411–419. [CrossRef] [PubMed]

Disclaimer/Publisher's Note: The statements, opinions and data contained in all publications are solely those of the individual author(s) and contributor(s) and not of MDPI and/or the editor(s). MDPI and/or the editor(s) disclaim responsibility for any injury to people or property resulting from any ideas, methods, instructions or products referred to in the content.

MDPI AG
Grosspeteranlage 5
4052 Basel
Switzerland
Tel.: +41 61 683 77 34

Journal of Clinical Medicine Editorial Office
E-mail: jcm@mdpi.com
www.mdpi.com/journal/jcm

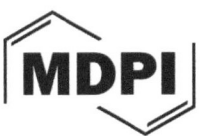

Disclaimer/Publisher's Note: The title and front matter of this reprint are at the discretion of the Guest Editor. The publisher is not responsible for their content or any associated concerns. The statements, opinions and data contained in all individual articles are solely those of the individual Editor and contributors and not of MDPI. MDPI disclaims responsibility for any injury to people or property resulting from any ideas, methods, instructions or products referred to in the content.

www.ingramcontent.com/pod-product-compliance
Lightning Source LLC
LaVergne TN
LVHW072353090526
838202LV00019B/2531